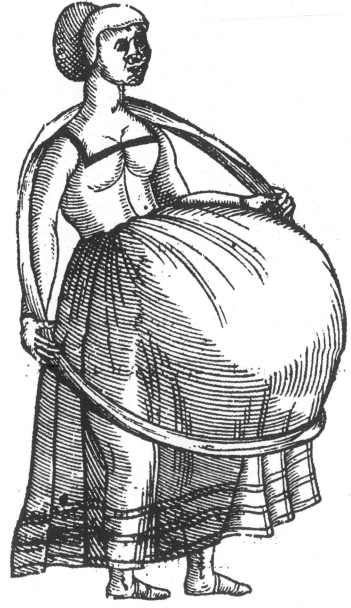

Lib. 4. de gener. ani. cap. 4.

SOURCE: Ambroise Paré, *Les Œuvres d'Ambroise Paré, Conseiller et Premier Chirurgien du Roy, Neufiesme Edition.* (Lyon: Claude Rigaud et Claude Obert, 1633)

THE LADIES DISPENSATORY

Containing
The Natures, Vertues, and
Qualities of all HERBS, and
SIMPLES usefull in *Physick.*
Reduced
Into a Methodicall Order, for
their more ready use in any sick-
nesse, or other accident of the Body.

The like never published in English.

WITH
An Alphabeticall Table of all the
Vertues of each Herb and Simple.

London. Printed for R. *Ibbitson,* to be sold by
George Calvert at the halfe-Moon in
Watlingstreet. 1652.

EDITED BY BALABAN, ERLEN, & SIDERITS

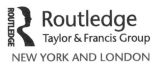
Routledge
Taylor & Francis Group
NEW YORK AND LONDON

First published in 2003 by
Routledge
711 Third Avenue,
New York, NY 10017, USA
www.routledge-ny.com

Published in Great Britain by
Routledge
2 Park Square, Milton Park,
Abingdon, Oxfordshire OX14 4RN
www.routledge.co.uk

First issued in paperback 2016

Routledge is an imprint of the Taylor and Francis Group, an informa business

Library of Congress Cataloging-in-Publication Data

Sowerby, Leonard.
  The ladies dispensatory/[Leonard Sowerby]; edited by Carey Balaban, Jonathan Erlen and Richard Siderits
      p. cm.
  Includes bibliographical references.
  ISBN 0-415-93533-4 (hb.)
    1. Therapeutics—Early works to 1800. 2. Materia medica—Therapeutic use—Early works to 1800. 3. Herbs—Therapeutic use—Early works to 1800. 4. Medicine, Popular—Early works to 1800. 5. Women—Health and hygiene—Early works to 1800. I. Balaban, Carey David, 1954- II. Erlen, Jonathan. III. Siderits, Richard, IV. Title.

  RM84.S69 2002
  615′.1′094209032—dc21

                                                              2002028483

ISBN 13: 978-1-138-97415-9 (pbk)
ISBN 13: 978-0-415-93533-3 (hbk)

Acknowledgments

The editors wish to thank Toby A. Appel, Historical Librarian, Cushing/Whitney Medical Library, Yale University, and her library for loaning their original copy of *The Ladies Dispensatory* for this project. Some of the illustrations were reproduced from a copy of the 1633 edition of John Gerard's *The Herbal or General History of Plants* in the collection of the Hunt Institute for Botanical Documentation at Carnegie Mellon University. The editors thank Charlotte Tancin, Librarian and Senior Research Scholar, for making this material available for our use. The other illustrations were reproduced from a 1633 edition of *Les Œuvres d'Ambroise Paré, Conseiller et Premier Chirurgien du Roy* ([Ninth Edition], Lyon: Claude Rigaud et Claude Obert, 1633), except for a variant on the illustration of aconite from the 1634 edition of *The Workes of that Famous Chirurgion, Ambroise Parey*, translated by Thomas Johnson (London: Thomas Coates and R. Young, 1634); copies of both works are from the collection of the Falk Library of the Health Sciences, University of Pittsburgh. We wish to thank John Symons of the Wellcome Institute of the History of Medicine in London for his assistance in locating biographical information about Leonard Sowerby. This work is dedicated to the editors' wives, without whose support and understanding this project would not have been completed: Naomi Balaban, Judith Ann Erlen, and Nancy Obis Siderits.

Introduction

In seventeenth-century England, primary health care was most commonly provided by a variety of lay people, including domestic healers (mothers, fathers, and housewives), local wise women, clergymen, midwives, and gentlewomen.[1] During the Protectorate of Oliver Cromwell (1648–59), there was an outpouring of self-help medical publications for the lay public in England. In contrast to the period between 1640 and 1648, when only 15 significant popular medicine titles were published, Charles Webster[2] documents the publication of 163 self-help titles in English during the period between 1649 and 1659. This flurry of activity reflects a major surge of public interest in both medicine and preventive health among the literate public, who could be cast in the roles of both lay patients and health-care providers.

The role of health-care provider required the self-help practitioner to both diagnose the disease and prepare the appropriate medicines. Since remedy texts such as Leonard Sowerby's *The Ladies Dispensatory* (1652) do not discuss diagnostic criteria, one must presume that the nosology of the disorders was either common knowledge or based on well-established texts such as Andrew Boorde's *Breviary of Helthe* (1547).[3] Once the diagnosis was determined, the medication

---

[1]Ronald Sawyer, "Patients, Healers and Disease in the Southeast Midlands, 1597–1634," (PhD. diss., University of Wisconsin—Madison, 1986), pp. 126–192; Mary E. Fissel, *Patients, Power, and the Poor in Eighteenth-Century Bristol* (Cambridge: Cambridge University Press, 1991), pp. 16–36.

[2]Charles Webster, *The Great Instauration: Science, Medicine and Reform, 1626–1660* (London: Duckworth, 1975), pp. 270–273.

[3]Andrewe Boorde, *The Breviary of Helthe* (London, 1547; facsimile edition of British Museum Shelfmark: C.122.d.I., Amsterdam: Da Capo Press, 1971).

could then be selected from the list of remedies, that were gleaned from four earlier authorities[4]: Gerard with Johnson,[5] Goræus, Fuchsius, and Dioscorides. In this sense, Sowerby's readership could be characterized as practitioners of *Empirical Medicine*, defined by Steven Blancard [Blankaart] (Professor of Physic from Middleburg in Zealand from 1650 to 1702) as:

> *Empirica Medicina*, Quacking, curing the sick by guess, without Reason, the Use of Anatomy, or knowing the Causes of Distempers, but to certain Symptoms only prescrib'd such Medicines as they had experience'd in such like cases before.[6]

However, it is important to note that, unlike alternative or popular self-help remedies in our contemporary society, that often deviate from "modern, standard medical practice," the self-help patient of mid-seventeenth-century England received Empiricist remedies that were consistent with standard medical practice of that day (e.g., *Pharmacopœia Londinensis*[7]).

The popularity of remedy texts in mid-seventeenth-century England suggests a wide acceptance of self-help medicine among the lay public. Insight into the popularity of self-help medication can be gleaned from contemporaneous utopian works. For example, Samuel Hartlib's *Macaria* (1641), in a dialogue between a Traveler and a Scholar, described the ideal of combining the functions of an Empiricist Physician and a Parson to cure both body and soul:

> *Sch.* But you spoke of health, how can that be procured by a better way than wee have here in England?
> *Trav.* Yes very easily; for they have a house, or Colledge of experience, where they deliver out yeerly such medicines as they find out by experience; and all such as shall be able to demonstrate any experiment for the health or wealth of men, are honourably rewarded at the publike charge, by which their skill in Husbandry, Physick, and Surgerie, is most excellent.
> *Sch.* But this is against Physicians.
> *Trav.* In *Macaria* the Parson of every Parish is a good Physician, and doth execute both functions, to wit, *cura animarum, & cura corporum*; and they think it as absurd

---

[4]*The Ladies Dispensatory*, Introduction.

[5]John Gerard, *The Herbal or General History of Plants. The Complete 1633 Edition as Revised and Enlarged by Thomas Johnson* (Facsimile of edition published by Adam Aslip, Joice Norton and Richard Whitakers, London, 1633; reprint, New York: Dover Publications, 1975).

[6]Stephen Blancard [Blankaart], *The Physical Dictionary. Wherein the Terms of Anatomy, the Names and Causes of Diseases, Chirurgical Instruments, and their Use are Accurately Described* (London: John and Benjamin Sprint, 1726), p. 141.

[7]Nicholas Culpeper, *Pharmacopœia Londinensis: or the London Dispensatory: further adorned by the studies and collections of the Fellows, now living of the said Colledg* (London: Printed for Peter Cole, 1653).

for a Divine to be without the skill of Physick, as it is to put new wine into old bot-
tles; and the Physicians being true Naturalists, may as well become good Divines, as
the divines do become good Physicians.

Sch. But you spoke of grat facilitie that these men have in their functions, how can
that be?

Trav. Very easily: for the Divines, by reason that the Society of Experimenters is
liable to an action, if they shall deliver out any false receit, are not troubled to trie
conclusions, or experiments, but onely to consider of the diversitie of natures, complexions, and constitutions, which, they are to know, for the cure of soules, as well
as bodies.

Sch. I know divers Divines in England that are Physicians, and therefore I hold well
with this report, and I would that all were such, for they have great estimation with
the people, and can rule them at their pleasure?[8]

From this perspective, any individual educated in the healing arts and reli-
gious precepts could be regarded as a qualified healer of body and soul. Perhaps
this laudable goal could also be achieved by lay readers of self-help texts.

Despite the popularity of these works, no less an authority than Nicholas
Culpeper (1615–1654) expressed his disdain for the implicit Empiricist approach
to medicine in the following passage from his landmark 1652 publication, *The
English Physician*:

First, To the Vulgar. Kind Souls, I am sorry it hath been your sad Mis-hap to have
been so long trained in such *Egyptian* Darkness, even Darkness which to your Sor-
row may be felt: The vulgar Road of Physick is not in my Practice, and I am therefore the more unfit to give you Advice, and I have now* [*Galen's *Art of Physick*]
published a little Book which will fully instruct you, not only in the Knowledge of
your own Bodies, but also in fit Medicines to remedy each Part of it when afflicted.[9]

However, the passage continued with instructions on the appropriate use of self-
help books such as *The Ladies Dispensatory*:

1. With the Disease, regard the Cause, and the Part of the Body afflicted; for Example, suppose a Woman to be subject to miscarry through Wind, thus do:

---

[8]Samuel Hartlib, *A Description of the Famous Kingdome of Macaria; Shewing its Excellent Government: Wherein the Inhabitants live in great Prosperity, Health, and Happinesse; the King obeyed, and
the Nobles honoured; and all good men respected, Vice punished, and vertue rewarded. An Example
to other Nations. In a Dialogue between a Schollar and a Traveller* (London: Francis Constable,
1641), pp. 5–7.

[9]Nicholas Culpeper, *The English Physician Enlarged with Three Hundred and Sixty-Nine Medicines
Made of English Herbs* (London: E. Ballard, L. Hawke and Co., 1770), p. 386.

1. Look Abortion in the Table of Diseases, and you shall be directed by that, how many Herbs prevent Miscarriage.
2. Look Wind in the same Table, and you shall see how many of those Herbs expel Wind.

These are the Herbs Medicinal for your Grief.

2. In all Diseases, strengthen the Part of the Body afflicted.

3. In mix'd Diseases there lies some Difficulty, for sometimes two Parts of the Body are afflicted with contrary Humours, as sometimes the Liver is afflicted with Choler and Water, as when a Man hath the Dropsy and the Yellow Jaundice; and this is usually mortal.

In the former, Suppose the Brain to be too cold and moist, and the Liver to be hot and dry; thus do:

1. Keep your Head outwardly warm.

2. Accustom yourself to the smell of hot Herbs.

3. Take a Pill that heats the Head at Night going to bed.

4. In the Morning take a Decoction that cools the Liver, or that quickly passeth the Stomach, as is at the Liver immediately.[10]

These instructions clarify the rationale for popular use of books like *The Ladies Dispensatory*. Once a disease was identified, the cure could be identified easily from reference works composed of lists of remedies nested within a table of diseases.

SOURCES FOR *THE LADIES DISPENSATORY*

Relatively little is known about the life of the compiler of *The Ladies Dispensatory*. Records of the Stationers' Company (London)[11] indicate that Leonard Sowerby had been a bound apprentice to Katherine Perry, widow, for seven years as of January 10, 1649, but there is no record of his becoming a free man. He was the son of Peircivall Sowerby, farrier, of Saint Martin's in the Fields. In addition to *The Ladies Dispensatory*, Donald Wing (W2812) lists a 1661 publication by a Leonard Sowersby, of Turnstile, near the New Market, in Lincoln's Inn Fields—

---

[10]Ibid., pp. 386–387.
[11]Donald F. McKenzie, *Stationers' Company Apprentices, 1641–1700* (Oxford: Oxford Biographical Society, 1974), p. 130.

an English translations of John Willis' *Mnemonica; or, the art of memory*.[12] This limited biographical information suggests that Leonard Sowerby was probably in his early twenties in 1652, at the time of publication of *The Ladies Dispensatory*.

In his Introduction, Sowerby acknowledged that his sources were Gerard with Johnson,[13] Goraeus, Fuchsius, and Dioscorides. The author expressed a particular debt to the legendary first-century A.D. herbalist, Dioscorides, asserting:

> Against my Authour Dioscorides, I do not so much as presuppose any Objection, who having learned most Languages, and seen many Countries, with good entertainment, will I presume finde as good reception in England, and be esteemed correspondent to his worth, and the credit he hath acquired among all learned men.[14]

The structure of *The Ladies Dispensatory* demonstrates a heavy reliance on Dioscorides's *De Materia Medica (Of Medicinal Matter)*.[15] Margin notes (reproduced as footnotes in this edition) provided direct cross-references between the common names of many medicinal ingredients and terms from Dioscorides's *Materia Medica*. Under each disease heading, the order of presentation of remedies follows closely Dioscorides's classification scheme. The original index, organized alphabetically by simple ingredients, is effectively a summary (or outline) of their medicinal uses from the author's sources.

The adoption of a large number of remedies from Dioscorides's *Materia Medica* is obvious in the Table of Medicinal Ingredients (included in this edition as an appendix). A minority of remedies were not included in the original Dioscorides. Under each disease heading, however, these materials were listed in the appropriate order for Diocorides's classification of medications. For example, the English term 'Weesil' in *The Ladies Dispensatory* refers to the "Gale katoiokidios" of Dioscorides.[16] Book II.27 lists medicinal applications of salted weasel carcasses, ashes of burned weasels, and a weasel stomach stuffed with coriander and weasel blood. These remedies appear in *The Ladies Dispensatory* in their appropriate order, and a related medication that was not in Dioscorides, a weasel scrotum stuffed with coriander, was placed in the same locations as other remedies using weasels. A similar example is provided by the Bastard Satyrion (Bird's nest or Goose-nest), which Gerard (1545–1612) stated "is not vsed in

---

[12]Donald Goddard Wing, *Short-title catalogue of books printed in England, Scotland, Ireland, Wales, and British America, and of English books printed in other countries, 1641–1700* (New York: Index Society, 1945–51).

[13]Gerard, *The Herbal or General History of Plants.*

[14]*The Ladies Dispensatory*, p. xxxi.

[15]*The Greek Herbal of Dioscorides, illustrated by a Byzantine A.D. 512, Englished by John Goodyer A.D. 1655, edited and first printed A.D. 1933*, ed. R.T. Gunther (New York: Hafner Publishing Co., 1959).

[16]Ibid., Book II.27.

Physicke that I can finde in any authoritie."[17] This remedy is listed in the appropriate location for a form of satyrion as a remedy for causing and hindering "standing of the yard."[18] In modern terms, *The Ladies Dispensatory* represented a popular, updated, self-help edition of some of the information from Dioscorides's *Of Medicinal Matter*.

The Ladies Dispensatory also appears to include information from at least one major source not cited in Sowerby's brief introduction. Most notably, there is an extensive section describing treatments for stings and bites of venomous animals, bites from nonvenomous animals, and poisoning, using terminology that is virtually identical to terminology in Chapter 21 in the 1634 translation of the works of Ambrose Paré that is attributed to Thomas Johnson.[19] Several illustrations of these venomous animals have been reproduced in an appendix to this volume. The inclusion of information from such a widely available work is not extraordinary. However, given the prominence of Dr. Thomas Johnson (d. 1644) as a botanist, member of the Apothecaries' Company, and Royalist Army colonel during the English Civil War,[20] it seems unlikely that his edition of Gerard would be cited while his edition of Paré ignored.

INTENDED AUDIENCE OF *THE LADIES DISPENSATORY*: WOMEN'S MEDICINE, HOUSEHOLD COMPLAINTS AND MALE VENEREAL DISEASE

The Ladies Dispensatory has several noteworthy features that give insight into the interests of its intended audience. As expected from the title, remedies were included for gynecologic problems ("Simples serving for the Matrix"), breast complaints ("Simples serving for the Teats, or Duggs"), personal hygiene and cosmetic applications ("Simples serving to embellish the Body"), and a wide variety of common diseases and injuries. The extensive list of remedies for poisons, animal bites, and stings include substances in the *Materia Medica* so that drug overdoses could be treated effectively. In addition, there is an extensive list of remedies for maladies of the male genitalia. It is clear, then, that the book provided reasonably encyclopedic coverage of the standard health problems encountered by a typical household in mid-seventeenth-century England.

---

[17]Gerard, p. 229.

[18]*The Ladies Dispensatory*, p.74.

[19]Ambroise Paré. *The Workes of that Famous Chirurgion Ambrose Parey: Translated out of Latine and Compared with the French*, trans. Thomas Johnson (London: Thomas Coates and R. Young, 1634), pp. 775–813.

[20]*The Dictionary of National Biography: founded in 1882 by George Smith; edited by Sir Leslie Stephen and Sir Sidney Lee; from the earliest times to 1900* (London: Oxford University Press, 1959–60), vol. X, pp. 935–936.

As one might expect from a popular compendium based on earlier sources, the disease categories lack systematic rigor. For example, there are no cures for "the whites" (white menstrues or leukorrhea) in the medications for the matrix, and separate lists of remedies are given for intermitting fevers and two of its constituent disorders, tertian and "quartane" fevers. It is also peculiar that there are no remedies for diseases such as the green sickness (chlorosis), measles, smallpox, and syphilis, that were prevalent and well described in medical texts of that era.

A similar lack of systematic rigor is apparent in the classification of effects of medications cited in *The Ladies Dispensatory*. For example, the section entitled "Simples serving to evacuate Humours, either upward, or downward" comprises a curious mixture of subsections on medications that purge humors (choler, phlegm, and melancholy) and subsections on emetics, medications for dropsy, and medications "to loosen the Belly." From the perspective of the categories of the actions of "Simples" in Nicholas Culpeper's 1653 edition of the *Pharmacopœia Londinensis*, Sowerby's section confounds humoral and nonhumoral effects. Culpeper classified drug actions in terms of (1) temperature (degree of heat, coldness, moisture, and dryness), (2) site of action (e.g., head, spleen, liver, bladder, or brain), and (3) other properties (e.g., binding, opening, cleansing, breaking wind, or purging humors).[21] Significantly, the terms *purging* and *evacuating* were reserved for an action strictly at the abstract humoral level. In *The Ladies Dispensatory*, however, the terms were used more concretely for any pharmaceutical action of purging or evacuating.

One distinctive feature of *The Ladies Dispensatory* is the inclusion of distinct lists of medications to induce abortion, to expel the afterbirth or a dead fetus, and to provoke a woman's terms. These separate categories reflect effects described by Dioscorides, which, in John Goodyer's mid-seventeenth-century translation,[22] were expressed in terms such as killing "Embrya," "casting out," "drawing out," or "expelling" the "Embrya," "menstrua," and "secondines" [afterbirth]. Most of the medications that were recommended by Dioscorides were cited as producing more than one of these effects. These medications had been published periodically in the botanical and "professional" pharmaceutical literature in Europe,[23] but Sowerby's presentation of a separate list of abortifacients in a popular work is significant because it appears to be a mid-seventeenth-century lay user's guide to medical abortion. In particular, this aspect of *The Ladies Dispensatory* suggests that the topic of medical abortion was not forbidden in mid-seventeenth-century England and, in fact, that the identity and use of abortifacients was common knowledge.

[21]*Pharmacopœia Londinensis*, p. 36.
[22]*The Greek Herbal of Dioscorides*.
[23]John M. Riddle, *Eve's Herbs: A History of Contraception and Abortion in the West* (Cambridge, Mass.: Harvard University Press, 1997), pp. 35–63, 140–148.

The order of abortifacient drugs in *The Ladies Dispensatory* (Table 1) shows a strong influence of Dioscorides's classification of *materia medica*. The first thirty-seven abortifacients include thirty-five from this earlier source. They are listed almost exclusively in their order of appearance in Dioscorides, with only one intercalated item ("perfume of vultures feathers") that is not included in the classical source and one displaced item (decoction of great Dragons [Book II.196] is placed before Pepper [Book II.189] and Sow-bread root [Book II.194]). However, vultures feathers and vultures dung were included in a form of incense to hasten birth and ease delivery and were considered to be interchangeable for removing hair in William Salmon's 1693 *The Compleat English Physician.*[24] Thus, one could argue that the classification order of Dioscorides was preserved by Sowerby's substitution of an equivalent medicine for vulture dung. The final eight items in the abortifacients are a second list, ordered by their appearance in Dioscorides, but including only three medications that the earlier work considered effective in "expelling embrya." The list also included four remedies that Dioscorides recommended to speed delivery[25] and one remedy to help "women having hard labours."[26] However, it must be noted that the list of Dioscoridean abortifacients in *The Ladies Dispensatory* was incomplete. Missing medications include Flower-de-luce of Illyria,[27] a rosewood (*Aspalathus*) pessum,[28] bark of Sweet Bay roots,[29] hare's rennet,[30] Cress,[31] Soapwort,[32] Round Aristolochia,[33] Sage,[34] Calamint,[35] Candy Alexander,[36] Camomile,[37] White hellebore,[38] Scammony,[39] Thymelæa,[40] Colocynthis,[41] Briony,[42] and Filix foemina roots.[43] Because these materials were recommended for other effects, the criteria for their exclusion from the abortifacient list is unclear.

[24]William Salmon, *The Compleat English Physician, or The Druggist's Shop Opened,* 1692, p. 632.
[25]viz; Woodbind seed, Jasper stone, Eagle-stone, and Samian stone. *The Greek Herbal of Dioscorides,* Bk IV. 14, V.160, V.161, V.173, pp. 410, 655, 656, and 658.
[26]Root of Alexandrian Bayes; *The Greek Herbal of Dioscorides.* Bk IV.147, Gunther p. 537.
[27]Ibid., Book I.1, p.6.
[28]Ibid., Book I.19, p. 20.
[29]Ibid., Book I.106, p. 58.
[30]Ibid., Book II.85, p. 113.
[31]Ibid., Book II.185, p. 194.
[32]Ibid., Book II.193, p. 201.
[33]Ibid., Book III.6, p. 238.
[34]Ibid., Book III.40, p. 274.
[35]Ibid., Book III.43, p. 278.
[36]Ibid., Book III.79, p. 312.
[37]Ibid., Book III.154, p. 379.
[38]Ibid., Book IV.150, p. 541.
[39]Ibid., Book IV.171, p. 572.
[40]Ibid., Book IV.173, p. 574.
[41]Ibid., Book IV.178, p. 578.
[42]Ibid., Book IV.184, p. 583.
[43]Ibid., Book IV.187, p. 588.

REMEDIES IN *THE LADIES DISPENSATORY*: SIMPLE AND COMPOUND MEDICATIONS IN MID-SEVENTEENTH-CENTURY ENGLAND

Medicines in the seventeenth century were classified broadly as *simples* and *compounds*. Culpeper defined simples as leaves of herbs, flowers, seeds, roots, and barks and their juices, describing them as "medicines which consist in their own nature, which authors vulgarly call Simples, though something improperly; for in truth, nothing is simple but pure elements: all things else are compounded of them."[44] The *Pharmacopoeia Londinesis* had a similar definition, reserving the term "Simples" for individual roots, barks, woods, herbs, flowers, seeds, gums, rosins, juices, living creatures (or their parts), products "belonging to the sea" (e.g., ambergris or coral), metals or stones.[45] However, this work also included two forms of distilled medications: simple distilled waters and "simple waters distilled after being digested beforehand." The common feature of these simple medications appears to be a single active ingredient.

Compounds, on the other hand, formed a diverse category of medications. Blancard defined *Composita* as a term that included two types of drugs: medicines "which are made up of many simple ones" and "certain Chymical Compositions; as divers Spirits mix'd, the volatile oleous Salts, Tinctures, Balsams, Essences, Powders, &c."[46] The former category included standard medicines such as simple expressed oils (e.g., almond oil), distilled vinegar, decocted or infused oils, herbed vinegars and wines, ointments, cerecloths, plaisters, spirits, compound distilled waters, decoctions, syrups, lohochs, juleps, preserves, conserves, sugars, powders, electuaries, pills and troches containing single or multiple active ingredients.[47] The compound medicines varied greatly in complexity. Some of these medications clearly had only one active ingredient. Simple distilled waters were prepared by distilling a suspension of one simple medication in water[48]; preserved roots, stalks, flowers, barks, fruits, and pulps were also prepared generally from one simple medication mixed with water and sugar, in a manner similar to present-day jams and candied fruit.[49] Other compound medications were a mixture of simples with similar effects, defined in terms of either properties of classical elements (hot, cold, dry, or moist), effects of pairs of elements that constituted "complexions" of humors (e.g., choler is

---

[44]Nicholas Culpeper, *Culpeper's Complete Herbal: Consisting of a Comprehensive Description of Nearly all Herbs with Their Medicinal Properties and Directions for Compounding the Medicines Extracted from Them.* (London: W. Foulsham, 1923), p. 405.
[45]*Pharmacopœia Londinensis*, pp. 35–54.
[46]Blancard, p. 99.
[47]*Culpeper's Complete Herbal*, pp. 405–415; *Pharmacopœia Londinensis*, pp. 62–185.
[48]*Pharmacopœia Londinensis*, pp. 58–59.
[49]*Pharmacopœia Londinensis*, p. 118; Culpeper, *Culpeper's Complete Herbal*, pp. 411–412.

hot and dry),[50] direct effects on specific humors (e.g., purging phlegm or melancholy), or organ-specific effects (e.g., cooling the liver). For example, the *Aqua Mirabilis* from the *Pharmacopoeia Londinensis* was compounded from eight ingredients that were termed hot and dry in the second or third degree[51]: cloves, galanga, cubebs, mace, cardamon, nutmeg, ginger, and juice of sullendine (celandine). *The Skilful Physician* states that these compound medications were believed to "avoid that general defect of all hath hitherto come forth of this useful Subject, especially in the Cure Of Internal Distempers, by varying the Administrations according to the Complexion, Strength, and Constitution of the Patient."[52]

Some compounds could be selected for similar organ-specific or humoral effects, rather than properties of heat, cold, dryness, and moisture. One example is a remedy from *The Skilful Physician* to "avoid the Stone," which is a compound of four simples: Pellitory of the wall, parsley leaves, parsley seed, and lemon juice.[53] The former three ingredients are either "good against difficulty making water," or "take away stoppings," "provoke urine," or "dissolve the stone," reflecting an empiricist perspective, whereas the latter ingredient thins "gross and slimy humors."[54] From the perspective of heat, cold, dryness, and moisture, however, this remedy is compounded from one cold (first degree) and moist simple (Pellitory of the wall[55]), one cold and dry simple (lemon juice[56]), and two hot and dry simples (parsley and parsley seed[57]), yielding a temperate but dry medication. Evidence of the same trade-off can be seen in remedies included in *The Ladies' Dispensatory*. For example, a remedy "against long worms"[58] consisted of roots of Carline thistle (a hot and dry herb that was said to drive away worms[59]) and a second hot and dry herb (organy) that was believed to provoke the terms and resist poison,[60] both taken in decoction of Castorium, another hot medication. Finally,

---

[50]See John Goeurot, *The Regiment of Life, Whereunto is added a treatyse of the Pestilence, with the Booke of Children Newly Corrected and Enlarged* (London, 1546; facsimile edition, Bodleian Library [Oxford] Shelfmark 8°.P.24 Med., Amsterdam/Norwood, NJ: Walter J. Johnson, Inc./Theatrum Orbis Terrarum, Ltd, 1976), pp. 1–1v; Sir Thomas Elyot, *The Castel of Helth Corrected and in some places augmented* (London: 1641; facsimile edition, New York: Scholars' Facsimiles & Reprints, 1937), p. 2.
[51]*Pharmacopoeia Londinensis*, pp. 36, 40, 45, 47, 68–69; Gerard, pp. 62, 816, 1070, 1535, 1537, 1542, 1549.
[52]Carey Balaban, Jonathon Erlen, and Richard Siderits (eds), *The Skilful Physician* (Amsterdam: Harwood Academic Publishers, 1997), p. 13.
[53]*The Skilful Physician*, p. 146.
[54]Gerard, pp. 331, 1014, 1465.
[55]*Pharmacopoeia Londinensis*; Gerard p. 331.
[56]Gerard, p. 1465.
[57]Gerard, p. 1014.
[58]*The Ladies Dispensatory*, p.60.
[59]Gerard, p. 1158.
[60]Gerard, p. 667.

"White Turbith, Epithyme, Salt, and Vinegar, of each a like quantity" were recommended for purging melancholy,[61] a humoral disorder. Gerard described turbith as a drug that purges thick phlegm with a slow time course,[62] whereas epithyme "relieveth them which be melancholicke" by purging "siege, flegme, and melancholy."[63] Other properties of these medications do not appear relevant to the remedy.

The introductory note in the *Ladies Dispensatory* characterizes the book as a collection of *"pure, Elementary Simples; not compounded of a hodgepodge of sophisticated Drugs (like the* Cadmeian Progenie*) one oppugning the other."* This claim is perplexing because Sowerby included a large number of medications that qualify as compound medicines. These remedies included an extensive list of ingredients that are compounds per se, including Physical Wines, Decoctions, Electuaries, Oils by Infusion and Decoction, Ointments, Chemical Oils and Liniments (see Appendix: Table of Medicinal Ingredients). The remedies also included medicines that were compounded from variable numbers of simples. Most of these remedies were mixtures of up to four simples, prepared for either topical or internal use. For example, topical remedies *"Against Morphew, and other blemishes of the face"* include (1) "liniment made of Ben, and urine," (2) "daffodill rootes applyed with nettleseeds, and vinegar," and (3) "liniment made of briony, bitter vetches, earth of chio, and fenugreek." Compound medications for internal use included "chalcitis distilled with Juice of Leeks" as a medicine *"To staunch the bleeding at the Nose,"* "Rue boyled with dry Dill, drunk" as a cure for *"belly-ach and wormes"* and "Juyce of water Basill distilled with Brimstone and Niter" as a treatment *"Against paines of the Eares."* Many of these compound remedies, such as the prescription of a drink of turnsole seeds and leaves, hyssop, niter, and garden cresses for round worms, were unaltered from Dioscorides and Gerard.[64] A majority of the compounds from the extensive list of decoctions, electuaries (mixture of powered herbs and clarified honey), and oils were also listed in the earlier works (see Table of Medicinal Ingredients). These medications contradict the author's assertion that *The Ladies Dispensatory* contained only elementary simples.

Given the obvious presence of compound medicines in the lists of remedies, the modern reader is tempted to dismiss the author's claim that *The Ladies' Dispensatory* is a collection of simples as a form of disingenuous false advertising. However, there are alternative explanations. One obvious possibility is that Sowerby did not use the term *Simples* in a literal sense; rather, the term connotes

[61]*The Ladies Dispensatory*, p. 152.
[62]Gerard, p. 415.
[63]Gerard, pp. 574–575.
[64]*The Greek Herbal of Dioscorides*, Book IV.194, p. 598; Gerard, p.336; *The Ladies Dispensatory* p. 61.

other properties of the medications, such as ease of digestion or lack of extreme side effects. This usage of the term *Simples* would be consistent with the following passage from Francis Bacon's 1526 utopian work, *New Atlantis*, that described an idealized view of medications:

> We have dispensatories or shops of medicines; wherein you may easily think, if we have such variety of plants, and living creatures, more than you have in Europe (for we know what you have), the simples, drugs, and ingredients of medicines, must likewise be in so much the greater variety. We have them likewise of divers ages, and long fermentations. And for their preparations, we have not only all manner of exquisite distillations, and separations, and especially by gentle heats, and percolations through divers strainers, yea and substances; but also exact forms of composition, whereby they incorporate almost as they were natural simples.[65]

Bacon's words are echoed by the still-prevalent popular belief that *natural elementary simples*, or "medicines unmix'd and uncompounded,"[66] were superior to more elaborate pharmaceutical preparations. However, Bacon's words also provide an explanation for Sowerby's inclusion of compounds in a compendium of simples: Although these medications are technically compounds, they are incorporated by the patients as easily as simples.

A second explanation for the seemingly contradictory presence of compounds in a book of simple medicines is that the author is merely informing the reader that the remedies are all described in terms of their constituent simples. In other words, *The Ladies Dispensatory* presents recipes for medicines in terms that were readily accessible to (and understandable by) the lay practitioner. "Plain language recipes" stand in contrast to remedies that were mixtures of complex drugs with Latin names. A prime example of one such remedy is a regimen "to comfort the Spirits of one that is weak" from *The Skilful Physician*,[67] that instructed the patient to take a spoonful of "Syrrup de Corticibus Citri" containing "three or four drops of Aqua Coelestis." The preparation of both of these medicines is described in the *Pharmacopoeia Londinesis*.[68] The ingredients of *Syrupus de corticibus citri* were dried citron peels, scarlet grain (granorum kermes), sugar, and oriental musk. *Aqua Coelestis*, though, was an extremely elaborate compound. The first step in compounding it was to prepare an infusion of more than thirty simples in Spirit of Wine for fifteen days. A distillate of the infusion was then prepared, and

[65]Henry Morley, *Ideal Commonwealths, Comprising More's* Utopia, *Bacon's* New Atlantis, *Campanella's* City of the *Sun and Harrington's* Oceana. (Port Washington, N.Y.: Kennikat Press, 1968), pp. 132–133.
[66]Blancard, p. 99.
[67]*The Skilful Physician*, p. 38.
[68]*Pharmacopœia Londinensis*, pp. 68, 69, 104.

the final product was made by adding three more simples (Yellow Sanders, Musk, and Ambergris), six compound powders (Powder of Diambra, Powder of Diamosen [Diamoschum] dulce, Powder of Aromaticum Rosatum, Powder of Diamargariton frigidum, Powder of Diathodon Abbatis, and Powder of Electuary of Gemmis), and one compound julep (clear Julep of Roses). Because each of the compound powders in this formula contained more than twenty ingredients,[69] it is obvious that remedies using *Aqua Coelestis* could be criticized as "a hodgepodge of sophisticated Drugs (like the *Cadmeian Progenie*) one oppugning the other."[70]

A third explanation for Sowerby's characterization of *The Ladies Dispensatory* as a book of elementary simples is that the medications were simple to prepare. Even the recipes for compound medicines from *The Ladies Dispensatory* could be prepared easily at any hearth. In contrast to the remedies in the 1653 edition of the *Pharmacopœia Londinensis*, *The Skilful Physician*, and Conrad Gesner's 1559 *Treasure of Euonymus*,[71] no compound remedy in *The Ladies Dispensatory* requires chemical distillation with specialized colanders or limbecks. The most basic of these compound medicines were decoctions, prepared by boiling [or "sodding"] the simple medication in either water or wine, with the possible inclusion of a sweetener such as sugar or honey. Syrups and lohocs were prepared by adding sugar to the decoction and boiling the mixture until the viscosity increased appropriately. Electuaries were a base of honey that contained either powdered herbs or a decoction. Herbs were steeped in wine or vinegar to produce their "physical" [medicinal] counterparts. Oils were produced by either simple expression or by a combination of infusion and decoction (boiling). Ointments and liniments were made by steeping or boiling the ingredients in oil or in an aqueous base. Perfumes were either the smoke or fragrance of the ingredients. From this perspective, Sowerby and his audience might have regarded the term *Simples* as synonymous with "naturally" rather than "chemically" prepared medicines. Alternatively, *Simples* might have been defined operationally in the popular genre as any remedies from Dioscorides, Fuchsius, Goræus, and Gerard.

---

[69]*Pharmacopœia Londinensis of 1618 Reproduced in Facsimile, with a Historical Introduction by George Urdang* (Madison: State Historical Society of Wisconsin, 1944), pp. 148–156 [pp. 53–61 in the 1618 text].

[70]*The Ladies' Dispensatory*, Introduction.

[71]Conrad Gesner, *The Treasure of Evonymus, cotyninge the vvonderfull hid secretes of nature, tochinge the most apte formes to prepare and destyl Medicines, for the conseruation of helth: as Quintessece, Aurum Potabile, Hippocras, Aromatical wynes, Balmes, Oyles, Perfumes, garnishyng waters, and other manifold excellent confections. Wherunto are ioyned the formes of sondry apt Fornaces, and vessels, required in this art. Translated (with great diligence, & laboure) out of Latin, by Peter Morvving felow of Magdaline Coleadge in Oxford.* (London: Iohn Daie, 1559; facsimile edition of copy from Beinecke Rare Book and Manuscript Library, Yale University, New York: Da Capo Press/Theatrum Orbis Terrarum Ltd., Number 97, The English Experience, 1969).

[72]Doreen E. Nagy. *Popular Medicine in Seventeenth Century England* (Bowling Green, Ohio: Bowling Green State University Popular Press, 1988), Chapter 4.

A SURFEIT OF CHOICES: MEDICINAL OPTIONS
IN *THE LADIES DISPENSATORY*

The Ladies Dispensatory offered the lay practitioner a list of medicinal options that greatly exceeded the number of remedies available in works such as Culpeper's *The English Physician,* the *Pharmacopœia Londinesis,* or *The Skilful Physician.* Since *The English Physician* was limited in its scope to a small set of herbs, one expects the list of remedies to be a limited subset of those in books such as *The Ladies Dispensatory.* What is surprising, though, is the relatively limited overlap between remedies in *The Skilful Physician* and *The Ladies Dispensatory* (Figure 1). If we consider all "simple" ingredients except juices that are used in the two books, only 21 percent are found in both works. More than half (51 percent) of the *materia medica* from the two books are found in *The Ladies Dispensatory* (LD) but not in *The Skilful Physician* (SP). The remaining 28 percent of simple medications are found only in *The Skilful Physician.* Because virtually all of these simples appeared in works such as Dioscorides, Gerard, and the *Pharmacopœia Londinesis,* the authors of each book appear to have selected different subsets of *materia medica* for popularization.

Given the current emphasis on finding the most efficacious treatments, the modern reader might be perplexed by the multiplicity of remedies listed in the seventeenth-century self-help genre. The seemingly encyclopedic listing of potential treatment options in *The Ladies Dispensatory* is, in fact, a representative characteristic of this genre. For example, Doreen Nagy[73] cites a 1655 book by Philiatrios that contains more than 1,700 remedies. What was the appeal of these compendia to the lay public in mid-seventeenth-century England?

An obvious reason for the popularity of these works is that a large variety of potential remedies would be a buffer against a local or seasonal lack of availability of one remedy or ingredient. However, the medical practices and utopian literature suggest that interest in these books reflected more profound considerations as well. For example, there was a perception that multiple individual factors, such as the complexion, temperament, and horoscope of the patient could determine the efficacy of medications. Culpeper's *The English Physician,* for example,

---

[73]Culpeper, *The English Physician,* p. 387. In astrology, the sky was divided into 12 sectors, termed *houses,* arranged in an anticlockwise direction from the *ascendant,* or East. The planet (sign of the zodiac) that occupies a given house was termed its *ruler* or *lord.* In Culpeper's system of medical astrology, the first house (the sign ascending) represented the life and health of the patient, the sixth house represented the sickness, and the tenth house, if a "strong" sign, designated a potent treatment. Hence, these astrological guidelines for treatment represent a balance of drug actions with the patient's horoscope. The treatment is selected to be (1) compatible with the constitution and temperament of the patient (i.e., the ascendant), (2) "antipathetical" to the sickness (i.e., the sixth house), and (3) compatible with the astrologically determined potency of medicines on that day (i.e., the tenth house). For a comprehensive exposition of these factors, see Graeme Tobyn, *Culpeper's Medicine: A Practice of Western Holistic Medicine* (Shaftsbury, Dorset, UK: Element Books, 1997).

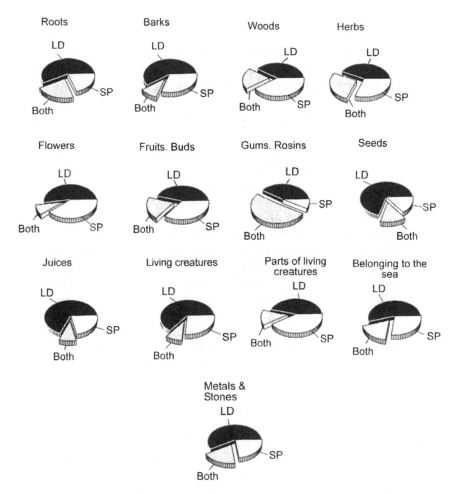

Figure 1

implores the reader to select medicine that is "Antipathetical to the Lord of the Sixth," of the same "Nature as the Sign ascending" and, "if the Lord of the Tenth be strong, make Use of his Medicines."[74] The patient was also urged "to fortify the griev'd Part of the Body by Sympathetical Remedies."[75] A large number of choices of medications would therefore provide the lay reader with adequate degrees of freedom to balance these factors in selecting a treatment. Perhaps this explains Bacon's view in the *New Atlantis* that the availability of a large variety of medicines represented a utopian ideal.[76]

[74]Ibid., p. 387.
[75]Morley, *Ideal Commonwealths*, pp. 132–133.
[76]Gerard 1633, p. 4.

In the final analysis, however, it is likely that an expectation of a large variety of remedies was a corollary of a prevalent concept of divine providence. The 1597 dedicatory note from John Gerard's *History of Plants*[77] clearly articulated the idea that spiritual delight could be derived from the contemplation of the providence that was implicit in the diversity of plant life:

> Among the manifold creatures . . . that have in all ages diversely entertained many excellent wits, and drawn them to the contemplation of the divine wisdome, none hath provoked mens studies more, or satisfied their desires so much as Plants hath done, and that upon just and worthy causes: For if delight may provoke mens labour, what greater delight is there than to behold the earth apparelled with plants, as with a robe of embroidered work, set with Orient pearles, and garnished with great diversitie of rare and costly jewels? If this varietie and perfection of colours may affect the eye, it is such in herbs and floures . . . if odours or if taste may worke satisfaction, they are both so soveraigne in plants, and so comfortable, that no confection of the Apothecaries can equall their excellent vertue. But these delights are the outward fences: the principal delight is in the minde, singularly enriched with the knowledge of these visible things, setting forth to us the invisible wisdome and admirable workmanship of almighty G-d. [orthography modernized]

This intuitive appreciation of divine wisdom was also viewed by Gerard as a noble pursuit, leading to wisdom, security, and health through an understanding of the uses of "Simples":

> in the expert knowledge of herbes, what pleasures still renewed with varietie? what small expence? what securitie? and yet what an apt and ordinary meanes to conduct man to that most desired benefit of health? . . . The drift whereof is a ready introduction to that excellent art of Simpling, which is neither so base nor contemptible as perhaps the English name may seem to intimate: but such it is, as altogether hath been a study for the wisest, an exercise for the noblest, a pastime for the best.[78]

From this perspective, compendia of simples such as *The Ladies Dispensatory* would constitute a reference guide to (or executive summary of) eternal, divinely ordained secrets for maintaining and restoring health.

---

[77]Gerard 1633, p. ¶3

Table 1

Abortifacient Medications: Other Uses

ABORTIFACIENTS	EXPEL AFTER-BIRTH (from 25 total)	EXPEL A DEAD CHILD (all remedies)	PROVOKE TERMS (from 114 total)
Castorium the weight of two drams taken with Penniroyall. [i]	Castorium the weight of two drams drunk with Penniroyall.		Bitumen drunk in wine with Castorium. Castorium the weight of two drams drunk.
Milke of a Bitches first Litter drunk [ii]			
Unwashed wooll applyed in a Suppositary [iii]			Unwashed wooll used as a pessary.
Dung of wild she Goates taken with some sweet and aromaticall thing [iv]			Dung of she Goates nourished on mountaines, drunk with some odorant thing.
Perfume of Vultures feathers. [v]			
Broth of Cich pease supped [vi]			
Decoction of Lupines, fomented with myrrhe and hony. [vii]			
Great water Parseneps used as other Kitchen herbs. [viii]			Great water Parsnep eaten as other pot-hearbs.
Decoction of great Dragons surringed. [ix]			
Pepper drunk. [x]			
Roots of Sow-bread fastened to the thigh. [xi]			

(continued)

Table 1 (*continued*)

Abortifacient Medications: Other Uses

ABORTIFACIENTS	EXPEL AFTER-BIRTH (from 25 total)	EXPEL A DEAD CHILD (all remedies)	PROVOKE TERMS (from 114 total)
Stalkes of Ivy leaves applied in a Suppositary with hony.[xii]			
Gentian roote used in a Suppositary.[xiii]			
Rootes of great Centaury used in a Pessary.[xiv]			Roots of great Centaury drunk, or the juyce used as a suppositary.
Juyce of small Centaury surringed.[xv]			
Penniroyall drunk.[xvi]	Pennyroyall drunk.		Penniroyall drunk.
Dittany drunk, used in a pessary, or perfumed.[xvii]		Dittany drunk, and applied in a suppositary.	
Decoction of Time supped.[xviii]	Decoction of Time drunk.		Decoction of Time, and of Summer Savory drunk. Wild Time drunk.
Decoction of summer Savory drunk.[xix]	Decoction of Summer Savory drunk.		Decoction of Time, and of Summer Savory drunk.
Root of Plowmans Spicknard fresh gathered, used in a Suppositary.[xx]			Decoction of the rootes of Plowmans Spikenard drunk.
Root of Hercules All-heal cut sharp at the end, put into the naturall place of women[xxi]			Hercules All heale drunk in wine.
Seed and root of Mountaine Siler drunk.[xxii]			

(continued)

Table 1 *(continued)*

Abortifacient Medications: Other Uses

ABORTIFACIENTS	EXPEL AFTER-BIRTH (from 25 total)	EXPEL A DEAD CHILD (all remedies)	PROVOKE TERMS (from 114 total)
Galbanum with myrrhe taken in wine, or perfumed. [xxiii]		Galbanum drunk with Myrrhe, and wine.	Galbanum perfumed, and used as a suppositary.
Wild Basill [xxiv] drunk.			Wild Basill drunk.
Decoction of Germander [xxv] drunk.			Decoction of Germander drunk.
Juyce of water Germander the weight of a dram drunk.			Juyce of water Germander drunk, or the hearb used as a suppositary.
Decoction of Mugwort fomented beneath. [xxvi]	Decoction of Mugwort bathed.		Decoction of Mugwort used as a Bath.
Flowers and leaves of Fleabane [xxvii] drunk.			Flowers and leaves of Flea-bane drunk.
Seed of Wall-flowers [xxviii] the weight of two drams taken in wine.	Wall-flowers the weight of two drams taken in wine.		Seed of Wall-flowers the weight of two drams taken in wine.
Leaves of Wild Buglosse [xxix] taken in wine.			
Roots of Madir, [xxx] used in a Suppositary.	Roots of Madir used in a suppositary.		Roots of Madir applied below.
Leaves of Beane Trefoile drunke in sod wine; or worne about the necke, so soone as the woman is delivered. [xxxi]	Leaves of Beane Trefoile drunke in sod wine.		Leaves of Beane Trefoile bruised, and drunk in sod wine.
Roots of Orkanet applyed. [xxxii]			

(continued)

Table 1 (*continued*)

Abortifacient Medications: Other Uses

ABORTIFACIENTS	EXPEL AFTER-BIRTH (from 25 total)	EXPEL A DEAD CHILD (all remedies)	PROVOKE TERMS (from 114 total)
Juyce of Mandragore surringed.[xxxiii]			Juyce of Mandragore, the weight of halfe an obol applied below.
Sweet Chervill drunk.			Sweet Chervill[xxxiv] drunk.
Leaves of Turnsole put into the naturall place of Women.[xxxv]			Turne-sole leaves, applied beneath.
Perfume of Brimston taken below.[xxxvi]			
Seed of yellow Carrot drunk.[xxxvii]			
Gum ammoniacum drunk.[xxxviii]			Gum Ammoniacum drunke.
Woodbinde seed the weight of a dram taken in wine.			
Roote of Alexandrian Bayes the weight of six drams taken in sweet wine.			
Allome used in a suppositary.[xxxix]			
Jasper stone fastened to the thigh.			
The Eagle stone used in the like manner [fastened to the thigh].			
The Samian stone worne about the neck			

(*continued*)

Table 1 (continued)

Abortifacient Medications: Other Uses

ABORTIFACIENTS	EXPEL AFTER-BIRTH (from 25 total)	EXPEL A DEAD CHILD (all remedies)	PROVOKE TERMS (from 114 total)
		Decoction of Sage drunk.	Decoction of Sage drunk.
	Decoction of Hore-hound drunk.	Decoction of Hore-hound drunk.	
		Decoction of Coltsfoot drunk.	

Note: Shaded remedies are listed in Dioscorides for the same purpose.

i "KASTOROS ORCHIS. Castoreum of Beaver. The Castor is a living creature of a double nature, being nourish for ye most part in ye waters with ye fishes & Crabs. The stones thereof are good against ye poisons of serpents. It is good also to cause sneesing, & generally, it is vsefull for many purposes. For two dragms thereof being dranck with Pulegium [= Penniroyal], doe provoke the menstrua, & doe cast out ye Embryons and the secondines." Dioscorides, Bk II.26, p. 99.

ii "Some say that the milke of a bitch when shee doth first whelp, doth do away with haire being anointed on, & that being dranck, it is an Antidot against Poy sonous medicines, & that it is a caster out of dead Embryos." Dioscorides, Bk II.78 [Gala gunaikos=Woman's milk entry], p. 110.

iii Wool fat or lanolin: "But that is best which is not made cleane with ye Radicula, & is smooth, smelling of unwasht wool, and which being rubbed with cold water in a shell growes white & hath nothing in it hard or compacted, as that which is counterfaited with Cerat or Adeps . . . being applied in woll [wool], it driues out the Embrya & the Menses." Dioscorides, Bk II.84, p. 113.

iv "And the berries of ye goates especially of such as live vpon the mountaines, being dranck with wine do cure the yellow jaundise. But being dranck with spices, they move ye Menstrua, & cast out the Embrya." Dioscorides, Bk II.98, p. 122.

v "And the dung of a Vultur being suffumigated is reported to draw out the Embrya." Dioscorides, Bk II.98, p. 123. Salmon (English Physician, p. 632) pre-scribes the fumes of a mixture of vulture dung, assafoetida, vulture feathers, ox-horn shavings and cow's to hasten birth and facilitate delivery. Feathers and dung are also listed as having similar efficacies as depilatory agents.

vi "Cicer that is set, or sown, is . . . expelling ot ye Menstrua & the Embrya." Dioscorides, Bk II.126, p. 136.

vii "It [decoction of lupines] bringeth down the menses, and expelleth the dead child if it be laid to with myrrh and honie." Gerard, 1633, p. 1218. "being given in a pessum with Myrrh & hony doth extract the menstrua & the Embrya." Dioscorides, Bk II.132, p. 144.

viii Sium maius latifolium (Gerard, p.256). "SION TO EN ODASIN. Sium aquaticum . . . expel ye Embrya, and ye menstrua." Dioscorides, Bk II. 154, p. 167.

ix“And Collyries also are formed of it with Hony for fistulas, & for ye drawin out of the Embrya. . . . The smell of ye roote, or of the herbe, is destructiue of late conceptions, as also thirtie graines of the seed being dranck with Posca (are of ye like effect).” Dioscorides, Bk II. 195, p. 206.

x“It is good also being either dranck, or anointed on, for periodicall rigors (of feuers) . . . & it driues out ye Embrya. And being applied as a Pessum it seems to be a hinderer of conception after coniunction.” Dioscorides, Bk II.189, p. 199.

xiHanging the root “about women in extreame trauell with childe, causeth them to be delivered incontinent, and taketh away much of their paine. . . . It is not good for women with childe to touch or take this herb, or to come neere vnto it, or stride ouer the same where it groweth for the natural attractiue vertue therein contained is such, that without controuersie they that attempt it maner abouesaid, shall be deliuered before their time.” (Gerard, p.845).

“KUKLAMINOS Cyclamen graecum. . . . They say that if a women great with childe doe go over ye roote, that shee doth make abortion, and being tyed about her it doth hasten the birth.” Dioscorides, Bk II.194, p. 203.

xii“KISSOS. . . . And the Corymbi being small beaten, & giuen as a Pessum, doe moue the menstrua. . . . And the Pediculus foliorum, being moystened with hony, & put into ye vulua, doth expel the menstru, & the embrya.” Dioscorides, Bk II. 210, p. 225.

xiii“But ye roote being layed to as a Collyrie doth cast out ye Embrya.” Dioscorides, Bk III.3, p. 235.

xiv“KENTAURION MAKRON. . . . It [the root] expells also ye menstrua, & ye Embra, being shaved into the form of a Collyrie, & applied to ye Vulua, the juice also doth do ye same things.” Dioscorides, Bk III.36, p. 240.

xv“KENTURION MIKRON. . . . Feverwort. . . . Ye juice also is good for eye medicines . . . & in a pessum it is extractive of ye menstrua & ye Embrya.” Dioscorides, Bk III.9, p. 241.

xvi“boiled in wine and drunken, prouoketh the monthly termes, bringeth forth the secondine [after birth]xvi, the dead childe and the vnnaturall birth.” (Gerard, p. 672). “But being drunk it expelleth ye menstrua, & ye seconds, & ye Embrya.” Dioscorides, Bk III.36, pp. 270–271.

xvii“DIKTAMNON. . . . doeth all things that the sative Pulegium [Penny-royall], but more forcibly, for not only being drank but also being applied and suffumigated it expells the dead Embrya.” Dioscorides, Bk III.37, p. 271.

xviii“THUMOS. . . . But ye decoction of it with honey . . . expells ye worms and ye menstrua, & ye Embrya, & ye secondines.” Dioscorides, Bk III. 44, p. 278.

xix“THUMBRA. . . . It can perform all ye things as Thyme, being taken after ye like manner, & it is fitting for ye use in health.” Dioscorides, Bk III.45, p. 281.

xx“BAKCHARIS. But one of ye tender roots being applied as a Pessum draws out ye Embryo, & ye decoction of it is good by way of Insession for women in child-bed.” Dioscorides, Bk III.51, p. 286.

xxi“Root of Hercules All-heale [Panax herculinum]: “PANAKES HERAKLEION. . . . ye root being shaven and laid to ye Vulua draws out ye Embryo.” Dioscorides, Bk III.55, p. 292.

xxii“The naturall plants of Seseli, being now better knowne than in times past, especially among our Apothecaries, is called by them Siler montanum and Seseleos.” Gerard, p. 1049.

"SESELI MASSALEOTIKON. . . . ye seed & the root . . . being drank they cure ye strangurie, . . . & they move ye mestrua, & ye Embryo." Dioscorides, Bk III. 60, p. 296. The same effects are reported for "Sesili aithopikon" and "Sesili Peloponnesiakon" (pp. 297–98).

xxiii"Galbanum is ye liquor of ye Ferula growing in Syria, which some call Metopium . . . being either applied or suffited, it expels ye menstrua, & ye Embryo." Dioscorides, Bk III.97, p. 330.

xxiv"Clinopodium. "But ye herb & the decoction of it is drank. . . . And it drives out ye menstrua, & embryo." Dioscorides, Bk III.109, p.340.

xxv"Chamaedrys. "CHAMAIDRUS. . . . But it must be gathered when great with seed; being newly taken, & soe sodden with water, & given for a drink, it hath power. . . . It expells also ye menstrua & embryo." Dioscorides, Bk III.112, p.343.

xxvi"ARTEMESIA MONOKLONOS. . . . But being sodden they are good to be put into womanish insessions for ye driving out of ye menstrua, & ye secondines, & ye Embryo." Dioscorides, Bk III.127, p.357.

xxvii"Conyza. "KONUZA. . . . & ye flower & ye leaves are drank with wine for ye expulsion of ye menstrua & ye casting out of ye Embryo." Dioscorides, Bk III.136, p.366.

xxviii"LEUKOION. . . . But ye seed of it being drank with wine, the quantity of 2 dragms, or applied as a pessum with honey doth draw out ye menstrua, & ye secondines, & ye Embrya." Dioscorides, Bk III.138, p. 369.

xxix Onosma. "The leaves of this being drank in wine expel ye Embryo." Dioscorides, Bk III.147, p. 375.

xxx"Ye root put up as a Pessum, expels ye Embryo, & ye menstrua, & ye secondines." Dioscorides, Bk III.160, p. 386.

xxxi Anagyris. "It is given to drink ye quantity of a dragm, in Passum for ye Asthma, & ye casting out of ye Secondine, & ye menstrua, & ye Embryo." Dioscorides, Bk III.167, p.392.

xxxii"Orkanet; Alkanet, Anchusa (Gerard, pp. 799–801). "Anchusa . . . being given as a Pessum it draws out ye Embrya." Dioscorides, Bk IV. 23, p. 421.

xxxiii"Ye juice . . . being put up to of itself, as much as half an Obolus, it expels ye menstrua, & ye Embryo, & being put up into ye seat for a suppository, it causeth sleep." Dioscorides, Bk IV.76, p. 473.

xxxiv Myrrhis. Dioscorides, Bk IV 116, p. 509.

xxxv"Ye leaves smeared on . . . move also ye menstrua, and expel ye Embrya, being beaten small, & so applied." Dioscorides, Bk IV.193, p.596.

xxxvi"Being suffumigated it draws out ye Embryo." Dioscorides, Bk V.124, p. 644.

xxxvii"Daucus. . . . But ye seed of them all hath a warming faculty, being drank, expelling of ye menstrua, ye embryo & ye urine." Dioscorides, Bk III. 83, p. 316.

xxxviii"And being drank it brings down ye belly, & drives out ye Embryo." Dioscorides, Bk III. 98, p. 340.

xxxix"Allom of Melo also co-operates with inconception, being laid before conjuction to ye mouth of the matrix, and it expels ye Embrya." Dioscorides, Bk V. 123, p. 643.

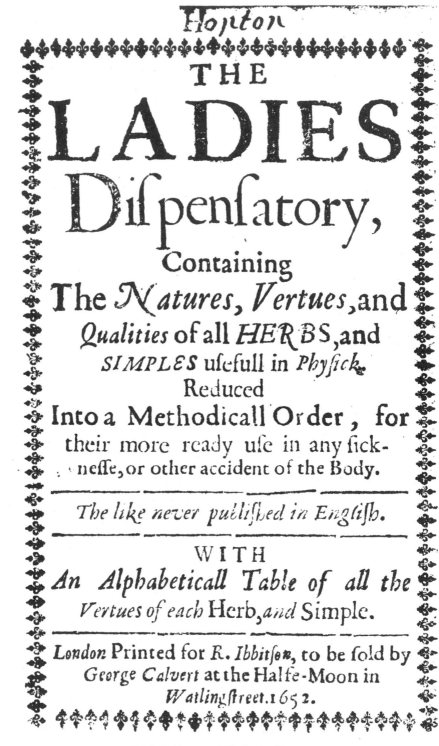

Hopton

THE
LADIES
Dispensatory,

Containing

The *Natures, Vertues,* and *Qualities* of all *HERBS,* and *SIMPLES* usefull in *Physick*. Reduced Into a Methodicall Order, for their more ready use in any sicknesse, or other accident of the Body.

The like never published in English.

WITH

An Alphabeticall Table of all the Vertues of each Herb, *and* Simple.

London Printed for R. *Ibbitson,* to be sold by *George Calvert* at the Halfe-Moon in *Watling street.* 1652.

Original title page of *The Ladies Dispensatory*

TO
His very good Friend
Mr. Gabriel Taylor.

Sir,

I Here present unto you, the painfull delivery of a long travaile; I hope you wil hold my boldnesse excused, that I have presumed to send it forth into the World under your Name; as that also you will bee pleased to accept this as a tribute, of the Affection and Ingagements, due unto you from me, for those many favours I have received of you, and which still oblige me to remain.

Yours,
to serve you wherein
he may,
LEONARD SOVVERBY.

To the Reader.

Courteous Reader,

After much revolving, writing, and blotting out, I resolved in my selfe to have said nothing unto thee, but fearing thou mightest be prejudiced against me, I have thought good to premise the helpes and Authors, I have had and followed, which are, Gerard *with* Johnson, Goraeus *and* Fuchsius, *men of excellent knowledge, and well esteemed in this kind of learning.*

Against my Authour Dioscorides, *I do not so much as presuppose any Objection, who having learned most Languages, and seen many Countries, with good entertainment, will I presume finde as good reception in England, and be esteemed correspondent to his worth, and the credit he hath acquired among all learned men.*

The work doth sufficiently commend itself, being the first and only peece of this kinde in our English tongue, containing almost as many Medicines as lines, &those consisting of pure, Elementary Simples; not compounded of a hodgepodge of sophisticated Drugs (like the Cadmeian Progenie*) one oppugning the other.*

Thus hoping thou wilt pardon the errors (from which no man is exempted) of this Collection, and accept of my paines, and good will; I Remaine,

Thine,
Leo. Sowerby.

The Ladies Dispensatory

SIMPLES SERVING FOR THE HEAD.

Against paines of the Head arising from Cold.

ROotes of Flower-de-luce of *Illyria*, applied with Vinegar and Oyle of Roses.

Oyle of wilde Olives[1] applyed.

Oyle of Almonds applyed.

Seed of *Agnus Castus* applyed like a Poultis.

Bitter Almonds bruised, and applyed like a Poultis on the fore-head, and cheeks, with vinegar, or oyl of roses.

Cramp-fish applyed alive.

New-shorne unwashed Wooll, applyed with vinegar, and oyl of roses.

[2]Water-minte bruised, and laid to the fore-head and temples.

Juyce of the leaves, or of the berries of Ivie, applyed with vinegar and oyle of roses.

Aloes applyed on the fore-head and cheekes, with vinegar and oyle of roses.

Minte bruised and laid to.

Wild Time boyled, then moystned in vinegar and oyle of roses and applyed.

Leaves of [3]Plow-mans Spikenard bruised, and laid to.

---

[1]Anointed, or layed to any way outwardly.
[2]Sisymbrium, or Water-cresses.
[3]Baccharis.

Rue laid to with vinegar, and oyle of roses.

Anise taken in drinke.

[4]Meddow-parsnep laid to with Rue

[5]Sow-fennell laid to with vinegar, and oyle of roses.

[6]Gith laid upon the fore-head, small fleabane laid to.

The tender leaves of [7]Beane-Trifoly, the weight of a dram taken in wine.

[8]The roote which smelleth like roses, laid to fresh with a little oyle of roses.

A chaplet of [9]Horse-tongue.

Leaves of [10]Periwinckle bruised, and laid to.

Juyce of wild Cowcumbers, dropped into the nose with milke.

Leaves and berries of Kneeholme, drunke in wine.

Scammonie applyed with vinegar, and oyle of roses.

Perfume of Sea-water, received as a stove, the head being covered.

Against paines of the Head, proceeding from heate.

OYle of Wild Olives applyed.

Oyle of roses applyed as a linement.

Flowers of privet laid to with vinegar.

The infusion of dry Roses well pressed, applyed.

Seed of *Agnus Castus* layed to.

Purslaine laid to.

Melilot layed to with vinegar, or oyle of roses.

Roots of Water-Lilly drunk, or put to the nostrils.

Rose-wort[11] layed on the fore-head, and on the temples, with oyle of roses.

Juyce of Poppy[12] applyed on the fore-head with oyle of roses.

Fleawort[13] layed to with oyle of roses, vinegar, or water.

A chaplet of Horse-tongue.

Great Housleeke layed to with oyle of roses.

Leaves of morell, or Garden Night-shade applyed.

---

[4]Spondilium.

[5]Peucedanum.

[6]*Nigella Romana* of the Apothecaries.

[7]*Anagyris.*

[8]*Rhodia radix*, Rosewort.

[9]*Hippo-glossum.*

[10]Chamce-daphne.

[11]*Rhodia radix.*

[12]Otherwise Opium.

[13]Psyllium.

Leaves and branches of Vine layed to.
Serpentine Marble worne about the neck, or arme.

To purge the Braine.

IUyce of Cole-wort, of wind-flowre, of Beets, of Celandine, of Sow-bread,[14]
or of Onions snuffed up the nose.
Pellitory of Spaine, and Staphis-acre chewed long.
    Coloquintida in pils.
    Dry Grapes chewed with Pepper.
    Vitriol snuffed up the nose, and put into the nostrils with Cotton.

To mittigate the Head-ach.

THe sent of oyle of Storax.
    Yellow Olives, Acornes, Phenician Dates, or Wall-nuts often eaten.
    Arbute berries, and branches of herbe Ferula eaten.
    Rootes of Spicknell taken abundantly.
Juyce of Worme-wood drunk.

Against the Lethargy.[15]

SEed of *Agnus Castus* layed to with vinegar, and oyle of roses.
    Castorium dropped into the nostrils with vinegar and oyle of roses.
    Boyled onions eaten.
    Mustard layed to, the head first shaved.
Medow Parsnep[16] used in perfume, or applyed on the head with oyle olive.
Sow-fennell layed to with vinegar and oyle of roses.

To provoke sleepe.

ROote of Flower-de-luce of *Illyria* drunk.
    Amomum[17] put upon the fore-head.
    Bitter Almonds eaten.
    Seed of *Agnus Castus* drunk.
    Lettice eaten.
    Aloes applyed alone, or with oyle of roses.
    The sent of Plow-mans spikenard.
    Seed of Aethiopian reed drunk.

---

[14]*Cyclamen.*
[15]The drowsie or sleepy evil.
[16]Spondilium.
[17]In place of which the greater Galingall may be taken, saith Fuchseus.

Five or six heads of wildPoppy,[18] boyled in three Cyathes of wine to the consumption of halfe, drunk.
Decoction of the heads or leaves of poppy drunk, or applyed.
Seed of Henbane drunk, or layed to.
Rinde of the roote of sleepy Night-shade, the weight of a dram taken in wine.
Decoction of Mandragore roote the measure of a Cyath, drunke with wine.
The smell of Mandragore apples.
Juyce of Mandragore used in the manner of a suppositary.

To cause horrible dreadfull Dreames.

BEanes eaten.
Lentils eaten.
Seed of Devils-bit,[19] the weight of a dram drunk.
Seed of great Bind-weed[20] the weight of three oboles drunk, with as mych venemous Tree Tre-foile.[21]

To cause Sneezing.

MVstard-seed bruised, and put to the nose.
The sent of sneezing-wort-flower.
The rootes of Sope-wort, bruised and put to the nose.
Powder of the roots of Crow-foot,[22] snuffed up the nose.
Spurge Laurell taken up the nose.
Powder of the roote of white Hellebore, snuffed up the nose.

Against Vertiginosities.[23]

SEed of Baulme drunk
SOw-fennell layed to with vinegar, and oyle of roses.
The smell of Galbanum.
Briony roote the weight of a dram drunk every day a whole yeare.
The tender branches of black Briony[24] boyled and eaten.
Squil wine drunk.
Squil vinegar drunk.

[18]Red poppy growing in Corn.
[19]Pycnocomon;
[20]Convolvulus major.
[21]*Dorycnium.*
[22]*Ranunculus*, called about *London* Butterflower.
[23]Swimmings and giddinesse of the head.
[24]*Vitis nigra.*

Against the Apoplexie.[25]

BRiony roote the weight of a dram, drunke every day a whole yeare.

Against the Falling-sicknesse.

GRaines of Paradise[26] drunke with water.
  Gum-Lac drunke.[27]
  Baulme-seed drunk.
  Perfume of Bitumen surnamed Naptha discovereth the Disease.
  Seeds of the Aspe Tree taken in vinegar Dry figgs eaten.
  The perfume of *Unguis odoratus.*
Curd of a Hare[28] drunk.
  The outward skin of a Weesils cod; farced with Coriander, dryed and
    eaten.
  The bloud of a Weesil drunk.
  Liver of an Asse rosted, eaten fasting.
  An Asses hoofe burned, drunk.
  The bonie excrescence growing on the Cronet of a Horses hoofe[29]
bruised, and drunk in vinegar.
  Stones found in the belly of the Swallowes first brood, tyed in a peece
    of Buck-skin, and worn about the neck.
  Whey drunk till it have loosed the belly.
  Curd of a Sea-calfe drunk.
  Gall of a Beare taken like an Electuary.
  Gall of a Tortoise put in the nose.
  Bloud of a Land Tortoise drunk.
  Storkes dung drunk with water.
  Plantain boyled with Lentils eaten.
  Mustard-seed bruised and put to the nose.
  Pepper long chewed.
  Squil drunk.
  Agarick the weight of a dram taken with Oxymel.[30]
  Root of Sea-holly[31] drunke in water.
  Seed of wild Rue drunk.
  Roote and seed of mountaine Siler taken in drink.

---

[25]Or dead Palsie.
[26]*Cardamomum.*
[27]*Cancamum.*
[28]*Coagulum*, that whereby milke is turned and brought into curds.
[29]Lichenes.
[30]A composition made of vinegar, hony, and water.
[31]*Eryngium.*

Sow-fennel laid to the head with vinegar and oyle of roses.
Gum *Sagapene*[32] drunk.
Benzoin taken in hony and vinegar.
The smel of Labdanum.[33]
Gum Armoniacum[34] taken with hony like an Electuary.
Seed and leaves of Trefoile drunk.
Flea-wort taken in vinegar.
Small Anthyllis[35] taken in Oxymel.
Bettony leaves taken in drink.
Five-leaved grasse[36] taken in drinke the space of thirty dayes.
Seed of Spatling-poppie drunke in honied water.[37]
Black Hellebore drunk.
Juyce of Hippophestus,[38] the weight of three oboles drunk.
Briony the weight of a dram drunk every day for a yeare.
Branches of black Briony Boyled[39] and eaten.
Honyed vinegar[40] drunk.
Squil wine, or Squil vinegar drunk.
The specular Stone[41] powdered, and drunk.
The Eagle Stone[42] in powder, applyed with oyntment of privet, or
Gleucinum,[43] or some other hot oyntment,
Naxian Stone[44] drunk.

Against the Frensie.

OYle of Saffron sprinkled on the head, put in the nose, or annointed.
Agnus Castus dropped into the nose with oyle of roses and vinegar.
Sparagus drunk in white wine, wild Time layed to with oyle of roses and
vinegar.

---

[32]It distils from a certain herbe in Media.
[33]A fat clammie matter, a kinde of Cistus.
[34]Issuing from the Cyrenian ferula.
[35]Sea pimpernell after *Gerrard*.
[36]Or cinque foile.
[37]*Aqua mulsa*, water mingled with hony.
[38]Thought to be a kinde of Fullers Teasell.
[39]*Vitis Nigra*.
[40]Hony mingled with vinegar.
[41]A stone cleare like glasse.
[42]Found in Eagles Nests.
[43]Oyle comming before the Olives be thorow prest.
[44]A kinde of Whetstone brought from Cyprus.

Perfume of meddow Parsnep,[45] or the herbe layed to the head with oyle.
Sow-fennell[46] applyed with oyle of roses and vinegar.

Against inflamations of the braine.

PArings of Gourds laid on the fore-part of the head.
    Parings of Pompions[47] layed on the fore part.
    Leaves of Turne-soile,[48] layed on the fore-head.
    Vinegar applyed on the forehead.

Against Melancholly.

SEed of Basill drunk.
    Black Hellebore drunk.
    Bettony leaves drunk.
    Dodder[49] drunk.

To prevent Drunkennesse.

SAffron taken fasting in sod wine[50]
    Juyce of Pomegranats drunke.
    Juyce of Mirtle-berries drunk.
    Coleworts eaten after meales.
    Wormewood eaten fasting,

Against Catharres and Rheumes discending from the head.

OYle of Flower-deluce put in the Nostrills.
    Storax applyed, or the perfume of it.
    Perfume of Bitumen.
    Cinnamon taken in drinke.
    Rootes of Spicknell bruised and taken with hony like an Electuary:
     especially when the rheumes oppresse the Stomach.
    Filbirds rosted, and drunk with a little pepper.
    Root of great Draggons rosted in embers, or boiled, eaten.

---

[45]*Spondilium.*
[46]*Peucedanum.*
[47]*Popon.*
[48]*Heliotropium.*
[49]*Epithymum.*
[50]*Sapa.*

Gum Dragant taken with hony, like an electuary.

Hysope, figs, rue and hony boyled in water, the decoction drunk.

Golden mothweed,[51] the weight of three obols drunke in wine and water.

Henbane seed the weight of one obol, drunk with seed of poppy.

To fortifie the brain.

WOod of Aloes.[52]

Against the Scurfe, and Vlcers flowing in the head.

FRankincense and Niter to rub the Ulcers.

Milk of garden and wild fig-tree, applyed with dry polenta.[53]

Stale urine to wash the Ulcers.

Fenegreek applyed.

Cich pease applyed.

Mallows used as a poultis with mans urine.

Ashes of garlicke incorporated in hony and laid to.

Fomentation with the decoction of Sowbread.[54]

Scalions applied with burned niter.

Melilot applyed with water and earth of Chio, or with wine and galls,

Bramble leaves laid to,

Rootes of Lillies burn'd and applyed with hony.

Maiden-haire bioled in lye

Sharpe brine rubbed on the Ulcers.

SIMPLES SERVING FOR THE SINEWES.

Against the Spasme.[55]

ILlyrian Flower-deluce drunk in vinegar,

Decoction of sweet-cane drunke.

Graines of Paradise drunke in water.

Root of Squinanth,[56] the weight of a dram, taken certaine dayes with the like weight of Pepper.

Costus taken in wine with wormwood.

---

[51]*Helychrisum.*

[52]Agallochum.

[53]Barly steeped in water, dried by a fire and after fryed for phisicall uses.

[54]Cyclamen.

[55]Shrinking of the Sinewes.

[56]*Squinanthum,* camells hay.

Baulme taken in water.

Elicampane taken with hony as an Electuary.

Oyntment of Marjerome used as a poultis.

Oyntment of Galbanum applyed,

Bdelium[57] applyed

Juniper berries drunk.

Fruit of cedar eaten.

Root of sea Purslaine,[58] the weight of a dram taken in honied water.

Ashes of fig-tree applyed with oyle.

Castorium laid to, and drunk

Wild time drunk.

Roots of Dragons rosted in embers, or boyled, eaten with hony.

Asphodill rootes the weight of a dram drunk.

Fruite of the Caper bush[59] drunke.

Rinde of the Caper plant drunk.

Bastard wild poppy,[60] applyed as a poultis.

Agaricke the weight of three obols taken in honied wine.

Rhaponticke[61] taken in drink

Galbanum taken in pills.

Gentian root the weight of a dram drunk.

Aristolochia rotunda[62] drunk.

Root of great Centuary[63] drunk in wine.

Seed of white thistle drunk.

Roots of Acanthium[64] drunk.

Seed of Suthernwood drunk in water.

Decoction of the root of Lady thistle[65] in wine drunk.

Organie eaten with figs.

Rootes of Sea holly[66] drunke with honied water.

Penniroyal drunke with water and vinegar.

Decoction of Calaminte drunk.

Roots of Plowmans spiknard[67] boiled in water, drunk.

---

[57]A Gum brought from Arabia and India.

[58]*Halimus.*

[59]*Capers.*

[60]*Argemone.*

[61]The best Rubarbe brought from Pontus.

[62]Round birth wort.

[63]Falsly put for the true Rhaponticke in shops.

[64]Cotton thistle.

[65]*Leucaeantha.*

[66]*Eryngium.*

[67]*Baccharis.*

Hercules Al heale applyed.
Rosemary roots applyed with meale of Darnel, as a poultis.
Sow-fennel[68] laid to with vinegar and oile of roses.
Wild Basil[69] taken in drink.
Decoction of Germander drunk.
Benzoin the weight of an obol taken in pils.
Serapinum[70] drunk.
Bettony leaves a penny weight taken in honyed water.
Roots of stinking Gladen[71] drunk in sod wine.
Comfry taken in honyed vinegar.
Flea-wort layed to.
Wild Time drunk, or applyed.
Decoction of Mullein drunk.
Briony eaten with hony as an electuary.
Squil wine drunk.
Germander wine drunk.
Wine of Goates organie.[72]
Satirioa rootes drunke in strong wine.
*Bastard St-Johns-wort drunk.
(*) [[Coris.]]

Against the Palsie, and resolution of the Sinewes.

SOw-fennel layed to with vinegar and oyle of roses.
Bark of the Caper plant drunk, also the fruit.
Rootes of Madir drunk.
Coloquintida taken in a Glister.
The first shootes of black Briony boyled and eaten.
Squil wine drunk.

Against trembling of the Sinewes.

BRaines of Hares fryed and eaten.
Castorium drunk, and applyed.
Cole-worts eaten.
Decoction of marsh mallowes drunk.

[68]*Peucedanum.*
[69]*Clinopodium.*
[70]Gum Sagapenum.
[71]Spatula taetida.
[72]Tragoriganum.

Against Rheumes fallen upon the Sinewes.

VVHeaten meale, incorporated in juyce of Henbane, and applyed.
  Barly meale incorporated in vinegar, and layed to.

Against Aches, and weaknesses of the Sinewes.

OYle Sycionium[73] aplyed.
  Oyle of Bayes applyed.
  Eleomelie[74] applyed.
  Oyle of privet.
  Oyle comming before the Olives be thorow pressed applyed.
  Oyle of Galbanum.
  Oyle of great Marjerome.
  Bdelium put in a poultis.
  Lexive of the ashes of Fig-tree applyed with oyle.
  Castorium drunk and applyed.
  Hedge-hogs eaten.
  Vipers flesh boyled and eaten.
  Decoction of Burnet[75] drunk.
  Sow-fennel applyed with vinegar and oyle of roses.
  Laser,[76] the weight of an obol taken in pils.
  Small centaury taken in drink.
  Roots of Lillies rosted in embers, incorporated in hony and applyed.
  Satirion root drunk in strong wine.
  Roots of marsh mallowes alone, or boyled in wine, or in honied water,
and used as a poultis.
  Scarlet graine layed to with vinegar, is good for cut sinewes.
  Leaves of Ground-sel applyed, is good for the same effect.
  Daffodil roots is also profitable.
  Juyce of Hyppophestus the weight of three obols taken.
  Sea-water fomented.
  Squil vinegar drunk.
  Wine of French Lavender[77] drunk.
  Wine of Time drunk.
  [*] Sesaminum layed to.
[*] [[An oyley graine.]]

---

[73]Made of wild Cowcumber roots and juyce, and oyle.
[74]A sweet fat liquor issuing from the trunks of certaine trees in Syria.
[75]Poterium, called by *Gallen* Neuras.
[76]The sap of Laser-wort called Benzoin, there is another sort named, Asa foetida.
[77]Stichas.

For cut sinewes.

SNayles bruised and layed to.
> Earth-wormes bruised and applyed.
> Butter layed to.
> Ground-sel leaves applyed as a poultis, with crums of Frankincense.
> Leaves of small Dragons applyed.
> Roots of Burnet[78] bruised and applyed.
> Lilly rootes incorporated in hony and layed to.
> Scarlet graine layed to with vinegar.
> Daffodil roots applyed.

To subtilize the Sinewes.

SEsaminum used as a poultis.
> Ashes of Vine branches applied with hoggs lard, or oyle.

SIMPLES SERVING FOR THE EYES.

To restraine falling of Haire from the Eye-lids.

FOmentation, with the decoction of spikenard.
> The moisture that Snails cast being pricked with a needle, laid upon the Eye-lids.
> The oylinesse of sheeps wool before it be washed layed to.
> Gumme and milk of Gum Succory[79] applyed.
> Bolearmonick layed to.

For sharpnesse of the Eyes, and Eye-lids.

BArke of the Frankincense Tree burned and layed to.
> Soote of Pitch[80] applyed.
> Juyce of Box thorne[81] layed to.
> Cutle bone powdered very small, and layed to.
> Gall of a Scorpeno,[82] or sea Urchin applyed.
> Gall of a sea Tortoise laid to.
> Gall of a Partridge applyed.

---

[78]Poterion.
[79]Chondrilla.
[80]Burned of purpose in a close pot.
[81]*Lycium.*
[82]A little dark green Fish found in the Marsellian Sea.

Gall of an Eagle applyed.

A white Pullets gall applyed.

Gall of a Hinde, or wilde she Goate applyed.

Powder of Mustard-seed incorporated in hony, and layed to.

Verjuyce applyed.

Scailes of brasse applyed.

Rust of Iron applyed.

Chalcitis[83] layed to.

Bloud-stone incorporated in hony,

Against the inflamations of the Eye-lids.

LEaves of great Marjerome layed to with polenta.

  Pimpernel applyed with polenta.

  Leaves of *Palma Christi* bruised, and applyed with polenta, like a
    poultis.

To make the Eye-lids thin.

AShes of Muskles washed as they wash lead, applyed.

  Ashes of *Unguis odoratus* applyed.

To heale the Itch of the Eye-lids.

IVyce of Onions layed to with the same weight of Spodium.[84]

  Milke of Fig-tree layed to.

To take spots and blemishes out of the Eyes.

OPobalsamum[85] layed to, and dropped into the eyes.

  Gum Lac[86] dissolved in wine, applyed.

  Myrrhe applyed.

  Bitumen named Naptha applyed.

  Ashes of Muskles washed, as they wash lead, applyed.

  Ashes of *Unguis odoratus* applyed on the eyes.

  Ashes of Snailes shels incorporated in hony applyed.

  Gall of a Scorpeno, or sea Hedge-hogge dropped into the eyes.

---

[83]A naturall caustick and corrosive Minerall, somewhat resembling brasse, and is full of long & shining veines.

[84]The shavings of Ivory, or Hartshorn (is commonly used for it) burned. Aloes applyed.

[85]Liquor of the Balsame tree.

[86]Cancamum.

The like may be done with the Galls of a sea Tortoise, of Partridge, of Eagle, of white Henne, or of wild she Goate.

Mans urine boyled in a Copper pot, applyed.

Milke of wild Lettice distilled into the eyes.

Juyce of Dragons applyed.

Juyce of Onions distilled into the eyes.

Ginger applyed.

Juyce of Spurge Time[87] applyed with hony.

Leaves of Bastard wild Poppy[88] applyed.

Gum Armoniack applyed.

Clary[89] layed to with hony.

Juyce of Melilot applyed with hony.

Salt applyed.

Flos salis[90] applyed.

Saphire stone applyed.

Scailes of brasse applyed.

To take skarres out of the eyes.

GUm Lac dissolved in wine, droped into the eye.

Myrrhe applyed.

Bitumen named Naptha applyed.

Rosin of Cedar layed to.

Ashes of Snailes applyed with hony.

Mans urine boyled in a Copper pot, distilled into the eyes.

Oyle of Fenegreeke, applyed with oyle of Mirtle.

Gum sapagene[91] applyed.

Juyce of Spurge Time[92] applyed with hony.

Verdigrease applyed.

Wine lees burned applyed.

Powder of Corral put thereon.

Bloud-stone layed thereon.

Saphire applyed.

Snayles burned in their shels, applyed with hony.

[87]Chamaesyce.
[88]Argemone.
[89]Orminum.
[90]A brackish foam or scum floating on certaine Lakes.
[91]Serapinum.
[92]Chamaesyce.

Against dimnesse and darknesse of Sight.

IVyce of sweet Cane dropped into the eyes.

Cinamon incorporated in other ocular Medicines, for to lay to the eyes.

Cinnamomum[93] put in the eyes.

Gum of Cherry-tree put into the eyes.

Infusion of Aeacalis[94] put in medicines prescribed to quicken the sight.

Juyce of Acacia[95] washed, and dropped into the eyes.

Three Pomegranat-flowers (how little soever they be) eaten, preserve one a whole yeare from blear-eyed-nesse.

Frankincense put in the eye.

Oyntment or dreggs of oyle of saffron[96] applyed.

Small shavings of Ebonie, infused in good wine, and applyed as a Collyrie.[97]

Juyce of Box-thorne put upon the eye.

Rosin of Cedar applyed.

Plum-tree Gum applyed.

Vipers flesh boyled and eaten.

Swallowes eaten.

Ashes of burned swallowes put in Collyries.

Fish-grease applyed.

Juyce of Fennel dropped into the eyes.

The galls of a Scorpeno, or Hedge-hogge of the sea, of Partridge, of Eagle, of white Hen, or of wild she Goat, distilled into the eyes.

Mans urine boyled in a Copper vessel, used as aforesaid.

Milk of wild Lettice used as before.

Juyce of the root of great Dragons.

Juyce of Onion dropped into the eyes.

Juyce of Melilot.

Juyce of Celandine boyled with hony in a copper vessel, applyed.

Juyce of Chelidony[98] dropped into the eyes.

Juyce of small Centaury.

Rue eaten frequently.

Verjuyce distilled into the eyes.

Hercules All-heale applyed.

[93]Cinamon of the Antients.
[94]The seed of an herb growing in AEgypt, much like the seed of Tamarisk.
[95]Or of sloes.
[96]Crocomagma.
[97]Any liquid medicine.
[98]Othoma.

Juyce of the roots and leaves of Rosemary dropped into the eyes.
Benzoin applyed with hony.
Juyce of Baulme distilled into the eyes with hony.
Juyce of Hore-hound applyed with hony.
Powder of Pumise-stone put into the eyes.
Flos salis put into the eyes.
Wine-lees burned, put into the eyes.
Marchasite-stone[99] put on the eyes.
The stone Thyites[100] put on the eye.
The stone Geodes[101] applyed.
The Saphire stone applyed.

To take a Web out of the Eye.

POwder of Cutle-bone applyed.
Liquoris powder put in the eye.

For hurts and fresh wounds of the Eyes.

VVOmans milke dropped into them with Frankinsence.
Bloud of Ring-doves, of Pidgeons, of Turtle-doves, or of Partridges applyed.
Leaves of Stoebe[102] applyed as a Poultis.
Bloud-stone put into the eyes with milke.

For Ulcers of the Eyes.

SOote of Frankinsence,[103] or of Turpentine, or of Butter applyed.
Barke of the frankincense Tree.
Myrrhe cast in the eye.
Ashes of Harts-horne well washed, applyed.
Liniment of Amylum,[104] especially when the ulcers are hollow.
Antimonie put in the eye.
The stones Galactitus,[105] Samius,[106] also the Saphire distilled into the eyes with milke.

[99]A minerall that smells like Brimstone the best is pure white like silver.
[100]A greenish stone which steeped in liquor yeelds a white humour.
[101]A round stone of the colour of rusty Iron, containing within it a yellowish earth.
[102]Thought of some to be scabious.
[103]Burned of purpose in a close pot.
[104]Fine Wheat-flower steeped in water, then streined, & let stand till it settle at the bottome, then drained off the water and dryed in the Sun.
[105]Called the milk-stone.
[106]A whitish stone found among the Samien earth.

Against Erosions happening in the corners of the Eyes.

FAt or oylinesse of new shorne unwashed wool applied.
    Verjuyce dropped into the eye.

Against Fistulaes, and hollow ulcers of the Eyes.

OLd Walnuts bruised and layed to.
    Decoction of Mirtle dropped into the eyes.
    Raw mallowes chewed, and applyed with a little salt.
    Plantaine applyed as a Poultis.
    The second kinde of *Auricula murie*[107] applyed.
    Leaves of Plow-mans Spikenard applyed as a Poultis, at the beginning of
      the malady.
    Cammomel applyed.
    Leaves of Morel[108] chopped small applyed; or the juyce layed to with the
reddest of a Hens dung.
    Haver grasse applied.
    Flowers of wild (Grape-bearing) Vine[109] applied.
    Alexandrian Tutie, or Calamine[110] applied.
    Scailes of brasse applied.
    Powder of Antimonie put into the Fistula.

To retire the eyes standing too farre forth of the head, and to take away spots, or buds that grow in the eyes.

BEane meale incorporated in white of Egges, with roses and frankincense,
      applied as a Poultis.
    Bramble leaves bruised and applied.
    Saphire stone applied.

Against Inflamations of the eyes.

AMomum layed to with dry Grapes.
    Soote of Frankincense, or of Pitch, applied as a Liniment.[111]
    Cyprus apples layed to with Polenta.
    Mirtil-berries applyed with Polenta.

---

[107]Mouse eare.
[108]Garden Night-shade.
[109]Oenanthe.
[110]A certain yellow minerall substance.
[111]Any thin oyntment.

Quince-flowers used as a poultis.

Cheese applied.

Sugar distilled into the eyes.

Sesaminum boyled in wine applied.

Purslaine layed to with polenta.

Endive applied alone, or with dry polenta.

Parings of Gourds applied.

Roots of Wind-flower[112] applied.

Mouse-eare, applied with polenta like a poultis.

Juyce of Gentian applied.

Sothern-wood boyled with Quinces, or with bread, used as a poultis.

Melilot put in poultisses, prescribed for inflammations.

Leaves of Plow-mans spikenard applyed.

Leaves of Housleeke applied.

Parsley applied with bread, or polenta.

Flowers of the Raspis-bush applied with hony.

Leaves of Burnet applyed with polenta.

Juyce of Poppie incorporated in the yolke of an egge, then rosted in embers, and layed to with saffron.

Seed and leaves of Henbane applied with meale, or polenta.

Fresh leaves of Mandragore applied with polenta.

Leaves of Mullein, which beareth yellow flowers layed to.

Starre-wort[113] applied.

Sweet Violet leaves applyed.

Leaves of *Palma Christi* applied with Polenta.

For paines of the Eyes.

YOlke of an Egge rosted in embers, applyed with oyle of roses, and oyle of saffron.

Sesaminum boyled in wine applied.

Juyce of Basill dropped into the eyes.

Wormwood boyled in sod wine, applied.

Rue used as a Poultis with Polenta.

Root of Aconitum, surnamed Pardalianchus put in medicaments prescribed for the eyes.

For persons which are pur-blinde.

GRavie dropping from the Liver of a he, or she Goat, rosted.

Liver of a Wild she Goat, rosted, eaten.

---

[112]Anemone.

[113]Aster Atticus.

Gall of a wild she Goat applied.

Bloud of Stock-doves, of Pidgeons, of Turtle Doves, or of Partridges applied.

Against the Pinne, or Web in the Eyes.

GAll of a Scorpeno applied on the eyes.

Vipers grease incorporated in rosin of Cedar.[114]

Pure hony and old oyle.

Galls of Sea Tortoises, of Partridges, of Eagles, of white Hens, or of wild she Goats applied.

Beane meale kneaded in wine, applied.

Juyce of Onions dropped into the eyes.

Juyce of Sow-bread used as aforesaid.

Gum Sagapene applyed.

Gum Euphoribium applyed with Annise.

Against weaknesse of sight.

GUm-Lac dissolved in wine, distilled into the eyes.

Little balles found upon Poplar-trees when they first begin to bud,[115] bruised and applyed with hony.

Gall of a Scorpeno applyed.

Cole-worts eaten.

Mustard applyed with hony.

Time eaten.

Juyce of Pimpernel taken up the nose.

Summer savoury eaten with meate.

Worm-wood applyed with hony.

Juyce of Rue boyled in a Pomegranate shel, adding thereto juyce of fennel, and hony, dropped into the eyes.

Juyce of wild Rue distilled into the eye with wine, hony, chickens dung, and juyce of fennel.

Juyce of sleepy Night-shade applyed.

Flos salis applyed.

Against Catarres and Rhumes of the eyes.

SAffron applied with womans milk.

Frankincense applyed with the yolk or white of an egge.

Soote of frankincense applied.

[114]*Galen* approveth not this remedy.
[115]Pilulae.

Soote of pitch applied.

The tenderest leaves of great Maple[116] boyled in wine, applyed.

Shavings of Ebonie, powdered smal applied.

Juyce of the leaves of wild Olive-tree distilled into the eyes.

Harts-horne burned, washed, and applyed.

Soote of butter layed to.

Amylum applyed.

Tutie washed and applyed.

Beanes husked, chewed, and layed upon the fore-head.

Two drams of the seed of Water-basill, incorporated in foure drams of
   hony, applyed as a liniment.

Leaves of Burnet applyed with Polenta.

Scailes of brasse washed, and put in the eye.

Lead washed, applied.

The stones Galactites, Morochthus,[117] and Samius, put in the eye with
milke.

Sarcocalla[118] distilled into the eye.

Allome applyed.

Powder of Corrall applyed.

Powder of Pumeisestone applyed.

Powder of Bloud-stone.

Against Blear-eyednesse.

PUrslaine and the juyce applied.

Juyce of Plantaine dropped into the eyes.

Leaves of Housleeke applyed.

Powder of Chalcitis, but not without good advise.

Ashes of Sponges applyed, especially when the disease is dry.

Bloud-stone bruised, and applyed with milke.

Against dazeling of the Eyes.

POwder of Germander sprinkled on the eyes, or applyed with oyle.

Juyce of Melilot applyed with hony.

Black Hellebore put in Collyries prescribed for the eyes.

Verdigrease put in the eyes.

---

[116]Erroniously called, Sycamore.

[117]A stone wherewith Linnen Drapers use to whiten their cloth Colature of Henbane-seed applied.

[118]A bitter persian Gum.

SIMPLES SERVING FOR THE EARES.

Against paines of the Eares.

JUyce of Bay-berries incorporated in old Wine, and oyle of roses.

Juyce of Popler leaves, both this and the former must be dropped into the eares.

Labdanum applyed with wine.

Decoction of dry roses, boyled in wine, distilled into the eares.

Juyce of the leaves and barke of willow boyled with oyle of roses, in a Pomegranate shell, to annoynt the eares.

Juyce of sowre Pomegranats boyled with hony, dropped into the eares.

Opium[119] applied with oyle of Almonds, myrrhe, and saffron.

Serpents skin boyled in wine dropped into the eares.

Woodlice chopped small, and boyled in oyle of roses in a pomegranate shel, distilled into the eares.

The grease of a Foxes Lungs distilled into the eares.

Greene minerall Chalke boyled in Goose-grease dropped into the eares.

Grease of a Goose, or of a Fox, or of Hens, dropped into the eares.

Urine of a Bull, or of a wild Bore, boyled with myrrhe used as aforesaid.

Hony distilled into the eares with minerall salt.

Seed of Sesaminum put in the eares with oyle of roses.

Juyce of Beets used as aforesaid.

Juyce of Plantaine distilled into the eares when the peccant matter is hot.

Juyce of the parings of Gourds distilled into the eares with oyle of roses.

Juyce of great and small Dragons dropped into the eares.

Juyce of Leekes distilled with frankincense, vinegar, and milk.

Juyce or decoction of mustard.

Juyce of Ivie; and of the berries.

Wormwood perfumed, or applied with hony.

Juyce of greene Organie distilled with milk.

Juyce of Mint dropped into the eares.

Juyce of Melilot distilled with sod wine.

Juyce of Rue boyled in a Pomegranate shel.

Juyce of Sow-fennel, dropped into the eares with oyle of roses.

Juyce of Goose-grasse.[120]

Juyce of Hore-hound distilled into the eares with oyle of roses.

[119]The hardned juyce of Poppy heads.
[120]A small kinde of Burre.

Juyce of Hemp.
Juyce of Knot-grasse.
Juyce of wall Pellitory.
Juyce of water Basill distilled with Brimstone and Niter.
Colature of Henbane-seed distilled into the eares.
Juyce of Morell.
Juyce of Pimpernel.
Juyce of the leaves of wild Cowcumbers.
Salt dropped into the eares with vinegar.

Against interiour inflammations of the eares.

SAffron put in the eares.
Sesaminum put in the eares with oyle of roses.

Against Impostumes and swellings which grow behind the eares.

NEw shorne unwashed Wooll applied.
Dung of Goates nourished upon mountaines boyled in wine, or in vinegar
applied.
Lin-seed bruised, reduced to a Poultis.
Beane meale applied with hony and fenegreeke.
Herbe patience boyled and applied.
Plantaine applied as a plaister.
Seed of Banke Cresses[121] bruised, boyled, and applied.
Perfume of Hisope, also a poultis of the same.
Misseltoe incorporated in the same weight of wax and rosin applied.
Marsh Mallowes boyled, and reduced to a liniment.
Fleawort[122] applied with oyle of roses, water, or vinegar.
Leaves of Morell applied with salt.
Hedge-nettle[123] applied with vinegar.
Cimolian earth applied.

For eares full of ordure and filth.

MYrrhe incorporated in Opium.
Castorium, and Glaucium[124] put in the eares.
Frankincense distilled into the eares with sweet wine.

---

[121]*Erysimum.*
[122]*Psyllium.*
[123]*Galiopsis.*
[124]The juyce of an Herb growing in *Syria.*

Rosin of the Larch-tree, of the Pitch-tree, of the Firre-tree, or
  Turpentine put in the eares, with hony, and oyle of olives.
Juyce of Box-thorne[125] dropped into the eares.
Decoction of Sumack.
Juyce of mirtill-berries.
Juyce of wild Olive-tree leaves, dropped into the eares with wine.
Gall of a Bull distilled into the eares with milke of a Woman, or of a
  Goate.
Urine distilled into the eares.
Ladies Navell[126] distilled into the ears with Deers marrow.
Juyce of Asphodil roots alone, or with Frankincense, hony, wine, and
  myrrhe.
Juyce of Onyons.
Wormwood applied with hony.
Annise distilled into the earswith oile of roses.
Juyce of the flowers of meddow Parsenep dropped into the ears.
Juyce of Knot-grasse.
Decoction of Stoebe.
Juyce of Flea-wort,
Verjuyce distilled with hony.
Allome incorporated in juyce of Buckes horne,[127] dropped into the eares.
Flos salis put in the ears.

For eares that are bruised or crushed.

SCalions applyed with dry polenta.
  Brimstone applyed with wine, and hony.

For Vlcers of the eares.

NEw shorne unwashed wool applyed.
  Gal of a Hog distilled into the ears.

Against deafnesse of the eares.

DEcoction of Asphodil roots dropped into the eares with oile.
  Juyce of Onyons dropped into the eares.
  Black Hellebore put in the eares, not removing it for three days.
  Juyce of Briony distilled with hony.

[125]*Lycium.*
[126]*Umbilicus veneris.* Wal penniwort.
[127]*Coronopus*

The whitest kinde of verdigrease put into the ears through a Tunnel.

Perfume of Brimstone,[128] put into the ear by a Tunnell.

Against ticklings and noise of the ears.

ROsin of Cedar put into the ears.

> Juyce of Ivy berries distilled with old wine and oile of roses.
> Dry figs bruised and incorporated in Mustard seed, with some liquor, and put into the ears.
> Buls gall dropped into the ears.
> Hony applied with mineral salt brused small.
> Juyce of Leeks distilled into the ears with Frankincense, vinegar, and milk.
> Juyce of Onyons dropped into the ears.
> Mustard bruised and put into the ears with figs.
> Perfume of boyling vinegar, put into the ears through a Tunnell.

Against worms in the Eares.

ROsin of Cedar distilled with vinegar.

> Mans Urine boiled in a Pomegranat shell, distilled into the ears.
> Juice of the roots of the Caper bush, dropped into the ears.
> Juice of Calaminte.
> Juice of Fleawort.
> Vinegar dropped into the ears.

SIMPLES SERVING FOR THE NOSE.

To stanch bleeding at the Nose.

POwder of Frankincense cast into the nostrils.

> Snailes bruised with their shels and applied.
> Juice of Leekseed droped into the nostrils with powder of Frankincense.
> Rue bruised, applied.
> Leaves of Nettles applied with the juice.
> Cummin applied with vinegar.
> Pith of Fennel-giant put in the nostrils.
> Yellow Willow[129] herbe put in the nostrils.
> Juice of water Bettony[130] dropped into the nostrils.

---

[128]The smoak or steam.
[129]*Lysimachia*
[130]*Clymenum*

Flowers of stinking dead Netle put in the nostrils.
Juice of Shavegrasse dropped into the nostrils.
Vinegar drunk, and put in the nostrils.
Nose bleed yarrow applied.
Chalcitis distilled with Juice of Leeks.

To cause one to bleed.

DEcoction of the root of Chamelaeon thistle[131] drunk.

Against Pimples of the Nose, and Noli me tangere.

CYprus apples bruised with figs and applied.
        Roots of great Dragons applied.
        Benzoin applied with vitriol, or verdigrease, and filed plates of
brasse, resolved in vinegar: but first cut the pimples with sizzars.
        Verdigrease applied.
        Red Orpine[132] applied with oile of roses.

Against Cankers and Ulcers of the Nose.

ROOt of great Dragons applied,
        Juice of Ivie dropped on them.
        Best red Arsenicke applied with oile of roses.

Against stench of the Nose.

JUice of Ivie dropped into the Nose.

Against dropping and distillations of the Nose.

SEed of Gith bruised, and bound up in a cloth, to smel often.

To purge the Humors of the Braine by the Nose.

JUice of Onyons put in the nostrils.
        Juice of both kind of Organie put in the nostrils with oyle of flower-
        deluce.
        Juice of Sowbread dropped into the nose.

---

[131]*Crocodilium.*
[132]*Sandaracha*, red Arsenick.

To provoke sneesing.

BEaver stones put in the nose.
>Seed of Basill, or the juice put in the nose.
>Mustard seed, bruised, snuffed up the nose.
>Root of Crow-foot,[133] dryed powdered and snuffed up the nose.
>Flowers of sneesing-wort snuffed up the nose.
>Root of sope-wort put in the nose.
>Powder of white Hellebore.

SIMPLES SERVING FOR THE MOUTH AND TONGUE.

Against Cancers and corrosive Ulcers.

POwder of Gallingal roots put in the mouth.
>Decoction of rose-wood,[134] boiled in wine, held in the mouth, with which
also the mouth may be washed against maligne ulcers.
>Acacia put in the mouth.
>Juice of Plantain held in the mouth.
>Wash the mouth with the decoction of Capers boiled in vinegar.
>Juyce of Liquorice held in the mouth.
>Juyce of Organy held in the mouth.
>Sweet Violets applyed with hony.
>Finger Orchis[135] applyed.
>Cammomil chewed.
>Juyce of Snake-weed[136] held in the mouth.
>Juice of Caltraps[137] taken with hony, like an electuary.
>Decoction of Bramble held in the mouth.
>The mouth washed with the decoction of Cinkefoile roots.
>Wash the mouth with the second kind of verveine and wine.
>Staphis acre applyed with hony.
>Flowers of Labruske[138] in powder, sprinkled upon the ulcers.
>Allome applyed with hony.
>Burned salt applied with Polenta.

To sweeten the Breath.

MAstick chewed.
>Myrrhe chewed.

---

[133]*Ranunculus* Butter flower.
[134]*Aspalathus* an aromatical wood used by perfumers.
[135]*Serapias.*
[136]*Bistorta Britanica.*
[137]*Tribulus.*
[138]Wilde (grape bearing) vine.

Citrons chewed.

Anise chewed.

Wild Oates boiled with roses held in the mouth,

For sharpenesse of the Tongue.

THe tongue rubbed with Minte.

Seed of Sumacke and hony used as aforesaid.

SIMPLES SERVING FOR THE TEETH.

To make the Teeth clean.

POwder of purple fish shel, of the Calamary fish shel, of Muskle shel, of *unguis odoratus*, and of Snailes shell, used in dentrifices.

Cutlebone, and Harts horn used to rub the teeth.

Decoction of Plantain root to wash the teeth.

Rub the teeth with round Aristolochia.

The fifth kind of Halcyonium,[139] the pumeise stone, the Arabian stone,[140] and the stone Samius used in dentrifices.

For the Tooth ach.

THe teeth often washed in the decoction of the leaves of pine tree, or of pitch tree.

Rosin of Cedar put in the hollow of the tooth.

Bark of Sycamore boyled in vinegar, wash the mouth in the said decoction.

Wash the mouth in the decoction of Tamarisk boyled in wine.

Lees of oyle boyled in a Copper vessell till it be thick like hony, to wash the mouth therein, with vinegar, wine, or honied wine.

The mouth washed with the decoction of the bark of Mulberry-tree.

Milk of Figge-tree put in the hollow of the tooth with wool.

The mouth washed in the decoction of Serpents skin boyled in vinegar.

The indented prick of the Forke-fish applyed upon the tooth.

The mouth washed in the decoction of Frogs boyled in water and vinegar.

Liver of a Lizard put into the hollow of the tooth.

Earth-worms boyled in oyle, distilled into the opposite ear, on the other side of the diseased tooth.

The mouth washed in the decoction of Sorrell.

Decoction of Sparagus roots held in the mouth.

---

[139]A kind of seafoam indurate called also *Spuma maris*.

[140]A white stone, clear & transparent like glasse, for which (as some say) it was formerly used.

Juyce of Asphodill roots dropped into the ear, opposite to the affected tooth.

Decoction of heart of Pine, of Garlick, and of frankincense held in the mouth.

Decoction of the root of Cammock[141] boyled in water and vinegar, to wash the mouth therein.

Lotion of the mouth, with the decoction of the seed of Capers.

Also the bark of the Caper bush, and the root chewed, is good for the same.

Roots of Dittander[142] hanged about the neck, after the opinion of some.

Roots of Crowfoot applied.

Juyce of Pimpernell,[143] distilled into the opposite ear.

Five kernels of Ivie-berries, boyled in oyle of roses, in a pomgranate-shel, dropped into the ear, on the other side of the diseased tooth.

Decoction of black Chameleon-thistle held in the mouth.

The mouth washed in the decoction of white Thistle.[144]

Root of our Lady-thistle chewed.

The perfume of boyling Wormwood[145] taken at the mouth.

Decoction of Hisope boyled in vinegar held in the mouth.

Hercules All-heale put in the hollow of the affected tooth.

Decoction of Pellitory of *Spaine* boyled in vinegar held in the mouth.

Juyce of Sow-fennel put in the hollow of the grieved tooth.

Decoction of Gith, boyled in vinegar, with heart of pine, held in the mouth.

Benzoin put in the hollow of the tooth.

Galbanum applyed, and put in the hollow of the tooth.

The mouth washed with the decoction of Baulme.

Decoction of marsh Mallowes boyled in vinegar, held in the mouth.

Decoction of Bettony boyled in wine, or in vinegar.

Periwincle chewed.

Roots of Spatling-poppy[146] chewed.

Decoction of Cink-foyle root held in the mouth.

The mouth washed with the decoction of Henbane-roots, boyled in vinegar.

Decoction of sleepy Night-shade held in the mouth.

The mouth washed in the decoction of the roots of wild-meddow saffron.[147]

---

[141]Called also, Rest harrow.

[142]*Lepidium*, Pepper-wort.

[143]Anagallis.

[144]*Bedeguar Spina alba.*

[145]The steam or vapour.

[146]*Polemonia*, white Ben.

[147]*Colacum Ephemerum*, having dark red roots.

Lotion of the mouth with decoction of mullein.

Decoction of Arction[148] boyled in wine held in the mouth.

Decoction of wild Cowcumbers held in the mouth.

Lotion of the mouth, with the decoction of Coloquintida.

Decoction of Staphis acre boyled in vinegar, held in the mouth.

Milk of Spurge, named Caracias, put in the hollow of the tooth, defending it with wax, least the milk fall down into the throat.

Lotion of the mouth with hot vinegar.

Sory[149] put into the hollow of the diseased tooth.

To cause viciate teeth to fall out.

ROsin of Cedar put into the hollow of the tooth.

Lees of oyle boyled with verjuce till it be thick like hony, applyed on the tooth.

The indented prick found in the taile of the Fork-fish, put in the hollow of the tooth.

Roots of Crow-foot put in the hollow of the tooth.

Roots of black Chameleon-thistle, put in the hollow of the tooth.

To fasten loose teeth.

DEcoction of Mastick-tree held in the mouth.

The mouth washed in the pickle of Olives.

Oyle of wild Olives held in the mouth.

The mouth washed with the decoction of Sory.

Allome dissolved in vinegar, and hony, applied.

For teeth set on edge.

PUrslaine chewed.

To stay watering of the Gums.

POwder of Galingall applyed.

The expression of dry roses boyled in wine, put in Lotions for the mouth.

Pickle of Olives held in the mouth.

Oyle of wild Olives held in the mouth.

Galls applyed in any sort.

---

[148]Clote-burre.

[149]A mettall like to Melanteria, but thinner and more spungie.

Pomegranate-flowers infused in their decoction to wash the mouth.
Decoction of Plum-tree leaves, held in the mouth.
The mouth washed with Asses milk.
Dry Peni-royall burned, reduced to powder, and applied.
Decoction of Bramble held in the mouth.
The mouth washed in the decocti on of Staphis acre.
Verjuyce applyed with hony.
The mouth washed with vinegar.
Rust of Iron applyed.
Allome applyed in any sort.
Burned salt applyed with dry polenta.
Powder of Alablaster, or of Emerie[150] applied.

For rotten putrified Gums.

GUm Lac applied, is a singular remedy.
> Box-thorn bruised, applyed.
> Juyce of Plantaine held in the mouth.
> Liniment of Aloes, made with wine, or hony.
> Land or water Caltraps, applied with hony.
> Ashes of the flower of Labrusk, applied with hony.
> The mouth washed with vinegar.
> Powder of Chalcitis, or of Allome, or of Pumeise-stone, or of Verdigrease
>   applyed.

SIMPLES SERVING FOR THE NECK AND THROAT.

Against the Squinancie.

Aarre applied.
> Wine of Mulberries boyled in a Copper vessell, and re-boyled in the
>   Sunne, applyed with a little hony.
> Wood-lice applied with hony.
> Ashes of burned Swallowes, applied as a poultis with hony.
> Gall of a Bul applied with hony.
> Gall of a Tortoise applied.
> Vinegar gargalized.
> Hony gargalized.
> Juyce of Onions applyed.

---

[150]A black hard minerall substance, where-with Iron-worke is polished, and precious stones and glasse cut.

Pepper applyed with hony.

Wormwood applied with hony and niter.

Seed of Radish gargalized with vinegar, mingled with hony.

Decoction of Hisope boyled with Figs, gargalized.

Swallows salted and dryed, the weight of a dram taken with water.

Benzoin gargalized with honied water.

Sweet Violets boyled in water drunk.

Juyce of wild Cowcumbers applied with hony, old oyle, or the Gall of a
   Bull; This is an excellent remedy.

Liniment made of salt, hony, oyle, and vinegar.

Spanish Broome[151] steeped in water, then the juyce pressed out, and the
weight of an obol is to be drunk.

For inflamation of the jawes.

AShes of burned Swallows applied as a Poultis with hony.

Milk gargalized.

Frogs boyled in oyle, reduced to a liniment, to annoynt Apostumes of the
Neck, of the nape of the neck, or Chine.

Hony applyed.

Juyce of green Organy gargalized.

Juyce of wall Pellitory gargalized, and applyed without.

Juyce of both sorts of Nettles gargalized.

Powder of Chalcitis applyed.

Allome applyed.

Burned Salt applyed with hony:

Vinegar gargalized.

Aloes applyed with hony, or wine.

Juyce of Snake-weed[152] applyed.

Caltraps applyed with hony.

Juyce of Bramble-berries gargalized.

Decoction of dry Figs gargalized.

To put up and fasten the Vvula.[153]

BEnzoin applied with hony.

Decoction of Plum-tree leaves, boyled in wine gargalized.

Verjuyce applyed.

---

[151]*Spartium.*

[152]Britannica.

[153]The palate of the mouth.

Vinegar gargalized.
Verdigrease in very small powder applyed.

Against Rheumes of the throat.

DEcoction of Poppy-heads, reduced in forme of a Lohoch with hony,[154] this
composition must be often taken.
    Bdelium dissolved with fasting spittle, applied.
    Female Verveine gargalized with wine.
    Verjuyce applyed.
    Verdigrease powdered very small and applyed.
    Allome applyed.
    Vinegar gargalized.

Against sharpnesse of the Throat, and passage to the Lungs.

MYrrhe resolved under the tongue.
    Barly water gargalized.
    Amilum reduced to the forme of an Electuary.
    Juyce of Mustard gargalized.
    Juyce of Lichorice dissolved under the tongue.
    Gum Dragant taken with hony as an Electuary.
    Benzoin dissolved in water, taken as Lohoch.
    Wall-wort[155] chewed.
    Decoction of Cinkfoile roots gargalized.
    Aethiopian mullein[156] taken with hony, as an Electuary.
    Milk gargalized.
    Juyce of Box-thorn[157] bruised, and taken as a Lohoch.

SIMPLES SERVING FOR THE BREASTS AND LUNGS.

For those which spit, and vomite Bloud.

REere Eggs supped.
    Ashes of Harts-horne washed, and drunk with Gum Dragant.
    Water Bettony[158] drunk.

---

[154]A medicine more liquid then an Electuary.
[155]*Symphitum petreum.*
[156]*Athiopis.*
[157]*Lycium.*
[158]*Climenum.*

Juyce of wild Time the weight of two drams drunk in vinegar.
Dung of a wild she Goat mingled with wine, or water, drunk.
Wheat meale boyled very thicke, taken as an Electuary.
Amilum drunk.
Green pitch of Herb *Ferula* drunk.
Purslaine well boyled eaten.
Plantaine taken in any sort whatsoever, or the juyce.
Seed of Plantaine drunk.
Leek-seed drunk with the like weight of Mirtill-berries.
Agarick the weight of three obols drunk in honied water.
Rhapontick drunk, as before.
Juyce of Willow Herb drunk, and applyed.
Roots of great Centaury drunk.
Roots of white thistle drunk.
Roots of *Arabian* thistle drunk.
Aloes the weight of six scruples, taken in fresh water, or in whey.
Juyce of Knot-grasse drunk.
Pills of the juyce of Sage taken with hony.
Wall wort taken with water.
Juyce of Mint taken with vinegar.
Decoction of marsh mallows drunk.
Bettony leaves the weight of three obols taken in wine and water.
Roots of Comfry drunk.
Achilles yarrow[159] drunk.
Ten graines of Sea Grape[160] drunk in wine.
Roots of Burre dock drunke with Pine-apples.
Seed of Columbine[161] drunk.
Mayden-haire drunk.
Juyce of Vine leaves drunk.
Flowers of Labrusk drunk.
Verjuyce drunk moderately.
Powder of Corrall drunk.
Powder of the Bloud-stone, or of the stone Morochthus, or of Samian
   earth, drunk with the juyce of Pomegranats.

For the Tisick.

PIstachoes, or Pine-apple kernels eaten alone, or with hony.
   Turpentine alone, or taken with hony like an Electuary.

---

[159]*Achillea*, noble yarrow.
[160]*Tragos*.
[161]*Isopyrum*.

Tarre the measure of a Cyath, taken as an Electuary.

Juniper-berries drunk.

Bay-berries bruised, and taken with hony, or sod wine.

Decoction of dry Figs boyled with Hisope drunk.

Boyled river Crabs eaten with their broth.

Womans milk sucked from the Duggs.

Broth of all fat things good to eate.

Plantaine drunk.

Leekes boyled with hony.

Agarick the weight of a dram taken in sod wine.

Roots of banck Ursine drunk.

Leaves of Hore-hound, or the juyce drunk.

Bettony leaves taken with hony.

Sweet Chervill[162] taken in broth.

Flower of the Asian-stone[163] taken as a Lohoch.

For Apostumes of the Lungs.

SEed of the second kinde of Sow-bread drunk the space of forty dayes.

The perfume of Colts-foot taken at the mouth, breaketh all Apostumes in the body.

For difficulty and shortnesse of breath.

BAy-berries bruised, and taken with hony, or sod wine.

Decoction of dry Figs with Hisope, drunk.

Decoction of old Cocks supped.

Hisope wine drunk.

Plantaine boyled with Lentils, eaten.

Rhapontick drunk.

Honied water drunk.

Round Aristolochia drunk.

Roots of great Centaury drunk.

Decoction of Hisope, Figgs, Hony, and Rue, boyled in water drunk.

Decoction of *French* Lavender[164] boyled in water drunk.

Penniroyall drunk with hony and Aloes.

Squill reduced to an Electuary, the weight of three obols taken.

Decoction of Time boyled in hony, drunk.

---

[162]*Myrrhis.*

[163]The saltish mold, or hoare that groweth on that Stone.

[164]*Stichas.*

Summer Savoury taken as aforesaid.
Decoction of the roots of Plowmans Spikenard drunk.
Rue drunk.
Juyce of Sow-fennell supped in a reere egge.
Gith taken in wine.
Galbanum taken in pills.
Decoction of Hore-hound, or the juyce drunk.
Fever-few taken with Oximel.[165]
Leaves of Beane Trifoly[166] drunk in sod wine.
Seed of Wood-binde[167] drunk with wine.
Decoction of Maiden-haire drunk.
Black Maiden-haire[168] drunk.
Juyce of wild Cowcumbers is a very good remedy for a short breath.
Juyce of stinking deadly Carrot[169] drunk.
Briony taken with hony as an Electuary.
Red Arsenick taken in pills.
Brimstone used in perfume, or taken in a reere egge.
Agarick the weight of a dram taken.
Gum Lac drunk in water, or in honied wine.

Against a Cough.

ILlyrian Flower-deluce eaten.
Graines of Paradice drunk in water.
Cinamon eaten or drunk.
Perfume of sweet Cane alone, or with Turpentine.
An Electuary made of Elicampane and hony.
Storax or Bdellium taken in the manner of an Electuary.
Mastick drunk.
Juniper berries drunk.
Cedar berries eaten.
Seed of Christs thorn[170] drunk.
Labdanum mingled in medicines or implaisters.
Gum of Cherry-tree drunk in wine and water.
Bitter Almonds, reduced to an Electuary, with hony and milk.

[165]*Matricaria.*
[166]*Anagyris.*
[167]*Matrisilua.*
[168]*Polytrichum.*
[169]*Thapsia.*
[170]*Paliurus.*

Gum of bitter Almonds drunk in wine and water.

Filbeards drunk with honyed water.

Dry figs eaten.

Decoction of Germander drunk.

Water Germander[171] drunk.

Perfume of Colts foot taken at the mouth.

Perfume of virgins waxe.

Hony eaten.

The decoction of wheat meal, taken as an Electuary, with Mint and butter.

Decoction of Oatemeal eaten.

Linseed taken with hony and pepper.

Beanes eaten.

Boiled Raddish eaten, especially when the Cough is old.

Roots of great Dragons, rosted in the embers, or boiled, eaten.

Asphodill roots the weight of three drams drunk.

Boiled Garlick eaten, is good against old Coughs.

Seed of Banke Cresses,[172] taken with hony as an Electuary.

An Electuary of pepper.

An Electuary of Squill, and of hony, when the Cough is inveterate.

Root of great Centaury drunk, when the disease is old.

Electuary of Gum Dragant, and Hony.

Decoction of Hysope, boiled in water, with hony, figs and rue, drunk

French Lavender prepared as the Hisope.

Electuary of Organy and hony.

Goates Organy[173] prepared in the same sort.

Decoction of the roots of plowmans spikenard, drunk, when the Cough is of long continuance.

All-heal drunk in sweet wine.

Seed and roots of seselios of Marseilles, drunk.

Roots of Candy Alexanders eaten.

Seed of YellowCarrot[174] drunk, when the Cough is inveterate.

Juice of Sow-fennell taken in a reer egge.

Benzoin taken in the same sort.

Decoction of Horehound, or the Juice, drunk.

Galbanum taken in Pills when the disease is old.

Gum Sagapene eaten, when the Cough lasteth long.

---

[171]*Scordium*

[172]*Erysimum.*

[173]*Tragoriganum.*

[174]*Daucus.*

Juice of Wall Pellitory,[175] the weight of a cyath taken, when the Cough is old.

The hearb and root called Horse-tail drunk.

Decoction of Rushes drunk.

Poppy-heads boiled in water, to the consumption of one half, then add hony sufficient to make it into an Electuary.

Henbane seed drunk.

Decoction of Mullein drunk, when the Cough is inveterat.

Root of mountain horse-foot[176] steeped in wine, eaten

Electuary of Briony and of hony.

The pulpe of white grapes[177] dryed, eaten.

Honyed water drunk.

Stinking deadly Carrot[178] applied as a Liniment.

Hisope wine drunk.

Perfume of red minerall Arsenicke, and of Rosin, taken through a Tunnell.

Perfume of Brimstone, or brimston taken in a reer egge.

Against sharpnesse of the breast.

JUyce of Liquorice dissolved under the tongue.

Root of Mountaine Horse-foot steeped in wine, and taken after the manner of an Electuary.

To clear the voice.

MYrrhe dissolved under the tongue.

Electuary of hony, and of gum dragant.

Electuary of Storax.

Coleworts eaten.

Wine of Hisope drunk.

Against Pleurisies.

HOgs-lard washed in wine applyed.

Juyce of Hercules All-heal drunk.

Gum Sagapene applied as a cataplasme.[179]

---

[175]*Helxine parietaria*
[176]*Cacalia*
[177]*Caro.*
[178]*Thapsia.*
[179]A poultis.

Against paines of the Sides without a Feavor.

DUng of she Goates incorporated in oyle and waxe, applyed as a poultis.

> Liniment made of Barly meal boiled with melilot aud poppy heads, in honyed wine.
>
> Stems of green Coleworts burned, and incorporated in Hogs Lard, then applyed as a poultis.
>
> Decoction of the roots, of our Lady thistle, boiled in wine drunk.
>
> Asphodil roots the weight of a dram drunk in wine.
>
> Juyce of the roots of Gentian the weight of a dram taken.
>
> Round Aristolochia drunke in water.
>
> Root of great Centaury drunk.
>
> Benzoin taken in broth.
>
> Galbanum applyed.
>
> Leaves of Hore-hound applyed with hony.
>
> Leaves and seed of stinking Trifoly drunke.
>
> Ethiopian mullein drunk.
>
> Decoction of sweet cane[180] drunk.
>
> Costus drunk with wormwood and wine.
>
> Wood of Aloes[181] drunk in water.
>
> Myrrhe the greatnesse of a Bean taken.
>
> Bdellium drunk.
>
> Turpentine applied.
>
> Electuary of Briony, and of hony.

For inflamations of the Lungs.

BAsill applyed with dry polenta.

> Electuary of Nettle seed, and of hony.
>
> Electuary of Goats organy and hony.
>
> Golden tode flax[182] drunk.
>
> Honied water drunk.

For those which spit putrified matter.

ELectuary of Bank cresses and hony.

> Bettony leaves the weight of two drams, taken in four Cyathes of honied water.
>
> Rootes of Bur dock with pine apples.

---

[180]*Acorum.*
[181]*Agallochii.*
[182]*Chrysocome.*

Ethiopian Mullein drunk.

Wine of Hysope.

Red Arsenicke taken in honyed wine. I cannot approve of this Medicine.

Perfume of brimstone, or brimstone taken in a reer egge.

To helpe difficulty of breathing.

BAy berries taken in hony, or in sod wine.

Dry Beanes boyled with Hysope, drunk.

A young childs Urine drunk.

Rue drunk.

Seed of the second kind of Sow-bread, drunk.

Roots of great dragons rosted in the embers, or boiled, and reduced to an electuary.

Honied water drunk.

The hearb, or seed of meddow parsnep,[183] taken in broth.

Root or leaves of horse-taile drunk.

Seed of Sothernwood, and seed of Ciprus, bruised, drunk in water.

Decoction of hisope, boiled in water, with figs, hony, and Rue, drunk.

Decoction of Calaminte drunk.

Hysope wine drunk.

Decoction of Time, boiled in hony, drunk.

Summer savory drunke with hony.

Seselios of Marseilles drunk.

Decoction of black maiden-haire drunk.

Cummin drunk in water and vinegar.

Root of Candy Alexanders eaten.

Stinking deadly Carrot, applyed.

Gum ammoniacke drunk.

Leaves of Baulme reduced to an electuary.

Perfume of Colts-foot taken through a Tunnell.

Juice of Hippophestus the weight of three obols taken.

Oake of Jerusalem drunk, or reduced to an Electuary.

Seed of Woodbinde drunk.

Decoction of Maiden-hair drunk.

To expell excrements difficult to spit.

ILlyrian Flower-de-luce drunk.

All Curds[184] drunk.

---

[183]*Spondilium.*

[184]That part in Beasts (as in Calves) whereof Runnet is made.

Boyled Raddish eaten.
Leekes boyled with *French* barly.
Garden Cresses boyled in pottage.
Scallyons rosted in embers eaten.
Gum Ammoniack taken as a Lohoch.
Water Germander drunk.
Liniment of stinking deadly Carrot.
Electuary of Lin-seed.
Three obols of dryed Squil, reduced to an Electuary.
Dry hore-hound drunk, with powder of Flower-de-luce.
Wine of Hisope drunk.

Against Rheumes falling down into the Breast.

SEed of Bank-cresses taken as an Electuary with hony.

Against all maladies of the Breast.

LEekes boyled in hony eaten.
Juyce of Licorice drunk.
Electuary of Time, and Hony.
Electuary of Summer Savoury, and hony.
Electuary of the root of Seselios of Candy, and of hony.
Roots of Rosemary drunk.
Wall-wort boyled in honied wine drunk.
Juyce of Cinkfoile-seed drunk.

SIMPLES SERVING FOR THE HEART.

For swoundings of the Heart.

THe smell of Cowcumbers.
Penni-royall put to the nose with vinegar.
Buglosse drunk.

For panting and throbbing of the heart.

SUccory applyed alone, or with polenta.
Wormwood boyled in sod wine applied.
Bramble leaves applied.

Against hardnesse of the Mideriffe.

RHapontick drunk.
Worm-wood wine drunk.

Against inveterate inflamations of the precordiall parts.

VVAter Germander incorporated in Wax applyed.

SIMPLES SERVING FOR THE TEATS OR DUGGS.

For inflamations of the Duggs.

LIniment made of Frankincense, of Cimolian earth, and of oyle of roses.
    Quinces reduced to a poultis, or liniment.
    A poultis of Wall-nuts, of Rue, and of a little hony.
    Beane meale applied alone, or with polenta.
    Roots and leaves of Asphodills applied with wine.
    Seed of bank Cresses applied.
    Root of Liriconfancie,[185] applied in the manner of a poultis.
    Boyled Marsh-mallowes applyed.
    Kernells of Grapes applied with salt.
    Powder of the stone Ostracites,[186] applyed with hony.
    Powder of the stone Geodes, applyed with water.
    Samian earth applyed with oyle of roses, and water.

To draw forth the Duggs of Women lately delivered.

WHeat bran boyled in decoction of Rue, applyed.
    Leaves of Plow-mans Spikenard, applyed as a poultis.
    Leaves of Barren-wort[187] chopped small, applyed with oyle as a poultis.
    Henbane-seed bruised, and applyed with wine.
    Leaves of Palma Christi applyed.
    Kernels of Grapes applyed with salt.

To dissolve and mollifie hardnesse of the Duggs.

MEale of bitter Vetch[188] applyed as a poultis.
    Ground pine, applyed with hony.
    Kernals of Grapes bruised with salt, and applyed.

[185]Hemerocallise.
[186]A precious Stone brittle as a shell, resembling the *Agathe*, after some *Goraeus* faith, it is a kind of *Cadmia*.
[187]*Epimedium*.
[188]*Orobus*.

For ulcerated Duggs.

AShes of Unguis Odoratus applyed.
     Roots of Swallow-wort[189] applyed.

To resolve Milk curdled, and clottered in the Duggs.

TEn drops of Wax, of the greatnesse of a hirse graine swallowed.
     Beane meale applyed alone, or with polenta.
     Liniment made of meale of Lentils.
     Parsley, and the juyce applied.

To put the Milke away.

HEmlock applyed on the Duggs.

To increase Milk abundantly.

LEaves of Sea-purslaine[190] eaten with meat.
     Seed of *Agnus Castus* drunk.
     French Barley boyled with fennel-seed, eaten often.
     Decoction of Mallowes drunk.
     Juyce of Sow-thistle drunk.
     Lettice eaten often.
     Rocket eaten often.
     Wind-flower, and the branches boyled and eaten with *French* Barley.
     Anise drunk.
     Dry Dill-seed drunk, or the decoction of the tops.
     Fennell eaten.
     Gith drunk many dayes.
     Seed of Bind-weed,[191] Night-shade taken in broth.
     Periwinckle eaten.
     Roots of Vipers Buglosse[192] taken in broth, or with wine.
     Glaux[193] boyled with oyle, salt, and meale, taken as broth.
     Milk-wort[194] drunk.
     Juyce of Briony boyled with wheat, eaten, but this I doe not allow.

[189]*Asclepias.*
[190]*Halimus.*
[191]*Circea.*
[192]*Echium.*
[193]A kinde of Cytisus, or milke trefoile.
[194]*Polygala.*

To defend Milk from setling in the Breasts.

MInte applyed with polenta.
  Lees of Wine applyed with vinegar.

To keep the Duggs from growing.

HEmlock bruised, and applyed.
  Powder of the Naxion stone, applyed.

SIMPLES SERVING FOR THE STOMACK.

Against turnings of the Stomack, and to prevent vomitting.

INfusion of Quinces drunk.
  Spikenard, and Celtick Spikenard drunk in water.
  Dates eaten.
  Date-skinnes in powder, put in cataplasmes for the Stomack.
  The inward skin of a Chickens gizerne dryed, powdered, and drunke with
    wine.
  Amber drunk.
  Beanes boyled in vinegar and water, eaten.
  Twenty graines of Lentils bruised and eaten.
  French beanes eaten.
  Water-cresses drunk.
  Bramble Leaves applyed outwardly.
  Lettice eaten unwashed.
  Wild Lentils eaten.
  Dryed Squil drunk.
  Agarick the weight of three drams taken alone without any liquor.
  Juyce of Gentian roots drunk with water.
  Roots of our Lady-thistle drunk.
  Two or three sprigs of Mint, drunk with the juyce of sower Pomegranats.
  Peony-seed drunk in strong wine.
  Bettony chewed, drinking presently after wine mingled with water.
  Juyce of the leaves and branches of Vine, drunk.
  Wine of Mirtle drunk.
  Lees of wine applyed.
  Squil wine drunk.

Against waterishnesse and rheumes which fall downe into the Stomack.

JUyce of Box-thorn[195] drunk, or taken in pils.
  Raw Quinces eaten.

[195]*Lycium.*

Green Mulberries dryed to powder, sprinkled on meat.
Lexive of the ashes of Figtree, the measure of a Cyath taken.
Tamarisk drunk.
Galls bruised, and steeped in wine, or water, applyed.
Seed of Sumack sprinkled on meat.
Mirtle leaves bruised, and applyed with water.
Liniment made of the leaves of wild Olive-tree, and of dry Polenta.
Curd of a Hare, or of a Horse, the weight of three obols taken in wine.
Beanes boyled in water and vinegar eaten.
Meale of Aegyptian beanes, and the decoction of their huskes, taken
with honied wine.
Seed of Sorrell drunk in water, or in wine.
Plantaine boyled in vinegar, eaten with salt.
Seed of Jacynth drunk.
Bucks horn[196] boyled, eaten.
Rhapontick drunk.
Roots of white Thistle drunk.
Pith of green Ferula[197] drunk.
Juyce of Laserwort taken with kernells of Grapes.
Root of water Lilly dryed, drunk.
Juyce of water Bettony drunk.
Seed of water Plantaine,[198] the weight of an Acetabule taken in wine.
Ten graines of small Sea-grape[199] taken in wine.
Decoction of Poppy heads, reduced to an Electuary with hony; to make it
more effectuall you may adde juyce of Acacia, and of male holly-rose.
Deocotion of Grape kernels drunk.
Grape kernels reduced to powder, used instead of polenta.
Water wherein hot Steele hath been quenched drunk.
The stone Morochthus drunk.
Wine of Mirtle drunk.
Maiden-haire drunk in wine.
Black Maiden-haire drunk in wine.

To cause Vomitting.

BAy-leaves drunk.
     Snayles which stick to bryers and bushes eaten.
     Roots of Pompions dryed, the weight of a dram drunke in honied water.

[196]*Coronopus.*
[197]Fennell-gyant.
[198]*Limonium.*
[199]*Tragos.*

White Daffodill roots eaten.

Organie confected in the Sun, in a copper vessell, with onions, and seed of Sumack drunk. It must have stood in the Sun all the Dog-dayes, and as many other as amounteth to forty.

Bole-armonick of the Orient,[200] drunk.

Against paines of the Stomack.

CAmmels hay drunk.

Scalions eaten.

Rhapontick drunk.

Decoction of worm-wood boyled in sod wine, drunk.

Decoction of Melilot boyled in wine drunk.

The small leaves of Mugwort bruised, and applyed with oyle, in the manner of a poultis.

Roots of water Lilly applyed.

Branches of Groundsell boyled in sod wine, eaten, or drunk.

Powder of Alablaster incorporated in a seare-cloth.

Against gripings of the Stomack.

SPikenard, and Celtick Spikenard drunk in water.

Cammels hay[201] drunk.

Juyce of Sycamore drunk.

Pine apples eaten.

Womans milk supped.

Juyce of Sow-thistle drunk.

Penni-royall taken with vinegar and water.

Juyce of both kinds of Hawk-weed, drunk.

Water Germander the weight of two drams taken in honied water.

Peony-seed taken in old thick red wine.

Against inflammations of the Stomack.

PUrslaine applyed with dry polenta.

Sow-thistles applyed as a poultis.

Juyce of Wall Penni-wort[202] applied.

All kinds of Succory eaten in vinegar.

[200]Best, true bole.
[201]*Squinanthum.*
[202]*Umbilicus veneris.*

Juyce of Licorice drunk.

Parsley drunk.

Fennell drunk in faire water.

Knot-grasse applyed.

Leaves of Morell applyed.

Leaves of Spurge Laurell drunk.

Leaves and branches of Vine[203] applyed as a poultis.

Flowers of Labrusk applyed.

Against wind in the Stomack.

ROots of Spicknell[204] boyled in water, or bruised raw, and drunk.

Spikenard, and Celticke Spikenard drunk in water.

Castorium drunk.

Broth of old Capons.

Worm-wood drunk with Seselios, or Celtick Spikenard.

Seed and roots of Lovage[205] drunk.

Seed of Candie Alexanders drunk.

Against the Hickop, and Vexing.

SEed of Water-cresses drunke in wine.

Rhapontick drunk.

Round Aristolochia drunk.

Two or three branches of Minte drunk with juyce of sower Pomegranats.

Decoction of the seed and tops of Dill drunk.

Wild Cummin drunk in vinegar.

Madwort drunk, or carried in the hand, or distilled into the nostrils.

Decoction of Ceterach drunk.

Woodbine-seed drunk.

Samphire drunk.

Against sharpe belching.

AGarick the weight of a dram taken.

Goates Organie drunk.

Bettony leaves the greatnesse of a beane taken with clarified hony.

[203]Here, as in all places else, when vine followes, is meant the tendrils wher-with they catch hold of what is nextthem, to get higher.
[204]*Meum*, Bearewort.
[205]*Lygusticum.*

To resolve Milke and Bloud, fixed and clotted in the Stomack.

LExive of the ashes of Figge-tree, drunk.
Curds of Horses, of Hares, of Lambs, of Kids, of Hindes, of Calves, or of Buf[l]les the weight of three obols taken in wine.
Tops of golden Moth-weed, drunk in honied wine.
Benzoin drunk.

Against inflamations of the Stomack.

A Poultis of both kindes of Hawk-weed.
A poultis of the leaves and branches of Vine with polenta.
Sweet Violets applyed with polenta.

To procure an appetite.

PEpper eaten.
Vinegar used in sauce.
Worm-wood drunk.

To help Digestion.

ROcket eaten.
All sorts of Pepper eaten.
Ginger eaten.
Squill boyled in hony eaten.
VVorm-wood drunk, or applied on the stomack.
Goates Organie drunk.
Penni-royall drunk.
Roots and seed of Lovage drunk.
Seed of Seselios, of Marseilles drunk in wine.
Caraway[206] drunk.
Bettony leaves the greatnesse of a bean, taken after meales, with hony, well clarified.
Wormwood wine drunk.

Against the flowing downe of humours upon the stomacke.

MAiden haire drunk in wine.
Decoction of dry Peaches drunke.
Quinces infused, then pressed, drink the liquor.

---

[206] *Carvi.*

SIMPLES SERVING FOR THE LIVER.

Against stoppings and obstructions of the Liver.

SPicknard, and Celtick Spicknard, drunk in faire water.
>   Bark of the Bay tree, the weight of three obols taken in wine.
>   Leaves of Pitch tree, the weight of a dram taken in water, or in honied water.
>   Electuary of bitter Almonds, of milke, and of hony, the bignesse of a small nut taken.
>   Juice of Gentian rootes, drunk in water.
>   Agarick drunk.
>   Rhapontick drunk.
>   Sea Holly[207] taken in wine.
>   Decoction of Cammomill, drunk.
>   Leaves of ground Pine, drunk seven dayes together in wine.
>   Bettonie the weight of a dram taken in honied vinegar.
>   Egrimony, or the seed drunk.
>   Root of horned poppy drunk.
>   Red Oker[208] drunk.
>   Electuary of the juyce of Licorice.

Against the Jaundise.

SPikenard, and Celticke Nard, drunk.
>   Harts-horne burned, washed, and drunk.
>   Wood-lice drunk in wine.
>   Cich Pease boiled with Rosemary, eaten.
>   Roots of sharp pointed docks boiled in wine, drunk.
>   Seed of Orage drunke in honyed water.
>   Decoction of Sparagus roots, boiled with figs, and Cich pease, drunk.
>   Decoction of Rock Sampire, and of their seed and roots, drunk.
>   Electuary of Bank cresses.
>   Electuary of Squill and of hony, the weight of three obols taken.
>   Celandine root, drunk in wine with Anise.
>   Root of Meddow Parsenep, drunk.
>   Agarick the weight of a dram taken.
>   Rhapontick drunk.
>   Decoction or infusion of worm-wood, three cyaths taken every day.
>   Alloes the weight of a dram drunk.

[207]*Eryngium*
[208]*Rubrica Sinopica*, called also *Bolearmonick* but is not the true right *Bole*.

The whole body washed in the decoction of Organy.

Calaminte drunk in wine.

Wild fennell drunk.

Rosemary roots, taken in wine with pepper.

Decoction of Rosemary, drunk.

Gith bruised and put into the nose with oyle of flower-deluce.

Benzoin taken with dry figs.

Juice of Hore-hound dropped into the Nose.

Decoction of both kinds of poley drunk.

Leaves and flowers of fleabane drunk.

Decocton of Ceterach drunk.

Liverwort applyed with hony.

Decoction of Maiden-haire drunk.

Decoction of blacke Maiden-haire drunk.

Decoction of Cammomil, drunk.

Oxe eie[209] drunke, going out of a Bath.

Peony root drunk.

Seed of Jacynth drunk in wine.

Roots of Madir drunk in honied water.

Leaves of ground Pine, drunk, seven days together in wine.

Bettonie leaves taken in water.

Juyce of wild Cowcumbers, drunk.

Decoction of the roots of Orkanet drunk.

Juyce of Cinkefoile the weight of 3 Cyaths, taken certain daies
   together.

Decoction of Tode flax,[210] drunk.

A bath made with the decoction of Marigolds.[211]

Squill wine drunk.

Leaves of verveine one dram, fankincense three obols, old wine a hemine,
take of this composition fasting, forty daies together.

Boxthorn, boyled in vinegar drunk.

Decoction of Tamariske, drunk.

Winter cherries[212] drunk.

Leaves of Spurge Time,[213] the weight of three obols, taken six dayes
together in water.

Leaves and berrys of Butchers broom drunke in wine.

---

[209]*Buphthamum.*

[210]*Osyris.*

[211]*Chrysanthemum.*

[212]*Baccae Halicacabi*

[213]*Chamaesyce.*

Ashes of Harts-horne, two drams drunk.
Brimstone taken in a reer egge.

Against the Dropsie.

A Sarabacka drunk.

Cinnamon drunk.
Decoction of sweet Cane, drunke with the seed of Smallage.
Land Hedge-hogs eaten.
Snailes bruised with their shells, and applied, are good aginst dropicall tumours.
Lees of oyle applyed as a Poultis with a very hairy skin.
The Patients Urine drunk.
She Goats urine, drunk every day with Spicknard.
Ciches boyled with Rosemary, eaten.
Raddishes applyed as a poultis.
Plantaine boyled with Lentills.
Roots of Walwort boyled in wine, drunk.
Boyled Garlick eaten.
A poultis of Scalions, of hony and of Pepper, in powder.
Squill three obols taken with hony.
Juyce of Pimpernell drunke in wine.
Roots of Carline thistle, drunk in wine.
Broth made of wormwood, of figs, niter, and darnell meale.
Decoction of Maiden-hair, drunk.
Deoction of blacke Maiden-haire drunk.
A poultis of hysope, figs and niter.
Decoction of Polipodie[214] drunk.
Decoction of Organy boyled with figs drunk.
Decoction of Marjerome drunk.
Poultis of Rue and of figs.
Decoction of Rue taken with wine, or the whole body washed therein.
Seed of All-heale drunk.
Annise drunk.
Seed of candy Alexanders, drunk.
Juyce of Laserwort taken with dry figs.
Decoction of Germander drunk.
Decoction of both kinds of Poley drunk.
Sea navell-wort[215] the weight of two drams drunk in wine.

[214]*Oakefearn*
[215]*Androsace*

Bettony leaves drunk in water.

Juice of wild Cowcumber roots the weight of one obol and a half taken; or the weight of four drams and a halfe, of the rinde of the roots taken.

A Bath of sea water.

Roots of wild vine boiled in water, taken in two cyaths of wine, allayed with sea water.

Squill wine drunk.

Seed of Agnus Castus drunk.

Liniment made of dry figs, boiled in wine with wormwood, salt, and polenta.

The third kind of Spuma maris.[216]

Sand heated in the Sun, the dropsicall person put in it up to the neck.

To heat the Liver.

SPicknard and celticke Spicknard drunk.

Decoction of Amomum, drunk.

Leaves of Pine tree, or of Pitch tree drunk in water, or in honied wine.

For pains of the Liver.

DEcoction of common sweet cane drunk.

Decoction of Wormwood applyed with sod wine.

Woodbine seed, drunke in wine.

Against hardnesse of the Liver.

GUm ammoniacum applyed, and drunk.

SIMPLES SERVING FOR THE SPLEEN.

Against hardnesse of the Spleen.

RAw Quinces applyed in a poultis.

Root of Sycamore drunk and applyed.

Raddishes applyed as a poultis.

Coleworts eaten in vinegar.

Decoction of Germander drunk.

Meale of Lupines applyed.

[216]*Halcyonium.*

To open the Spleen.

CEltick nard drunk in wine.
    Maiden haire drunk.
    Black maiden hair drunk.

Against inflammations of the Spleen.

ILlyrian Flower-deluce drunke in vinegar.
    Common sweet Cane drunk.
    Celtick Spicknard drunk in wine.
    Mountaine Spikenard drunke in wine.
    Decoction of Tamariske boyled in wine drunk.
    Seed of Agnus Castus drunk.
Littany drunk, and applyed.
Lllyrian Flower-de-luce drunk in vinegar.
Common sweet Cane[217] drunk.
    Mountaine Spikenard, and Celtick Spikenard, drunk in wine.
    Decoction of Tamarisk boyled in wine drunk.
    Seed of *Agnus Castus* drunk.
    Seed of the second kinde of Sow-bread, drunk forty dayes together.
    Gum Sagapene drunk.
    Gum Ammoniacum the weight of a dram taken in vinegar.
    Germander drunk in vinegar.
    Garden Cresses drunk.
    Roots of the Pepper-plant applied.
    Decoction of both kinds of Poley drunk in vinegar.
    Juyce of Sow-bread applied.
    Capers the weight of two drams drunk forty dayes together in wine.
    Root of the Caper-bush, the weight of two drams drunk in wine.
    Dittander[218] applyed with Elicampane roots.
    Ivie leaves boyled in wine, or dryed, incorporated in bread, and applied.
    Wild Woad drunk and applied.
    Agarick the weight of a dram taken in honied vinegar.
    Rhapontick drunk.
    Roots of Candie Alexanders eaten in a sallad, or otherwise.
    Gentian roote the weight of two drams drunk.
    Round Aristolochia drunk.

[217]The false adulterated sweet Cane, a kinde of Corn-flag:
[218]*Lepidium*

Decoction of the root of Chameleon-thistle[219] drunk; this is very profitable.

Liniment made of Figgs, of Hisope, and of Niter.

Goates Organie drunk in vinegar.

Penni-royall applied with salt.

Sison[220] drunk.

Juyce of Sow-fennell drunk.

Liniment made of Misseltoe, boyled with Cole-worts, and the stone Gagates.[221]

Great Germander[222] drunk in water, or vinegar, or applied with Figs.

Roots of Wall-flowers[223] applied with vinegar.

Roots of water Lilly drunk in wine.

Leaves of Ceterach drunk, or the decoction of them drunk forty dayes together with vinegar, or the leaves applied with vinegar.

Seed of Rampions drunk.

Moon-fearn[224] drunk in vinegar.

Seed of Madir drunk in honied vinegar.

Leaves of the second kind of Spleen-wort[225] drunk in vinegar.

Bettony leaves taken in Oximel.

Roots of Spatling-poppy taken in water.

Seed of Woodbinde drunk in wine forty dayes together.

Seed of stinking Gladdon taken in vinegar.

Roots of Orkanet drunk in honied water.

All kinde of Nettles used in seareclothes.

Black Maiden-haire drunk.

Squill wine drunk often.

Ben drunk with honied water, and meale of bitter vetch.

Briony the weight of three obols drunk in vinegar, every day for thirty dayes, or applyed with Figgs.

Young shoots of black Briony boyled, and eaten.

Roots of male Fearne drunk.

Wine, or water wherein hot Steele hath been quenched drunk.

Third kinde of Halcyonium drunk.

Corrall drunk in water.

---

[219]*Crocodilium.*
[220]Bastard stone parsley after *Cordus.*
[221]*Goraeus* saith, it is jet.
[222]*Teucrium*
[223]Cheiri.
[224]Hemionitis.
[225]Lonchitis.

Liniment made of Asian Stone, of vinegar, and of unslecked Lime.
Scailes of Iron which fall from the Grind-stone drunk in vinegar.

SIMPLES SERVING FOR THE GUTS.

For the Collick.

ELectuary of bitter Almonds, of milke, and of hony, the greatnesse of a
    Filbeard taken.
    Snailes bruised with their shels, and a little Myrrhe, drunk.
    Rosted Larks eaten.
    A Hoggs heele burned to powder, drunk, when the disease is windy.
    Butter given in a Glister, when the Gut Colon is ulcerated.
    Dung of Poultry drunk in wine, or in vinegar.
    Decoction of Rue given in a Glister with oyle.
    Garden parsley[226] drunk.
    Coloquintida given in a Glister.
    Decoction of Bastard Saffron[227] given in a Glister.

For the Belly-ach and wormes.

ILlyrian Flower-de-luce drunk.
    Decoction of common sweet Cane drunk.
    Roots of Spicknell bruised, and reduced into an Electuary with hony.
    Graines of Paradise drunke in water.
    Lignum Aloes drunk in water.
    Wall-nuts burned with their shels, and applyed on the navell.
    Decoction of Figgs and Rue, given in a Glister.
    Leaves of Sea-purslaine[228] the weight of a dram, drunk in honied water.
    Saffron drunk.
    Seed of yellow Carrot[229] drunk.
    Roots of Rosemary drunk.
    Seed of Fenell-gyant drunk.
    Juyce of Sow-fennell taken in a reere egge.
    Decoction of Baulme glisterised.[230]
    Castorium drunk.

---

[226]*Petroselinum.*
[227]*Carthamum.*
[228]*Halymus.*
[229]*Daucus.*
[230]Given in a Glister.

Butter given in a Glister.

Wild time drunk.

Decoction of Calaminte drunk.

Sea Holly drunk.

Melted Wax drunk.

Ammeos[231] taken in wine.

Liniment made of VVheat bran boyled in the decoction of Rue.

Millet heated, and applyed on the belly in a little bagge.

Meale of bitter Vetch steeped in vinegar, applyed.

Seed of VVater-Cresses drunk in wine.

Pepper drunk with Bay leaves.

Electuary made of Squil, and ofhony

Rhapontick drunk.

Decoction of Marjerome drunk.

Roots of great Centaury drunk.

Rue boyled with dry Dill, drunk.

All-heale taken in wine.

Decoction of the seed and tops of Dill drunk.

Seed and roots of Lovage drunk.

Decoction of Cummin, given in a Glister with oyle.

Flowers, leaves, and seed of Spider-wort[232] drunk.

Cotten-weed[233] drunk.

Leaves and Flowers of Fleabane drunk.

Root of Peony drunk.

Winter Cresses[234] taken in vinegar.

Fomentation with sea water.

Ground pine drunk.

Decoction of Couch-grasse[235] drunk.

Leaves of Spurge Laurell drunk.

Salt heated & applied in little bags.

Niter drunk in honied water with Cummin.

Seed of Seselios of Marseilles drunk.

Roots of Swallow-wort drunk.

Beares eare[236] drunk alone, or with the like weight of yellow Carrot-seed.

A Hoggs heele burned drunk.

[231] A small seed like Cummin but lesse, brought from the Orient.
[232] *Phalangium.*
[233] *Centunculus.*
[234] *Pseudobunium.*
[235] *Gramen.*
[236] *Alisma.*

Decoction of Lin-seed given in a Glister.
Agarick the weight of two obols taken.

Against the Bloody Flix, and the Dysenterie.[237]

DEoction of Rose-wood glisterised.
    Myrrhe the greatnes of a Bean taken.
    Mastick drunk.
    Bark of the Pitch-tree drunk.
    Bark of Macer[238] drunk.
    Leaves and roots of Christs-thorne drunk.
    Hawthorn berries eaten, or drunke.
    Berries of Wild Eglantine[239] eaten.
    Leaves and flowers of Holly-rose[240] drunk.
    Juyce of Male Holly Rose, drunk.
    Ladanum drunk in old wine.
    Wild rose buds, unblown, drunk.
    Juyce of Box-thorn[241] drunk.
    Juyce of Acacia drunk.
    Decoction of Acorn shells drunk.
    The inward rinde of Ches-Nuts, drunk.
    Unripe Galls, bruised and drunke with wine, or water: or applyed with
the same liquors.
    Decoction of Sumack leaves given in a glister, or drunk.
    Seed of Sumacke used in place of salt.
    Decoction of the rinde or skin of Dates glisterised, or drunk.
    Kernells of four Pomegranats, dryed, and drunke; or fomented beneath.
    Leaves and seed of Mirtle drunk.
    Quinces eaten raw or boiled, or their juyce drunk.
    Peares domesticall or wild, eaten.
    Medlers eaten.
    Berries of the Lote Tree, eaten, or drunk.
    Dryed Services taken in any sort.
    Sloes eaten.
    Carobs eaten.
    Snailes rosted in their shells, in the embers, according to *Gallen*.

[237] A painfullwringing Flix, which breedeth ulcers in the Guts.
[238] An Indian root.
[239] *Rubus Canis.*
[240] *Cistus.*
[241] *Lycium.*

Fomentation with the pickle of the fish Silurus.[242]

Hares blood fryed, eaten.

Garum[243] given in a glister.

Harts-horn two drams, drunk.

Waxe taken in broth.

Milke wherein burning flints, have been quenched, glisterised.

Curd of a Hare, or of a Horse, the weight of three obols, drunke in wine.

Garden Sparagus, boiled or rosted in the embers, and eaten.

Roots of Idea[244] drunk.

Juyce of Marsh Mallowes boyled, drunk in wine or water.

Roots of Marsh mallowes drunk.

Harts tongue drunk.

Purslain well boiled, eaten.

Plantain given in a glister.

Juyce of Horse taile, drunk.

Goates Suet taken with Sumacke, and polenta, or glisterised.

Baulm drunk.

Small saxifrage[245] boiled, eaten.

Beans dressed with water and vinegar.

Root of Bear eare drunk, with the same weight of the seed of All-heal.

Seed of Sorrell drunke in wine, or in water.

Willow herb drunk.

Ten graines of small Sea-grape drunk in wine.

Leaves of Periwincle drunke in wine.

Decoction of Stoebe glisterised.

Seede of water plantaine drunke in wine.

Herb Speedwell boiled, drunk.

Roots of spatling Poppy taken in wine.

Leaves and seed of Egrimony drunk in wine.

Roots of water Lilly, dryed, and drunk in wine.

Housleek drunk in wine.

Blood of a hee Goat, of a she Goat, of a Hare, of a Hart, fryed and eaten.

Juyce of the leaves and branches of vine, drunk.

Decoction of Grape skins drunk.

Grape kernells reduced to meale, applyed as polenta.

---

[242] A fresh water fish like a Sturgeon.
[243] The pickle or brine of fish or flesh.
[244] It beareth leaves like Knee-holme, and is of a sharpe astringent taste.
[245] *Tragium.*

Dry white Grapes eaten alone or with their kernells.

Verjuyce given in a glister.

Wine of the flowers of Labruske drunk.

Wine of Quinces drunk.

Wine of Sumack drunk.

Lemnian Earth drunk.

Brine given in a glister when the guts are ulcerated, through the long continuance of the disease.

Water Germander the weight of two drams drunk in water.

Ivie flowers, so many as you can hold between three fingers, drunk in wine twice a day.

To bind the Belly.

CUrd of a Hare drunk.

Any Milk wherein burning flints have been quenched, drunk.

Cheese boyled, or rosted, eaten.

Dogs dung drunk in water in the canicular dayes.

Crust of wheaten bread eaten.

Liniment made of Barly meal, and of mirtil berries, or of wilde Pears, or of Pomegranat shells and wine.

Broth of Spelt-corn or of Oates or of Millet eaten.

Rice eaten,

Boiled Lentills eaten with their husks, especially if they be boyled in Vinegar or with other astringent things.

Seed of Sorrell or of sharpe pointed Docke, drunke in wine or in water.

Coleworts well boiled, eaten.

Black Beets boyled with their roots among Lentills, eaten.

Plantain boiled in vinegar, eaten with salt, or given in a glister. The seed also drunke in wine is very good.

Wilde or garden Succory, eaten.

Juyce of Gum Succory,[246] boyled, and drunk.

Wilde Lentills taken in any sort.

Stone Basill[247] drunke.

Annise drunk.

Seed and tops of Dill drunk.

Parsely eaten.

Harts tongue drunk.

Roots of Branke ursine drunk.

Wild Fennell drunk.

---

[246]*Chondrylla.*
[247]*Acynos.*

Rue drunk or eaten.

Satyrion[248] drunk in wine.

Peony roots boyled in wine drunk,

Decoction of Marsh Mallowes drunk.

Roots of Bears eare drunk.

Juyce of Knot-grasse drunk.

Periwincle drunk in wine.

Hare foot Trefoile[249] taken in wine, or in water, provided the party have no feaver.

Roots of stinking Gladdon taken in honied wine.

Leaves of Orkanet taken in wine,

Decoction of branches of Bramble, drunk.

Decoction of Cinkefoile rootes, drunke.

Red Darnell[250] drunk in strong wine.

Roots of Idea drunk.

Seed of Bull-rush, especially of sea Bull-rush, fryed and drunk in wine allayed with water,

Root of Milk vetch,[251] drunk in wine.

Root of Jacynth drunk in wine.

Seed of black Poppy drunk in wine.

Flowers and roots of Mullein, drunk.

Flowers of Labruske Drunk.

Wine of sowre Pomegranats drunk.

Red Oker given in a glister, or taken in a reer egge.

Lees of wine applyed.

Housleek drunk in wine.

Decoction of Maiden-hair drunk.

Decoction of blacke Maiden-haire drunk.

Vinegar mingled with meale.

Against inveterate Fluxes of the Belly.

BlLod of a he Goate, of a she Goate, of a Hare, or of a Hart, fryed in a skin and eaten.

To loosen the Belly.

CHerryes eaten.

Sweet Apples eaten.

[248]*Serapias* finger *Orchis.*
[249]*lagopus.*
[250]*Phenix.*
[251]*Astragalus.*

Peaches eaten.

Ripe Mulberries eaten.

Ripe figs eaten.

Sea Hedg-hog eaten.

Broth of Tellines,[252] Flions, Cockles,[253] and other small shell-fish supped with salt.

Cutlefish eaten.

The fish Silurus eaten.

Broth of Gudgeons supped.

Broth of all fish supped alone or with wine.

Broth of old Capons.

Milke supped.

Whey drunk.

New Cheese eaten.

Butter eaten, or supped.

Marrow of bones eaten.

Cich Pease eaten.

Herb Patience, Beets, Mallowes, Orage, White Beets, Sparagus, or Lettice, boiled and eaten.

Coleworts lightly boiled, eaten.

Goates Organy drunk.

Against wind in the Guts.

LIniments made of wheat meal; and of juyce of Henbane.

A Poultis made of Barly meale, of Fenegreek and of Lin-seed.

Seed of Basill drunk.

Rhapontick drunk.

Decoction of the seed and tops of Dill drunk.

Decoction of Cummin, given in a Glister with oyle.

Cummin seed steeped in oyle, and water, reduced to a Liniment with Polenta.

Juyce of Sow-fennell taken in a reer egge.

Decoction of Cammomil drunk.

Against long wormes.

GRaines of Paradise drunk.

Decoction of the root of Pomegranat tree drunk.

Walnuts eaten aboundantly.

---

[252]A smal shel fish.

[253]Not unlike a cockle, only having a whiter & smoother shell.

Decoction of the barke of the roots of Mulberry tree drunk.

Garlick eaten or drunk.

Roots of Carline thistle, the weight of an acetabule taken in the decoction of Castorium and of Organy.

Roots of Finger fearn, the weight of three drams drunk with hony.

Seed of Gith drunk, or applyed with water upon the Navel.

Vitrioll the weight of a dram taken in the manner of an Electuary with hony.

Seed and Leaves of Turnsole,[254] drunk with Hisope, Niter, and garden cresses.

Against round Worms.

MEale of Lupines taken as an Electuary with hony, or drunke with
    vinegar, pepper, and Rue.

Colewort seed drunk.

Juyce, or seed of Purslain drunk.

Garden cresses drunk.

Worm-seed-wort drunk.

Electuary of Hisope and of hony.

Minte drunk.

Decoction of Calamint taken with salt and hony.

Time drunk.

Summer Savory drunk.

Decoction of Rue drunk with oile.

Coriander seed taken in sod wine.

Third kind of Orcanet drunk with Hisope and garden Cresses.

Wormewood wine drunk.

Housleek taken in wine.

Roots of Fearn[255] the weight of three drams taken in wine, but before you take this medicine you must eate Garlick.

Against Fluxes caused by Laxative Medicines.

GIzernes of old Cocks salted and dryed in the shade, drunk.

Against wounds of the Guts.

LEaves and roots of Horse-taile drunk in water.

[254]*Heliotropium.*
[255]Common ordinary Fearn or brake.

Against Ulcers of the Guts.

ALL sorts of Milke wherein burning flints have been quenched, given in Glisters.

Powder of Saphire stone drunk.

SIMPLES SERVING FOR THE FUNDAMENT.

To heale Clefts and Chaps of the Fundament.

LIniment of Tarre.

Lees of oyle boyled in a Copper pot, to the consistence of hony, used as a liniment.

Seed of Agnus Castus applyed with water.

River Crabbs burned and applyed with sod hony.

Roots of Teasell[256] boyled in wine, bruised and applyed often.

Wall-flowers incorporated in Wax, applyed as a poultis.

Flowers of Labruske applyed.

Washed Lead applyed.

For Ulcers of the Fundament.

POwder of Frankincense incorporated in milke, applyed upon soft linnen folds.

Juyce of sower Pomegranats boyled with hony, used as a liniment.

Unwashed wool applyed, to incarnace and mollifie the ulcers.

Washed lead applied.

Against Apostumes of the Fundament.

RAw Quinces applyed as a poultis.

Yolke of an egge rosted in the embers, reduced to a liniment with oyle of roses and saffron.

Aloes applyed with sod wine.

Ashes of Dill seed burned, applyed.

Rosemary applied as a poultis.

Leaves of stinking Hore-hound rosted in the embers, applyed.

Bramble leaves applyed.

Wall Pellitory applyed.

Cinkefoile roots applyed.

Ashes of Vine branches, and of Grape-skins applied with vinegar.

Rust of Iron used in a liniment.

---

[256]*Virga pastoris.*

Washed lead applied.
Red Arsenick applied with oyle of roses.
Hoggs Lard applied.
Saffron put in Cataplasmes.

Against inflammations of the Fundament.

LIniment made of Melilot, Lentils, Quinces, dry Roses, bark of Pomegranate, and oyle of roses.
    Liniment of the juyce of Sow-thistle.
    A Poultis made of Melilot, meale of Fenegreek, Linseed, and of sod wine.
    Rosemary applyed.
    Liniment made of the boyled roots of marsh Mallowes.
    Poultis made of the roots of Comfry,[257] with groundsell leaves.
    Flowers and leaves of Groundsell, applyed with a little wine.

To resolve Tumours of the Fundament.

TArre layed thereto.

For the falling of the Fundament.

LEaves and juyce of the Mastick-tree applied.
    Decoction of Quinces fomented.
    Cramp-fish applyed.
    Liniment made of the juyce of Sow-bread, boyled till it be as thick as hony.
    Flowers of female Pimpernell applied.
    Star-wort[258] applied.
    Liniment or fomentation made with vinegar.
    Sharp brine fomented.

For a great desire of going to stoole, without doing any thing.

GListers of sheeps milke, of Goates milke, or of Cowes milke, wherein burning flints have been quenched.
    A Glister of the decoction of Fenegreek-seed.
    Lin-seed applyed in any sort.
    Liniment made of meale of bitter Vetch soaked in wine.

[257]*Consolida major.*
[258]*Aster Atticus.*

Against Warts growing on the Fundament.

GALL of wild shee Goates applied.
    Sheeps dung applyed with vinegar.
    Asa Fetida boyled in vinegar in a Pomegranate shell.
    Vinegar applyed.

To cause Emeroids come forth.

THe place rubbed with onions.

To stay the Flux of Emeroids.[259]

ALoes applyed with vinegar.
    Rosemary used as a poultis.
    Bramble leaves layed to.
    Liniment made of Dates.

To heale Emeroids.

SEed of Sumack applyed.
    Liniment made of Dates.
    Decoction of Rest-harrow drunk according to the opinion of some.
    Washed lead applyed.
    Liniment of the Arabian stone.[260]
    Purslaine well boyled applyed.

SIMPLES SERVING FOR THE REINES.

For paines in the Reines.

GRains of Paradise drunk in wine.
    French Spikenard drunk, and applied.
    Decoction of Amomum drunk.
    Liniment made of the roots of Reed Cane, and of vinegar.
    Gum Dragant, dissolved in sod wine, the weight of a dram, with ashes of
Hearts-horne washed, and a little of the best Allome; drink this composition.
    Juyce of Sow-fennell drunk.
    Dry white Grapes eaten.

---

[259]Bleeding or mattering.
[260]*Goraeus* saith, it is white marble.

Third kinde of *Spuma Maris* drunk.
Decoction of Fenell, bathed and fomented.
Pimpernell drunk.
Agarick the weight of a dram drunk.
Juyce of Licorice drunke in sod wine.
Seselios of Candie[261] drunk.
Sea pimpernell[262] drunk.
Peony roots drunk in wine.
Wall-wort[263] drunk in water.
Decoction of Orkanet boyled in water drunk.
Honied wine drunk.

For the Stone, and gravell of the Reines.

ALL sorts of Spikenard drunk, but Celtick Spikenard is best.
Bay leaves drunk, or the bark of the roote which is much more effectuall.
Gum of Cherry-tree drunk in wine.
Gum of bitter Almond-tree taken in sod wine.
Rinde of the roote of Rest-harrow drunk in wine.
Annise drunk.
Seed of wild Cummin[264] drunk.
Decoction of Mugwort fomented.
Decoction of Cammomill drunk, or used as a Bath.
Leaves of Fever-few drunk.
Decoction of marsh Mallows drunk.
Decoction of Beares eare drunk
Juyce of land, or water Caltraps drunk.
Roote of Bramble drunk.
Decoction of the roote of horned Poppie drunk.
Leaves and roots of wall Penniwort drunk.
Worm-wood wine drunk.
Maiden haire drunk.
Black Maiden-haire drunk.
Dry white Grapes eaten.
Honied wine often drunk.
Third kind of *Spuma maris* drunk.

---

[261] *Tordilium.*
[262] *Anthyllus.*
[263] *Symphitum Petreum.*
[264] *Consolida regalis.*

To heale Ulcers of the Reines.

ALL sorts of milk drunk.
Leaves and roots of Plantaine drunk in sod wine.
Dry white Grapes eaten.
Honied wine often drunk.

To remove obstructions of the Reines.

RHapontick drunk.
Worm-wood wine drunk.
Honied wine drunk.

SIMPLES SERVING FOR THE BLADDER.

To expell Urine.

DEcoction of common sweet Cane drunk.
Roots of Spicknell boyled in water, or bruised raw, drunk.
All sorts of Spikenard drunk.
Graines of paradise drunk in wine.
Asarabacca drunk.
Dry great Valerian drunk.
Indian leafe[265] drunk.
Cinamon drunk.
Cinnamomum drunk.
Costus drunk.
Squinanth drunk.
True sweet Cane drunke, with the seed of Couch-grasse, or Parsley.
Decoction of Rose-wood drunk.
Saffron drunk.
Decoction of Elicampane rootes drunk.
Dregs of oyle of Saffron[266] drunk.
Kernels of Pine apples eaten, or drunk in sod wine, with seed of
  cowcumbers.
Decoction of Mastick-tree drunk.
Berries of the Turpentine-tree eaten.
All kinde of Rosins, especially Turpentine swallowed.
Cyprus leaves taken in sod wine, with a little Myrrhe.
Cedar berries eaten or drunk.

---

[265]*Malabathrum.*
[266]*Crocomagma.*

Decoction of Bay leaves fomented.

Bark of Poplar tree, the weight of an ounce drunk.

Decoction of leaves and roots of Christs-thorne drunk.

Leaves of Mock-privet[267], drunk.

Ladanum drunk in old wine.

Gum of Aethiopian Olive-tree, and of other Olive-trees drunk.

Acornes drunk.

Decoction of the outward skin of Dates in powder, drunk.

Juyce of sower Pomegranats drunk.

Gum of Cherry-tree drunk.

Gum of the bitter Almond tree drunk.

Sea Hedge-hoggs eaten.

Land Hedge-hoggs salted and dryed, drunk in honied vinegar.

Earth-wormes bruised and drunk in sod wine.

Hony drunk.

French Barley eaten.

Ale drunk.

Broth of Cich pease supped.

Broth of bitter Vetch supped.

Decoction of Lupine roots drunk.

Boyled Cole-wort stalks eaten.

Radish eaten, and the seed drunk.

Skirrets eaten.

Sparagus lightly boyled.

Great water Parsnep taken in any sort.

Seed of Cowcumbers drunk.

Seed of both kinds of Rocket drunk.

Small Dragons drunk.

Boyled *French* beanes eaten, with their shels.

Asphodill roots drunk.

White Daffodill roots eaten, or the decoction thereof drunk.

Wild, and Garden Leekes eaten.

Boyled Onions eaten.

Garlick eaten.

Capers drunk forty dayes together.

Juyce of Pimpernell[268] drunk.

Decoction of Calamint drunk.

Decoction of Sage drunk.

---

[267] *Phillyria.*
[268] *Anagallis.*

Seed of Chamaeleon-thistle drunk.

Decoction of Time drunk.

Decoction of Summer Savoury drunk.

Wild Time drunk.

Rue taken in any sort.

Root of White-thistle[269] drunk.

Roots of Brank ursine drunk.

Rinde of the root of Rest-harrow drunk in wine.

Roots of Sea-holly drunk.

Worme-wood, or the decoction thereof drunk.

Decoction of Hisope drunk.

Organie drunk.

Decoction of Goats Organy drunk.

Wild Rue applyed on the groine.

Seed and root of Lovage drunk.

Seed of All-heale drunk.

Caraway seeds drunk.

Decoction of the seed and tops of Dill, drunk.

Smallage eaten raw, or boyled.

Parsley[270] drunk.

Decoction of Fennell drunk.

Gith drunk many dayes together.

Decoction of Poley-mountaine drunk.

Decoction of Mugwort used in fomentation.

Decoction of Cammomill drunk, or used as a Bath.

Gromell taken in white wine.

Root of Madir drunk.

Roots of Spleen-wort drunke in wine.

St. Johns-wort drunk.

Bettony leaves drunk.

Seed of Woodbinde drunk, is an excellent remedy.

Saxifrage drunk.

Roots of stinking Gladdon, the weight of three obols drunk, but the seed is much better.

Seed of Sea Bulrush fryed, and drunk in wine and water.

Perfume of Maudlein[271] with uncut leaves.

Winter Cherries eaten.

Seed of sleepy Night-shade drunk.

---

[269]*Bedeguar.*
[270]*Petroselinum.*
[271]*Ageratum.*

Leaves, berries, small stalks, and roots of Kneeholme drunk in wine.
Broome-seeds eaten.
The first spriggs of Briony boyled, and eaten.
Decoction of milke Trifoile[272] drunk.
Seed of yellow Carrots drunk.
Seed of Bastard St. Johns-wort drunk.
Juyce of Horse-taile drunk.
Leaves of Wall Penni-wort eaten with the roots.
Seed of Rampions, and of Winter-Cresses[273] drunk.
Roots of Milke vetch[274] taken in wine.
Roots of Jacynth drunk.
Young spriggs of black Briony boyled and eaten.
Juyce of the leaves of Spurge Laurell drunk.
Wine of Quinces, of Hisope, of Squill, or of Wormwood drunk.
Honied water drunk.

For those which pisse with difficulty and paine.

Punies[275] bruised and surringed up the yard.
Wood-lice drunk in wine.
Cigales[276] rosted, and eaten.
Perfume of Grasse-hoppers chiefly for women.
Ashes of Harts-horne well washed two drams.
Decoction of Mallowes bathed.
Purslaine eaten often.
Decoction of Sparagus rootes drunk.
Decoction of the rootes, leaves, and seeds of Samphire boyled in wine, drunk.
Decoction of Artificiall Vermillion[277] drunk.
Bastard Parsley eaten as other Garden herbs.
Decoction of great Marjerome drunk.
Decoction of the roots of Plowmans Spikenard drunk.
Seed of Basill drunk.
Roots of Candie Alexanders drunk.
Agarick the weight of a dram taken.

---

[272]Cytisus.
[273]Pseudobunium.
[274]Astragalus.
[275]A stinking worm so called.
[276]A kind of great flyes unknown in England.
[277]*Sandix*, it is made of burned Ceruse.

Juyce of Sow-fennell drunk.

Rhapontick drunk.

Juyce of Canary-grasse[278] taken in wine, or in water.

Nettle-tree bruised drunke alone in wine, or in sod wine with seed of
   Mallowes.

Ground Pine drunk.

Decoction of Carline-thistle drunk.

Seed of Southern-wood bruised, steeped in hot water, and drunk.

Seed of All-heale drunk, or applied on the groine.

Seed of Seselios of Candy drunk.

Roots of spatling Poppy drunk in water.

Seed of Bastard Stone Parsley[279] drunk.

Ammeos taken in wine.

Parsley-seed drunke.

Galbanum drunk.

Decoction of water Germander boiled in wine, or in water, drunk.

Second kinde of sea Pimpernell, the weight of two drams drunk.

Peonie drunk.

Decoction of marsh Mallows drunk with wine.

Decoction of the roots of Couch-grasse drunk.

Roots of Clote burres[280] boyled with the seed, drunk.

Maiden-haire drunk.

Black Maiden-haire drunk.

Third kind of *Spuma maris* drunk.

Powder of Blood-stone drunke in wine.

Powder of the Stone Morochthus drunk in water.

Powder of the Stone Judaicus,[281] the bignesse of a Cich-pease taken in
hot water.

Sponge Stones[282] taken in wine.

For the Strangury.

DEcoction of common sweet Cane drunk.

   Seed of Water-cresses drunke in wine.

   Hercules All-heale taken in wine.

   Seselios of Marseilles drunk.

[278]Phalaris.

[279]*Sison.*

[280]*Arction.*

[281]White stone in forme of an Acorn brought from *Syria.*

[282]Found in Sponges.

Seed of Wild Cummin[283] drunk.
Seed and root of Smallage, or of Parsley drunk in honied wine.
Polycnemon[284] taken in wine.
Wild Basill drunk.
Roots of Oenanthe[285] taken in wine.
Leaves and flowers of Flea-bane drunk.
Decoction of Spleenwort drunk.
Onions boyled with Sparagus roots drunk.
Red Fetchling[286] drunk.
Juyce of knot-grasse drunk.
Saxifrage boyled in wine drunk.
Roots of stinking Gladdon taken in honied wine.
Juyce, seed, and leaves of small Saxifrage[287] drunk.
Leaves, roots, and berries of Butchers Broome drunk.
Roots of Alexandrian bayes the weight of six drams drunk.
Tops of Golden mothweed[288] drunk in wine.

To heale Ulcers of the Bladder.

LEaves and berries of mirtle drunk.
　　All sorts of milke drunk.
　　Cowcumber-seed drunk in milke, and sod wine.
　　Dry white Grapes much eaten.

For wounds of the Bladder.

BUtter surringed.
　　Leaves of Horse-tayle drunk in water.

To void the stone of the Bladder.

THe izerne of Ossifragus[289] drunk at times.
　　Mice dung taken in honied wine with Frankincense.
　　Urine of a Boare drunk.
　　Decoction of the roots of sharpe-pointed dock drunk.

---

[283]*Consolida regalis.*
[284]A shrub having leaves like Organie, many branches, and small black berries.
[285]An herbe with great roots, rising in many round heads, growing among stones.
[286]Onobrychis.
[287]Tragium.
[288]Helichrison.
[289]Kind of Eagle so called.

Great water Parsnep boyled, or raw, eaten, or drunk, or the decoction of
them drunk.
Seed of Water-cresses drunk.
Decoction of Plow-mans Spikenard drunk.
Seed or rootes of Parsley drunk in wine.
Wild fennell drunk.
Gum Sagapene drunk.
Decoction of Maiden-haire drunk.
Decoction of black Maiden-haire drunk.
Gum issuing out of Vine-stocks drunk in wine.

To breake Stones in the Bladder.

GRaines of Paradise drunk, with a dram of the rinde of the roote of
    Bayes.
Bdellium drunk.
Gum of Cherry-tree drunk.
Decoction of Spleen-wort drunk.
Gromell[290] drunk in white wine.
Saxifrage drunk.
Decoction of Couch-grasse drunk.
Seed of small Saxifrage drunk.
Roots and berries of Knee-holme drunk.
Powder of the Stone Judaicus, falling there-from, being rubbed against
    another sharp stone, drunk in hot water.
Sponge Stones drunk.

For those which cannot keep their water.

SEEd of wild Rue fryed, and eaten.
    Red Darnell drunke in strong wine.

Against the Itch of the Bladder.

HErcules All-heale drunk in honied water, or in wine.
    Garden Brook-lime[291] drunk.

For those which pisse small clots of bloud.

SEEd of wild Cummin drunk.
    Tops of golden Moth-weed drunk in honied wine.

---

[290]*Milium solis.*
[291]*Cepaea.*

For persons which pisse bloud by reason of stones broken in the Bladder.

SHarp brine surringed up the yard or passage of the Urine, so soone as it
  is perceived.

SIMPLES SERVING FOR THE GENITALL MEMBERS AND SECRET PARTS.

To cause standing of the Yard.

COstus drunk in honied wine.
  Saffron drunk.
  Lin-seed taken with hony and pepper.
  Boyled Turnips eaten.
  Rocket much eaten.
  Seed of Rocket drunk.
  Roots of great Dragons rosted in embers, or boyled, drunk in wine.
  Asphodill roots eaten.
  Garden Cresses drunk, or eaten.
  Leek seed drunk.
  Boyled Scalions eaten.
  Garlick bruised with Coriander-seeds, eaten.
  Nettle-seeds drunk in sod wine.
  Roots of Ladies Bed-straw[292] eaten.
  Juyce of Mint drunk.
  Roots of All-heale eaten.
  Annise drunk.
  The rankest roots of Bastard Satyrion eaten, or drunk.
  Roots of Satyrion eaten.
  Clary drunk.
  The first and highest root of Corn-flag[293] drunk in wine.
  Reines of Skinke,[294] the weight of a dram drunk in wine.
  All sorts of Milke supped.

To augment Sperme and naturall Seed.

COriander seed drunk.
  Finally all Medicines good to cause standing of the Yard, are proper for
  this, except those which are excessively hot and dry.

---

[292]Gallium.
[293]Xyphion.
[294]A kind of small land Chrocodile divers parts whereof are of good use in physick.

To hinder standing of the Yard.

SEed of *Agnus Castus* drunk, or the leaves applyed on the Genitalls.
Purslaine eaten, or layed upon the Genitalls.
Seeds of Lettice drunk, defendeth dreaming of love in the night.
Decoction of the seed and tops of Dill frequently drunk.
Rue eaten and drunk often.
The leanest roots of bastard Satyrion drunk.
Hempseed taken frequently.
The second and lowest roote of Corn-flag[295] drunk.
Hemlock with the tops, applyed on the Genitalls, having first bruised
it; this is a very good receipt.

For those which lose their Seed.

ROots of water Lilly drunk.
Roots of Illyrian flower-de-luce drunk in vinegar.

For Ulcers of the secret parts.

NEw-shorne unwashed wooll applyed.
Liniment of the powder of Aloes, or the powder it selfe applied.
Juyce of Knot-grasse boyled in wine, and applied with hony.
Allome applied in any sort.
Flos salis, powdered, and sprinkled.

For inflammations of the Genitalls.

CIches boyled with bitter vetches applied.
Beanes boyled in wine, applied as a poultis.
Leaves of Groundsell, and the flowers, used as a poultis.
Liniment of Asphodill leaves and roots.
Cimolian earth applied.
A poultis of Melilot.
Liniment made of the stone Geodes.
Liniment of Rue, and of Bay leaves.
Liniment of Organie, of salt, and of leaven.
A poultis of Cummin, dry Grapes, and Bean-flower, or with wax.
Liniment of Coriander, dry grapes and hony.
A poultis made of Lilly roots cut in chives, with henbane, and
wheate-meale.

[295]Gladiolus.

Liniment of Samian earth, of oyle of roses, and water.
Henbane seed bruised and layed to with wine.

Against itching of the Genitalls.

DEcoction of Sage applied with wine.
 All Rosins, especially Turpentine applied.

Against hardnesse of the Genitalls.

SEEd of Bank Cresses[296] layed to.

For those which have no Prepuce.[297]

 IUyce of stinking deadly Carrot, applyed on the head of the member
  causeth a tumour, which mollified by fomentation of fat things, serveth
  in place of a fore-skin.
 Hony applied thirty dayes, upon the member after bathing.

For Corrisive Vlcers of the Genitall Members.

GAll of a Bul applyed with hony.
 Flowers of Labruske bruised and applied with hony, saffron, Myrrhe, and
  oyle of roses.

Against Warts growing on the genitall Members.

HEad of a Cackarell-fish salted, burned, and layed to.
 Gall of wild she Goates applied.
 Sheeps dung layed to with vinegar.
 Time applied as a poultis.
 Summer Savoury layed to.
 Powder of Pepper, Rue, and Niter, used in frication.
 Milke of Spurge applyed.
 Branches of Spurge Time[298] bruised, and applyed.
 Juyce of Mercury applyed.
 Seed of Turne-soile layed to.

---

[296]*Erysimum.*
[297]The fore-skin, or skin that covereth the nut of the yard.
[298]Chamasyce.

SIMPLES SERVING FOR THE MATRIX.

For the suffocation of the Matrix.

ROots of Spicknell bruised, and reduced to an Electuary with hony.
>   Juniper berries drunk.
>   Perfume of *Unguis odoratus.*
>   Punies put to the nose.
>   Bitumen smelled unto applied, or perfumed.
>   Curd of a Seale drunk.
>   Urine boyled in oyle of privet, given in a Glister, or surringed.
>   Juyce of Plantaine drunk.
>   Mustard-seed bruised, and put to the nose.
>   Agarick the weight of a dram taken.
>   Liniment of Rue incorporated in hony, applied to the fundament, and
>   secret parts.
>   Seed of Hercules All heale drunk in wine.
>   Roote of Mountaine Siler, with the seed, drunk.
>   Sow-fennell smelled to.
>   Gum Sagapene applied about the nostrils, to smell to.
>   Seed and leaves of stinking Trefoil drunk.
>   The black berries of Peonie, fifteen in number, drunk.
>   Roots of Beares eare drunk.
>   Bettony leaves the weight of a dram drunk.
>   Perfume of the stone Gagates.[299]

To provoke Womens monthly Purgations.

ILlyrian Flower-de-luce taken in wine, or used in fomentation.
>   Fomentation and Baths, with the decoction of Spicknell rootes, used
>   beneath.
>   Decoction of common sweet Cane fomented beneath.
>   Decoction of Gallingall roots fomented.
>   Roots of Asarabacca, the weight of six drams drunk in water.
>   Decoction of Valerian drunk.
>   Cinamon drunk.
>   Cinamomun drunk, or used with Myrrhe in manner of a Suppositary, or
>   pessarie.
>   Costus drunk.
>   Cammels hay[300] drunk.

[299]Jet.
[300]Squinanth.

Sweet Cane drunk, or used in fomentation.

Gum Lac drunk in honied water.

Decoction of Elicampane rootes drunk.

A poultis made of Myrrhe, and Worm-wood incorporated in juyce of Lupines, or in juyce of Rue.

Storax drunk, or applied.

Bitumen drunk in wine with Castorium.

Cedar berries drunk with pepper.

Decoction of Bay leaves fomented.

Leaves of Mock privet[301] drunk.

Seed of Agnus Castus, the weight of a dram drunk.

Gum of Olive tree drunk.

Bitter Almonds applied.

Milk of Fig-tree drunk with bruised Almonds.

Snayles and their shels bruised, put into the naturall place of women.

Castorium the weight of two drams drunk.

Juyce of Onions applyed on the secret parts.

Unwashed wooll used as a pessary.

Liniment made of the grease of a Goose, or of a Hen.

Dung of she Goates nourished on mountaines, drunk with some odorant thing.

Decoction of Lin-seed fomented.

Decoction of Lupines used as a suppositary with myrrhe and hony.

Radishes eaten, or the juyce drunk.

Asphodill roots drunk.

Decoction of sea-Holly drunk.

Decoction of Cole-worts supped, or the juyce applyed with Darnell meale as a suppositary.

Great water Parsnep eaten as other pot-hearbs.

Samphyre eaten, or the decoction drunk.

Roots of great Centaury drunk, or the juyce used as a suppositary.

Gum of Gum Succorie used with myrrhe as a suppositary.

Scandulaceum[302] drunk.

Milk of wild Lettice drunk.

Wild and Garden Leeks eaten.

Decoction of Garlick leaves used as a Bath.

Sow-bread drunk, or used in the manner of a suppositary.

Seed of Southern-wood drunk with water.

---

[301]*Phyltirea.*
[302]Some think it is *Volubilis major*, the greater Withiwind.

Seed and rinde of the Caper plant drunk.

Roots of Wind-flower used in a suppository.

Ivie berries bruised, and used as a suppositary or pessarie.

Penni-royall drunk.

Agarick the weight of a dram drunk in Oximel.

Organie drunk.

Worm-wood drunk, or applied beneath.

Goates Organie drunk.

Decoction of Sage drunk.

Ammeos drunk in wine.

Decoction of Time, and of Summer Savoury drunk.

Wild Time drunk.

Seed of Candie Alexanders drunk.

Decoction of great Marjerome drunk or applyed on the naturall place of
   women.

Decoction of the rootes of Plowmans Spikenard drunk.

Wild and garden Rue drunk and applyed beneath.

Hercules All heale drunk in wine.

Seed and roots of Lovage drunke, and applyed.

Seed of All-heale drunk.

Seed and roots of Seselios of Marseilles drunk.

Seselios of Candie drunk.

Fennell taken in wine.

Bastard stone Parsley[303] drunk.

Rosemary roots drunk.

Juyce of Sow-fennell drunk.

Parsley drunk.

Yellow Carret drunk.

Gum Ammoniacum drunke.

Gith drunk frequently.

Gum Sagapene drunk.

Benzoin drunk with Peper and Myrrhe.

Galbanum perfumed, and used as a suppositary.

Wild Basill[304] drunk.

Decoction of Germander drunk.

Lilly roots burned, and applied beneath with oyle of roses.

Decoction of Baulme used below as a Bath.

Seed and leaves of Trefoile drunk.

Decoction of both kindes of poley drunk.

Juyce of water Germander drunk, or the hearb used as a suppositary.

---

[303]Sison.
[304]Clinopodium.

Decoction of Mugwort used as a Bath.

Sweet Chervill[305] drunk.

  Flowers and leaves of Flea-bane drunk.

Roots of yellow Lilly applyed with wooll.

Leaves and berries of Knee-holme taken in wine.

Decoction of Wall-flowers[306] used as a Bath.

Seed of Wall-flowers the weight of two drams taken in wine.

Decoction of Cammomell drunk, or used as a Bath.

Peonie root the bignesse of an Almond taken.

Roots of Madir applied below.

Decoction of Maiden-haire drunk.

Black Maiden-haire drunk.

Leaves of Beane Trefoile[307] bruised, and drunk in sod wine.

St. Johns-wort drunk, and applyed beneath.

Seed of bastard St. Johns-wort drunk.

Leaves of all kinde of Nettles bruised, and applied with Myrrhe.

Bettony leaves the weight of a dram, taken in wine.

Seed of Blew Coventrie bels[308] drunk.

Juyce of Spurge Laurell leaves taken in wine.

The first roote of Corn-flag[309] applied beneath.

Seed, leaves, and juyce of small Saxifrage[310] the weight of a dram drunk.

Golden Tode-flax[311] taken in Metheglin.

Tops of golden Moth=weed drunk in honied wine.

Juyce of Mandragore, the weight of halfe an obol applied below.

Seed of Mandragore drunk.

Spurge of Laurell drunk.

White and black Hellebore applied beneath.

Young shoots of black Briony boyled as Sparagus, eaten.

Turne-sole leaves, applied beneath.

Wine of Squill, or of Worm-wood, or of Hisope drunk.

To restraine great excesse of Womens monthly Purgations.

SPikenard.

  Mosse of trees used in Baths.

---

[305]Myrrhis.
[306]Cheiri.
[307]Anagyris.
[308]Medium.
[309]Gladiolus.
[310]Tragium.
[311]Chrysocome.

Bark of the Frankincense-tree applied in a pessary.

Hawthorn berries eaten, or drunk.

Juyce of male Holly-rose[312] drunk, or put into the naturall place of women.

Seed of Sumack drunke, stay the whites of women.

Green Dates eaten.

Date-skins drunk.

Kernells of Pomegranats dryed in the Sun, powdered, and sprinkled on meat, or boyled and eaten.

Galls put in Baths, aud fomentations for the lower parts.

The inmost skin of Acornes drunk, or applied beneath.

Mirtill berries used in Baths, or fomentations.

Decoction of Quinces fomented.

Acacia drunk and applied.

Juyce of Box-thorne[313] used in manner of a Suppositary.

Decoction of Lote tree drunk, or fomented below.

Leaves of Mastick tree drunk, or applied in a suppositary.

Curd of Hares, of Kids, of Lambs, of Harts, of Calves, or of Hindes drunk, or used in a suppositary.

Harts-horne burned, and washed with some astringent liquor drunk.

Juyce of wild Olive-tree leaves, applied upon the naturall place of women.

Dung of she Goates nourished on mountaines, dryed, powdered, and applied with Frankincense, as a suppositary.

Roots of hearb Patience used as a suppositary.

Plantaine drunk, or fomented.

Juyce of Goates beard taken in wine, or used as a suppositary.

Leaves of Leekes boyled in sea water, and vinegar, bathed below.

Decoction of branches of Bramble, drunk.

Roots of Arabian-thistle eaten.

Wild Darnell drunk in strong wine.

Seed of horned Poppie drunk.

Yarrow used in a suppositary.

Roots of Idea drunk.

Decoction of Bramble drunk.

Leaves of Horse-taile drunk.

Suppositary of Minte.

Seed of sea Bul-rush fryed, and drunk in wine allayed with water.

Wild Basill drunk in wine.

Annise drunke, especially for the Whites.

---

[312]Hypocistis.
[313]Lycium.

Cummin used in a Suppositary with vinegar.

Seed and root of the water Lilly, which beareth yellow flowers, drunk with thick strong wine.

Peony berries twelve in number taken in strong wine.

Juyce of Willow herbe applyed in a suppositary.

Sorcerers Garlick[314] used in a suppositary with Darnell meale.

Juyce of Knotgrasse applied in a suppositary.

Decoction of Wallwort[315] drunk.

Juyce of Clymenum[316] drunk with wine.

Seed of Water Plantain, the weight of an Acetabule taken in wine.

Root of Blew Coventry bels[317] boiled and made into an Electuary, with hony.

Berries of small Sea Grape[318] ten in number taken in wine.

Henbane seed the weight of an obol taken in honyed water.

Juyce of Morel applyed with wool as a suppositary.

A suppositary of Mandragore-seed, of brimstone, and of wine.

Housleek used in a suppositary with wooll.

Decoction of Grape-skins drunke, and fomented.

Flowers of Labruske used in a pessary.

Verjuyce used in a pessary.

Rust of Iron applied in a suppositary.

Chalcitis used in a pessary with juyce of Leeks.

Lees of wine applyed on the groin, and on the secret parts.

Bloodstone taken in wine.

The stone Morochthus applied with wooll as a pessary.

Powder of the stone Ostracites,[319] the weight of a dram taken in wine.

Samian earth drunk with the flowers of wild Pomegranat tree.

To expell the after birth.

CAstorium the weight of two drams drunk with Penniroyall.

Seed of the second kind of Sowbread drunk.

Decoction of Garlick leaves used in fomentation.

Long Aristolochia drunke with myrrhe and pepper, or used as a Pessary.

Pennyroyall drunk.

Decoction of Time drunk.

[314]Moly.
[315]Symphitum petreum.
[316]By some called Saponalia.
[317]*Medium.*
[318]*Tragos.*
[319]A kind of artificial Cadmia.

Decoction of Summer Savory drunk.

Parsely seed drunk.

Decoction of Hore-hound drunk.

Decoction of wilde Hore-hound[320] drunk.

Decoction of Mugwort bathed.

Four pounds of Bindeweed night-shade,[321] bruised and infused a whole night in seven pounds of sweet wine: drink of this infusion 30 daies together.

Leaves, stalkes, and seed of Oenanthe taken in honyed wine.

Wall-flowers the weight of two drams taken in wine.

Roots of Madir used in a suppositary.

Leaves of Beane Trefoile drunke in sod wine.

Ground Pine used in a suppositary with hony.

Golden Tode flax[322] drunk in honyed water.

Black maiden hair drunk.

Briony used in a Suppositary.

Myrrhe drunk.

Juyce of Sow-fennel drunk.

Seed of Rampions drunke.

Seed of Candy Alexanders drunk.

Decoction of Maiden-haire drunk.

To cause abortion.

CAstorium the weight of two drams taken with Penniroyall.

Milke of a Bitches first Litter drunk.

Unwashed wool applyed in a Suppositary.

Dung of wild she Goates taken with some sweet and aromaticall thing.

Perfume of Vultures feathers.

Broth of Cich pease supped.

Decoction of Lupines, fomented with myrrhe and hony.

Great water Parseneps used as other Kitchen herbs.

Decoction of great Dragons surringed.

Pepper drunk.

Roots of Sow-bread fastened to the thigh.

Stalkes of Ivy leaves applyed in a Suppositary with hony.

Gentian roote used in a Suppositary.

Rootes of great Centaury used in a Pessary.

Juyce of small Centaury surringed.

---

[320]*Stachys.*
[321]*Circea.*
[322]*Chrysocome*

Penniroyall drunk.

Dittany drunk, used in a pessary, or perfumed.

Decoction of Time supped.

Decoction of summer Savory drunk.

Root of Plowmans Spicknard fresh gathered, used in a Suppositary.

Root of Hercules All-heal cut sharp at the end, put into the naturall
  place of women.

Seed and root of Mountaine Siler drunk.

Galbanum with myrrhe taken in wine, or perfumed.

Wild Basill drunk.

Decoction of Germander drunk.

Juyce of water Germander[323] the weight of a dram drunk.

Decoction of Mugwort fomented beneath.

Flowers and leaves of Fleabane drunk

Seed of Wall-flowers the weight of two drams taken in wine.

Leaves of Wild Buglosse[324] taken in wine.

Roots of Madir used in a Suppositary

Leaves of Beane Trefoile drunke in sod wine; or worne about the necke,
  but it must be taken away, so soone as the woman is delivered.

Roots of Orkanet applyed.

Juyce of Mandragore surringed.

Sweet Chervill drunk.

Leaves of Turnsole put into the naturall place of Women.

Perfume of Brimston taken below.

Seed of yellow Carrot drunk.

Gum ammoniacum drunk.

Woodbinde seed the weight of a dram taken in wine.

Roote of Alexandrian Bayes the weight of six drams taken in sweet wine.

Allome used in a suppositary.

Jasper stone fastened to the thigh.

The Eagle stone used in the like manner.

The Samian stone worne about the neck.

To hinder Conception.

LEaves of Willow taken apart, or with water.

Curd of a Hare, taken three days after the womans monthly purgation.

Menstruall blood applied on the naturall place.

---

[323]*Scordium.*
[324]*Onosma.*

Colewort flowers applyed in a pessary presently after the woman is delivered.

Sparagus rootes worne about the neck.

Pepper put into the naturall place, after a woman hath known a man carnally.

Ivy berries, the weight of a dram taken after their monthly purgation.

Hatchet Fitch[325] used in a Suppositary before the carnall knowledge of a man.

Rosin of Cedar applied on the mans member.

Powder of the stone Ostracites the weight of two drams, drunke foure dayes after the monthly purgation.

Scaleferne gathered in the night when the Moone doth not shine, fastened unto the womans belly, with the Milt of a Mule; according to the opinion of some.

Seed and leaves of Wood-bine drunk 36 dayes together,

Leaves of Barrenwort,[326] bruised and drunk 5 dayes together, presently after the monthly purgation.

The Lower root of Corne-flagge[327] drunk.

Roots of Brakes drunk.

Turnesole worn about the neck.

Rust of Iron drunk.

Minte applyed on the naturall place of women, before they know men carnally.

To cause Conception.

CUrd of a Hare used in a Suppositary, presently after the womans monthly purgation.

Perfume of darnell meale, myrthe, Frankincense, Bitumen, and Saffron taken beneath.

Seed of All-heale drunk.

To deliver a woman of a dead Child.

DIttany drunk, and applied in a suppository.

Decoction of Sage drunk.

Galbanum drunk with Myrrhe, and wine.

Decoction of Hore-hound drunk.

Decoction of Coltsfoot drunk.

---

[325] *Securidaca.*
[326] *Epimediu.*
[327] *Gladiolus.*

To preserve the Childe till the limitted time.

THe Eagle stone worn about the left arme.
The Samian stone worne about the neck.

For women in Labour.

ROOt of Dittany drunk.
Decoction of the Roots of Plow-mans Spicknard fomented.
Wild Fennell drunk.
Juyce of Sowfennell drunk.
Dry Peony roots drunk.
Decoction of Marsh Mallowes surringed.

Against loathing of meate of women with Child.

IUyce of the leaves and Tendrels of vine drunk.

Against inflammation of the Matrix.

DEcoction of Spicknard bathed.
Decoction of Squinanth to bath the secret parts.
Decoction of the leaves and seed of Agnus Castus, fomented.
Fresh Butter applyed.
Juyce of Sow-thistle applyed.
Agarick the weight of a dram taken in Oximell.
Decoction of Penniroyal to foment the privy parts.
A Poultis of Melilot, and of sod wine.
Gum of Hercules All-heale put into the naturall place of women with
  hony.
Decoction of Mugwort used as a bath.
Decoction of Wallflowers applyed in fomentation
Root of Sea Pimpernell laid to with milk and oyle of Roses.
Decoction of Feverfew bathed.
Decoction of Marsh Mallowes incorporated with Goose-grease; or in Hogs
  Lard, or in Turpentine, used as a Suppositary.

For Ulcers in the naturall places of women.

DEcoction of Rose-wood boyled in wine surringed.
Milke wherein burning flints have been quenched, surringed.
Unwashed wool applyed, both healeth and mollifieth.
Liniment of the Leaves of Fenugreek and vinegar.
Leaves of Swallow wort applyed.

To mollifie hardnesse of the naturall parts of Women.

A Poultis of Myrrhe, and Worm-wood, made with sap of Lupines, or with Rue.

Liniment of Storax.

Liniment of the grease of a Goose, or of a Hen.

Liniment of Bdellium.

Decoction of Mallowes surringed.

Labdanum used in a pessary.

Hercules All-heale put into Womens naturall places with hony.

Decoction of Elder, and of Wall-wort fomented.

Decoction of Fever-few used as a bath.

The expression of Fenugreek steeped in water, incorporated in Goose-grease, and used as a pessary.

Roots of Lillies applied.

Perfume of Maudlein[328] with uncut leaves.

Against Wind in the Matrix.

A Glister of Rue boyled in oyle.

Herbe Doves foot,[329] and the roots, the weight of a dram drunk.

Against falling and relapsing of the Matrix.

PErfumes, or fomentations made of Cinamon.

Juyce of Mirtill berries fomented.

Decoction of Quinces used in fomentation.

Decoction of Galls used as a Bath.

Acacia in a suppositary.

Juyce of male Holly-rose used in a suppositary.

Leaves of all sorts of Nettles applied.

Vinegar used in fomentation.

Against paines, and gripings of the Matrix.

LIniment of the grease of a Goose, or of a Hen.

Urine boyled with oyle of privet applied.

Decoction of Lin-seed surringed.

Decoction of Mallowes surringed, or used as a Bath.

Decoction of Purslaine surringed; this is a singular receipt against gripings of the Matrix.

[328]Ageratum.
[329]Geranium hearb Robert.

Rhapontick drunk.

Roots of great Centaury drunk.

Decoction of Dill used beneath in fomentation.

Verveine leaves incorporated in fresh Hoggs lard, or in oyle of roses used as a suppositary.

Decoction of Henbane-seed surringed.

Juyce of Mandragore applied in a pessary.

SIMPLES SERVING FOR THE ARMES AND LEGGS.

For the Gout of the Leggs, and Feet.

AMomum applyed.

Roots of Spicknell applied.

Liniment made of Aspen leaves, and of vinegar.

Raw fresh lees of oyle, used in fomentation.

Decoction of the leaves and bark of Willow fomented.

A poultis made of milk of Figtree, vinegar, and meale of fenugreek.

Snayles bruised with their shels.

Liniment made of the ashes of a burned Weesill, with vinegar.

Sea Lungs[330] chopped small and applied.

Liniment made of womans milk, of opium, and of wax.

Suet of Sheep, of she Goates, or of he Goates, incorporated with the beasts dung from which it was taken, and applied as a liniment.

Menstruall bloud applied.

Dung of wild she Goates applied with their suet.

A poultis made of Barlie meale, and of Quinces.

A poultis made of boyled lentils with polenta.

Decoction of Turnips to foment the diseased part.

A poultis made of Cole worts, of fenugreek, and of vinegar.

Liniment made of Succory alone, or with polenta.

Parings of Gourds applied.

Roots of Cuckow pinte[331] incorporated in Oxe dung, and applied as a poultis.

Asphodill roots the weight of a dram taken in wine.

Decoction of Sow-bread fomented.

Scalions applied alone, or with hony.

Liniment made of Hercules All-heale, and of dry grapes.

Poultisses of Rosemary, Darnell meale, and vinegar.

Water Germander applyed with water, or vinegar.

Liniment made of Wall-flowers, and of vinegar.

---

[330]A round spungie excresence of the sea.
[331]Aron.

Sea Navell-wort[332] applied.

Liniment made of the juyce of Wal-Pellitory, incorporated in wax, and suet of a he Goate.

A poultis made of the seeds and leaves of Henbane, and of polenta.

Housleek applied when the disease is accompanied with great heat.

Liniment made of Nettles.

Corraline applied.

Liniment made of wild Cowcumber rootes, and of vinegar.

Juyce of stinking deadly Carrot applied.

Ben applied.

A poultis made of the leaves of Elder, and of Wall-wort, incorporated in suet of a Bull, or of a he Goat.

A poultis of Briony incorporated in she Goates dung.

Liniment of Turne-sole leaves.

Dry Grapes, the kernels taken out,[333] applied with juyce of All-heale.

Stewes made of boyling vinegar, and of brimstone.

Liniment made of the rust of Iron.

Liniment of brimstone, water, and niter.

Salt and vinegar applied.

Liniment of Beane meale, and Asian stone.

Liniment made of Jet.

Bricks very well burned applied.

For the Sciatica.

ROots of Spicknell applied.

Elicampane rootes boyled in wine, applied.

Decoction of Illyrian Flower-de-luce given in a Glister.

Graines of paradise taken in water.

Asarabacca drunk, or glisterised.

Barke of Poplar tree, the weight of an ounce drunk.

Sciatica cresses[334] bruised and applied as a poultis.

Pickle of the Fish Silurus given in a Glister.

Pickle of all Fish glisterised.

Seed of Candie Alexanders drunk.

Dung of Oxen at grasse applied.

A poultis of Darnell meale boyled in honied water.

Liniment of meale of Lupines, and vinegar.

[332]Androsace.
[333]Or Raisins stoned.
[334]Iberis.

Gum Ammoniacum drunk.

Seed of S. Peters-wort[335] taken in water.

Decoction of Sparagus roots drunk.

Decoction of Marsh Mallowes drunk.

Mustard-seed bruised, and applied, with Figgs, letting it remaine till the place looke red.

Garden Cresses given in a Glister.

Seed of Bank Cresses glisterised.

Scalions applied alone, or with hony.

Capers drunk.

A poultis made of the leaves and roots of Dittander,[336] bruised and incorporated with Elicampane roots.

Agarick the weight of three obols, taken in honied vinegar.

Rhapontick drunk.

Seed of Tutsan St. Johns-wort[337] drunk, but you must drink water presently after the Medicine hath done its operation.

Decoction of great Centaurie given in a Glister.

Decoction of our Lady-thistle roots drunk.

Seed of Southern-wood drunke in water.

Roots of Madir drunk.

Penni-royall applied till the place be made red.

Green Calaminte bruised, and applied till the place be red.

A poultis of Time, Mans dung, and Polenta.

Summer Savoury prepared in the like manner.

Seed of wild Rue drunk forty dayes together.

Liniment of Hercules All-heale, and hony.

Liniment of *Asa Fetida* incorporated in wax, oyle of privet, and oyle of Flower-de-luce.

Euphorbium taken in some Aromaticall potion.

Lions leafe[338] given in a Glister.

Seed of St. Johns-wort drunk forty dayes together.

Leaves of ground Pine taken in water forty dayes together.

Bettony leaves drunk in water.

Roots of Spatling Poppy taken with water.

Roots of stinking Gladdon taken in honied wine.

Seed of wild Basill taken in wine, with myrrhe, and Pepper.

Decoction of Cinkfoile rootes drunk.

Tops of golden Moth-weed taken in wine.

[335]Ascirum.
[336]Lepidium.
[337]Androsaemum.
[338]Leontopetalum.

Decoction of the roote of horned Poppy drunk.

Decoction of the Aethiopian Mullein drunk.

Clote-burre[339] drunk in wine, or applied.

Leaves of Spurge Time,[340] the weight of three obols, taken in water thirty or forty dayes together.

Fresh Coloquintida glisterised, or used in frication.

Roots of wild Cowcumber, given in a Glister.

Infusion of Broome steeped in Sea water, given in a Glister.

A poultis of Scammonie boyled in vinegar, and barley flower.

Honied vinegar drunk.

Sory given in a Glister with wine.

Brine glisterised.

Adarca[341] applied.

Against the Gout of the hands, and paines of the joynts.

BRoth of old Cocks supped.

Liniment of Cole-worts, fenugreek, and vinegar.

Rue drunk, or used in a poultis.

Agarick the weight of a dram taken in honied vinegar.

Decoction of Cinkfoile roots drunk.

Liniment made of Fleabane, oyle of roses, and vinegar, or water.

Rootes of Mandragore applyed as a poultis with dry polenta.

A poultis of Nettles.

Black Hellebore drunk.

Sea weed applied fresh.

Liniment of the juyce of stinking deadly Carrot.[342]

Daffodill roots bruised and applied with hony.

Honied vinegar drunk.

Honied wine frequently drunk.

For bruised joynts.

LIniment of Vine branches burned to ashes, and incorporated in grease, or in oyle.

Against knobs and nodosities growing on the joynts.

ROots of wild Hemp boyled and applied.

Liniment made of Oker.

---

[339]Arction.

[340]Chamaesyce.

[341]A salt blackish foame cleaving to reeds, and other marsh hearbs in dry seasons.

[342]Thapsia.

To heale Kybes on the heeles.

FRankinsence applied with grease of a Hogge, or of Goose.
Tarre applied.
Acacia applied.
Decoction of Mirtill berries fomented.
Burned Figgs incorporated in a Cerot, and layed to.
Liniment of the ashes of burned river Crabbs, and hony.
Sea Lungs chopped small, and applied to, fresh.
Ashes of burned Asses hoofe, incorporated in oyle, applyed.
Beares grease annoynted.
Juyce of wall Penni-wort applied.
A plaister made of Lentils, Melilot, dry roses, pomgranate shels,
   Quinces, and oyle of roses.
Decoction of bitter vetch used in fomentation.
Decoction of Turnips fomented.
Decoction of Beets bathed.
Leaves of great Dragons boyled in wine, applied.
Oyle boyled in the hollow of an Asphodill roote, applied.
Decoction of Sow bread fomented, or oyle boyled with a little wax, in
the hollow of the rootes of Sow-bread.
Burned Squill applied.
Decoction of Crow-foot bathed.
Clote burre applied with wine.
Allome dissolved in water.

Against blisters and inflammations of the feet, caused by the shooes.

LIghts of Lambs, of Beares, or of Hoggs applied.
Soles of old Shooes burned, and applied.
Juyce of Onions incorporated in Hens grease, and applied.

To heale clefts, and chaps of the Feete.

LIniment made of the ashes of river Crabbs, and of sod hony.
Squill boyled in oyle, applied with rosin.

Against Ulcers which grow on the ends of the Fingers, and divide the skin from the Nayles.

IUyce of Pomegranats applied.
Mirtill leaves bruised, and applied.
Leaves of wild Olive tree bruised, and layed to.

Powder of Ivorie applied.
Aloes applied with sod wine.
Nayle-wort[343] chopped small, applyed.
Brionie boyled in oyle till it be soft, applied.
Flowers of Labruske, burned and applyed with hony.
Rust of Iron layed to.
Acacia applyed.
Leaves of Sumack applyed with hony, or vinegar.
Leaves of Hore-hound layed to with hony.
Cinke-foyle roots applied.
Milke of male Spurge applyed.
Vinegar applied.
Allome dissolved in water.
Salt applied.

Against Apostumes which grow in the roots of the Nayles.

FRankincense applyed with hony.
Shavings of Ivorie layed to.
Leaves of Nayle-wort applied.

To cause rough Nayles fall off.

TArre applied.
Lin-seed with the like weight of Garden-cresses, and hony.
Cyprus apples applied.
Liniment made of the roots of Herb Patience boyled in vinegar.
Roots and leaves of Crowfoot applied.
Liniment of the lesser Celandine.[344]
Misseltoe applied with powder of Orpine.
Allome sprinkled with water.
Liniment made of Brimstone and Turpentine.
Red Arsenick applied with pitch.
Lees of wine burned, and incorporated in rosin, applied.

To take away loose Nayles.

DRy Grapes[345] applied.

---

[343]Paronychia, white low-grasse.
[344]Scrophularia minor.
[345]Or Raisins.

For bruised Nayles.

SCallions applyed with dry Polenta.

To take away Cornes.

WHeaten leaven applied.

For Veines puffed and swelled with bloud.

ROots of Thistle[346] gentle applied on the diseased place.

Against paines of the sides.

ROots of Vipers Bugloss[347] drunk.
    Colts-foot applyed.

Against Kernells and Inflamations of the Groine.

HAre-foot Tre-foile applied.
    Starre-wort[348] fresh gathered, applyed.

Against burstings, and falling downe of the Guts.

CYprus apples applied.
    A poultis of Pomegranate Flowers.
    A poultis of wall-wort.
    Cinquefoile drunk.
    Leaves and rootes of Horse-taile drunk.
    A Cataplasme of Aloes.

Against Windy ruptures.

LIniment of the ashes of Vine branches.

---

[346]Cirsium.
[347]Echium.
[348]Aster Atticus.

SIMPLES SERVING GENERALLY AGAINST MANY MALADIES, AND FIRST OF THOSE WHICH SERVE AGAINST FEAVERS.

Against Tertian Feavers.

A Spider bruised in a cloth spread upon linnen, and applied on the fore-head, or Temples.

Earth-wormes boyled in Goose-grease, applied.

Three entire Plantaine roots drunk in three cyaths of wine, with as much water.

Three leaves, and as many berries of stinking Trefoile, bruised, and drunk.

St. Johns-wort drunk in wine.

The third knot or joynt (from the ground) of the stalke of female Verveine drunk, with the leaves which are upon it.

Three graines of Turne-sole drunk before the fit.

Juyce of Purslaine supped.

Against Quartane Feavers.

SEven Punies put in beanes made hollow, drunk.

Foure entire Plantaine roots drunk in foure Cyaths of wine, and as much water.

The worms which are found in Fullers Thistle, fastned to the arme, or worne about the neck in a little leather purse.

Wild Rue drunk in wine.

St. Johns-wort taken in wine.

Foure sprigs of Cinkefoile drunk.

The fourth knot or joynt of female Verveine (counting from the roote) drunk, with the leaves found thereon.

Foure graines of Turne-sole taken an houre before the fit.

Against long inveterate Feavers.

BRoth of old Cocks.

Agarick drunk.

Honied wine drunk, when the stomack is very weake.

Against Feavers Epiales.[349]

THree or foure leaves of Henbane drunk.

---

[349]A kind of Quotidian, in which is felt both heat and cold.

Against intermitting Feavers, returning at certaine times.

MUstard-seed sprinkled on meat.
>   Seed of Candie Alexanders drunk.
>   Pepper drunk.
>   Rue drunk.
>   Gum Sagapene drunk.
>   Cammomill given in a Glister.
>   Juyce of knot-grasse drunk an hour before the fit.
>   Cinkefoile drunke in water, or in wine, with a little pepper.

Against languishing Feavers.

PUrslaine applied on the mouth of the stomack, and on the sides.

Against shaking of Feavers.

PEpper drunk.
>   Agarick the weight of a dram drunk.
>   Round Aristolochia drunke before the fit.
>   Liniment made of Southernwood and oyle.
>   Decoction of Calaminte drunk.
>   Hercules All-heale applied.
>   Seed and roots of Candie Alexanders, drunk in sod wine.
>   Liniment of wall pellitory.
>   Benzoin taken in wine with frankincense and pepper.
>   Liniment of fleabane and oyle.
>   Seed of bastard St. Johns-wort drunk with pepper.
>   Seed and root of Buglosse drunk.
>   Liniment made of Wood-binde-seed, and oyle.

Against pestilentiall Feavers.

Sweet Chervill[350] drunk every day, twice or thrice a day.

SIMPLES SERVING AGAINST APOSTUMES, SWELLINGS AND TUMOURS.

Against inflammations and rednesse of any diseased part.

FResh Rose leaves, bruised, and applyed.
>   Liniment of bruised Acornes.

---

[350]Myrrhis.

Seed of Sumacke applyed with water.

A poultis of meale of Lupines, dry polenta and water.

Juyce of Wall-penniwort, anointed about the Tumour.

A poultis of Plantaine.

Asphodill roots layed to with dry polenta.

Vinegar applyed with unwashed Wooll, or Spunges.

Rhapontick applyed with vinegar, when the place hath been long
  inflamed.

Penniroyall applyed with polenta.

Leaves of Colts-foot, bruised, and applyed with hony.

A poultis of Feverfew.

Second kind of Spleen-wort applyed.

A poultis of the roots of wilde Hempe.

Knot grasse applyed.

A poultis of Caltraps.

Roots of stinking Gladon applyed with vinegar.

Yarrow[351] applyed.

A poultis of Wall-Pellitory.

Liverwort applyed.

Liniment made of female Verveine leaves, when the place hath been long
  inflamed.

Leaves and heads of Poppy applyed, or the heads onely with dry polenta.

Leaves and seed of Henbane applyed.

Fresh leaves of Mandragore applyed with Polenta.

Briony root boyled in wine, layed to.

Liniment of the leaves of Wall-wort, or of Elder, and Polenta.

Liniment of *Indian* leafe, to break apostumes.

Wheaten Bran boyled in good vinegar, applyed.

Wheate flower steeped in oyle and water, or in honyed water used as a
  Liniment.

A Poultis of Wheaten-bread, boyled in honyed water, with herbs proper
for the same effect.

Sesamum applyed.

Against Carbuncles.

LEaves of Privet applyed.

   Liniment of Tar, Hony, and dry Grapes, to breake the Carbuncles and
      remove the skars.

   Cyprus leaves bruised and applyed.

---

[351]*Achillea.*

Liniment of Savin leaves and wine, to breake the Carbuncles.

Dry ripe Olives applied to take away the skars.

Kernells of old Wall-nuts applyed.

Pidgeons dung incorporated in hony and Lin-seed.

A poultis of meale of bitter Vetch.

A poultis of meal of Lupines and vinegar.

Coleworts applyed with salt to break them.

Garden Cresses applyed.

Leeks applyed with salt.

Liniment of Hercules All-heal.

A poultis of Coriander, dry grapes[352] and hony.

Liniment of Asa foetida.

Milke of Male spurge applyed.

Dry Grapes cleansed from their kernels[353] applyed with Rue.

Against fellons, and small Apostumes.

WHeaten Leaven applyed.

Wall-pellitory applyed.

A poultis made of salt, dry grapes, and Hogs Lard, or hony.

Asphodill roots boyled in wine lees, applyed.

Leaves of Meddow Saffron[354] boiled in wine, applyed.

Liniment made of Nettle leaves.

Roots of Lyons Cudweed[355] worne about the neck.

Wild Cowcumber roots applyed with Turpentine.

Liniment made of the juyce of Scammony, hony and oyle.

Gum of Mulberry tree rootes, applyed.

Liniment of the juyce of stinking deadly Carrot, and hony.

Leaves of Devills bit[356] applyed.

Red Arsenick applyed with grease.

Liniment made of Asian stone, incorporated in Tar, or Turpentine.

Liniment of Cimolian earth, incorporated in vinegar.

To prevent Gangrenaes, and releive diseased parts, tending to St. Anthonies fire.

LEaves of Sumack applyed with hony and vinegar.

Juyce of Pomegranats applyed.

---

[352]Or Raisins.

[353]Raisins stoned.

[354]*Colchicum Ephemerum.*

[355]*Leontopodium.*

[356]*Pycuocomum.*

Old Wallnuts applyed.

Lye made of the ashes of Fig tree applyed with Spunges.

A poultis of Raddishes, salt, and darnell meale.

Meale of Ciches applyed with Barly and hony.

Liniment made of Lentils, Melilot, oyle of Roses, dry Roses, Pomegranat
shel, and salt water.

Meale of bitter Vetch applyed.

Coleworts boyled, used as a Cataplasme with hony.

Scalions applyed alone, or with hony.

Asa fetida applyed, having first scarified the place.

Leaves of stincking Nettle, with the seed, Juyce, and stalkes thereof,
applyed with vinegar.

Leaves of Mullein which beareth yellow flowers, applyed.

Milke of Male spurge applyed.

Liniment made of the root, Berryes and leaves of Briony, with salt.

Dry Grapes the Kernells taken out[357] applyed with salt.

Against the Holy fire, burning sharpe Inflammations, and St. Anthonies fire.

LIniment made of Saffron, mingled with refrigerative things.

Cyprus leaves applyed alone, or with polenta.

Leaves of Ramne thorne applyed.

Leaves of Privet applyed.

Roses layd to.

Juyce of Acacia laid to.

Leaves of Wild Olive tree bruised, and laid to.

Liniment made of Mirtell leaves, oyle of green Olives, and a little oyle
of roses or wine.

Menstruall blood applyed.

Wild she goats dung, boyled in wine, or vinegar, applyed.

Settlings of the parties Urine applyed.

A poultis made of Lentils, Melilot, dry roses, oyle of Roses, and
Pomegranat shells.

Liniment made of Mallowes boyled in oyle.

A poultis of Coleworts chopped and incorporated in polenta.

A poulits of Purslaine and Polenta.

Liniment made of Plantain, Cimolian earth, and Ceruse.

Leaves and roots of Succory applyed with polenta.

Liniment made of the leaves of Garden Woad.

A poultis of Stone Basill.[358]

---

[357]Or Raisons stoned.

[358]*Acynos.*

Liniment made of the juyce of Rue, Vinegar, Ceruse, and oyle of roses.
Liniment made of Coriander, bread, and dry polenta.
Liniment made of Lilly leaves; and vinegar.
Leaves of Colts-foot, bruised and applyed with hony.
A poultis made of the herb and flowers of Feverfew.
Knot grasse applyed.
Roots of Orcanet applyed with polenta.
The root of Wild Buglosse[359] applyed with polenta.
Raspis flowers applyed.
Wal-Pellitory laid to.
A poultis of boyled Cinkefoile roots.
Liniment made of Male Verveine and vinegar.
Poppy heads cut in peeces applyed with polenta.
Liniment made of the juyce of Morell, or of the leaves, incorporated in
  polenta.
Liniment made of Mandragore roots and vinegar.
Juyce of Hemlock applyed.
Juyce of Wall-Pennywort applyed.
Liniment made of Fleabane, or of its Mucilages.
Ducks meat applied.
Liniment made of the leaves of *Palma Christi*, and vinegar.
Housleek applyed.
Yarrow applyed.
Vinegar applyed.
Rust of Iron applyed.
Chalcitis applyed.
Liniment made of Salt and Vinegar or of Hisope.

Against the Shingles.

JUyce of Acacia applyed.
  Mirtill leaves applyed with oyle of green Olives, or with a little oyle
    of roses, and wine.
  Leaves of wild Olive tree, bruised, and laid to.
  Liniment made of Wild she Goats dung, boyled in wine or vinegar.
  A poultis made of Lentills, Melilot, oyle of roses, dry roses, and
    Pomegranat shels.
  Liniment made of the juyce of Wal-Pellitory and Ceruse.
  Plantaine applyed.

[359]*Lycopsis.*

Liniment of Cellandine and wine.

Bramble leaves applyed.

Liniment made of the juyce of Morell, Ceruse, oyle of Roses, and
  Lithargy.

Against Wheales, Pushes and red Spots.

LIniment made of the dung of she Goates, or of Sheepe, and vinegar.

  Coleworts chopped small, applyed with Polenta.

  Plantaine applyed in any sort.

  Cowcumber leaves applyed with hony.

  A poultis made of the leaves of Leeks and the seed of Sumack.

  Liniment made of Wormwood and water.

  Coriander seed applyed with dry graps[360] and hony.

  Misletoe applyed on soft linnen folds.

  Seed of Turnesole applyed.

  Dry Grapes, the Kernells taken out[361] laid to with Rue.

For the Kings Evill.

ILlyrian Flower-de-luce boyled and applyed.

  Liniment made of Tar, and Barly meale, boyled in a young childs Urine.

  Dry figs boyled and applied.

  Early figs[362] boiled and applied

  Boiled Vipers flesh eaten.

  Weesills blood applyed.

  Ashes of Asses hoofes steeped in oile, applyed.

  Dung, of Oxen at grasse applyed.

  A poultis of Barlie meale, and pitch, incorporated in a young childs
    urine.

  A Poultis made of Darnell meale, and Pidgeons dung boyled in wine.

  Liniment of Beane-flower, hony, and Fenugreek.

  Liniment made of Lentills boyled in vinegar with Melilot.

  Meale of Lupines applyed with vinegar.

  Herbe Patience boyled, applyed.

  Plantain applyed with salt, or the roots worne about the neck.

  Liniment made of Brimstone and Mustard.

  Garden Cresses applied with Brine.

  Pepper applyed with Pitch.

---

[360]Or Raisins.

[361]Raisins stoned.

[362]The first figs which being too forward do not thrive.

Coriander seed applyed with Beane flower.

Galbanum applied.

Goose grasse applied.

Leaves of Baulme applyed with salt, as a poultis.

Marsh Mallowes boiled in wine, or in honied water, applied.

Cinkefoile roots boiled, or chopped small, and applied.

Liniment made of Benzoin and waxe.

Juice of Wall Penniwort applied.

Fresh leaves of Mandragore applied with polenta.

The third kind of Housleek applyed.

Leaves, stalkes, seed, and juice of stinking Nettle used in a poultis

Four sprigs of Winter Cresses drunk with water, or applied.

Maiden-haire, applied.

Liniment made of Tiles, powdered and incorporated in a Sear-cloth.

Leaves and roots of the Caper-bush, bruised and applyed.

Against flat Apostumes, called in Greek Panos.

LIniment made of the leaves of wild Olive tree, and hony.

Dry figs, boiled and applyed.

Dung of Oxen at Pasture, applyed.

Meale of Lupines aplyed with vinegar.

Orage raw, and boyled applied.

Plantain laid to with salt.

Liniment made of Scallions boiled with polenta, and Hogs Lard.

Leaves of Garden Woad applyed.

Sea Holly worn about the neck.

Liniment made of Southernewood, or of Barly meale, incorporated in oile
   and water.

Stone Basill laid to.

Seed and flowers of Esculapius All-heal used as a poultis.

Coriander seed applied with Bean meal.

Gum Ammoniacum applied.

Red Fetchling[363] chopped small, applied.

Liniment made of the uppermost root of Corne-flag,[364] of Darnel meale
and fresh water.

Fleawort applyed with oyle of roses, or water, or Vinegar.

Leaves of Mandragore new gathered, applyed.

Liniment made of the leaves, seede, stalkes, and juyce of stinking
   Nettle.

[363]*Onobrychis.*
[364]*Gladiolus*

Roots of Clote burre applyed on the leaf with grease.

Devills bit[365] applyed.

Fleawort used in a poultis.

Wine Lees applyed.

To resolve all Apostumes and Tumours.

RIver Crabs applyed.

Lin-seed applied.

Meale of Fenugreeke used in a Poultis.

Leaves and roots of the Caper bush, bruised, and applyed.

Roote of Candy Alexanders applied.

Gum Ammoniacum applied.

Leaves and flowers of Oxe-eye,[366] incorporated in wax, applied.

Liniment made of fresh Mandragore leaves and polenta.

A poultis made of the juyce, leaves, stalkes, and seeds of stinking nettle.

Havergrasse[367] applied.

Drosse of brasse[368] applied with Turpentine, or wax.

Marcasite stone applied.

Alablaster burned, and incorporated in rosin, or in pitch.

Liniment made of Fullers earth.

Against hard, or almost unsensible swellings between the flesh and the skin, called Scirrhus.

BLoud of a Bull applied with polenta.

Liniment made of the dung of Oxen, at grasse, and vinegar.

Darnell meale boyled in wine, with Pidgeons dung.

Lin-seed boyled with niter and lye, of the ashes of Fig-tree.

Arse-smart[369] applied.

Roots of wild Hemp applied.

For Cankers.

LIniment made of the ashes of river Crabbs boyled in hony.

Seed of bank Cresses bruised, and applyed.

All sorts of Nettles applied.

Leaves, juyce, seed, and stalkes of stinking nettle applied.

---

[365]*Pycnocomon.*
[366]Buphthalmum.
[367]Aigilops.
[368]Dyphriges.
[369]Hydropiper.

To dissolve all swellings.

HOggs Lard applied.
    Cole-worts chopped small, and applied with polenta.
    Gourds applied.
    Seed of small Clote burre.[370]
    Liniment made of Scalions boyled with polenta and Hoggs grease.
    Lin-seed used in a poultis.
    Liniment of fenugreek seed
    Onions boyled, and applied with figgs, and dry grapes.
    Daffodill roots applied.
    Briony rootes boyled in wine applied.
    Leaves of Garden-woad applied.
    Roote of Candie Alexanders applied.
    Goates Organie applied with polenta.
    Minte applied in a poultis with polenta.
    Liniment made of the leaves of great Marjerome incorporated in Wax.
    Yellow Carrot applied.
    Rosemary roots used as a poultis.
    Gith applied with vinegar.
    Common Clary[371] applied with water.
    Flowers of Oxe-eye, incorporated in wax.
    Boyled marsh Mallowes applied.
    Roote of wild Hempe used in a poultis.
    Liniment made of the leaves of beane Trefoile.
    Knot-grasse used in a poultis.
    Liniment made of the roots of stinking Gladon and vinegar.
    Wall pellitory applied.
    Cinkfoile roots boyled, and used as a poultis.
    Leaves of female Verveine applied.
    Liniment made of oyle of roses, vinegar, and water.
    Leaves of meddow Saffron boyled in wine, applied.
    Leaves of Milk Trefoile[372] applied with bread.
    Roote of wild Cowcumber applied with polenta.
    Branches of Spurge Time bruised. and applied
    Seed of Devils-bit applied with polenta.
    Indian leafe applied.
    Wine lees, crude, applied alone, or with mirtle.

[370]Lappa min.
[371]Horminum.
[372]Cytisus.

Against Apostumes[373] which yeeld an oiley fat matter.

MArigold-flowers[374] bruised, incorporated in wax, and applied.

Against Apostumes[375] which yeeld matter like Hony.

LIniment made of herbe Patience, oyle of roses, and saffron.
    Melilot applied with water.
    Raisins stoned, and applied with Rue.

Against swellings caused by Blowes.

COleworts chopped small, applied with Polenta.
    Liniment made of Gourds applied.
    Arse-smart applied.
    Liniment made of Time, or of Summer Savoury.

Against bruises, and prints of strokes.

NEw Cheese applied.
    Unwashed Wooll steeped in oyle, and vinegar.
    Beane-flower applied with hony, and fenugreek.
    Meale of Lupines applied.
    Raddish applied with hony.
    Ashes of Garlick layed to with hony.
    Mustard applied.
    Arse-smart applied.
    Sneesingwort, and the flowers applyed.
    Scalions applied alone, or with the yolke of an egge.
    Rhapontick applied with vinegar.
    Aloes applied with hony.
    Asa fetida applied.
    Worm-wood applied with hony.
    Hot sea water fomented.
    Hisope with hot water.
    Calaminte with wine.
    Leaves of great Marjerome dryed, applied with hony.
    Wild Cummin chewed, and layed to with hony and raisins.

---

[373]Steatomata.
[374]Chrysanthemum.
[375]Melicerides.

Ammeos with hony.

Vinegar and hony.

Juyce and roots of stinking deadly Carrot incorporated in the like weight of frankinsence and wax, applied as a poultis; it must remaine only two houres on the part offended, which must be often fomented with Sea-water.

Briony roote boyled in oyle till it be soft, applied.

Liniment of salt and hony.

SIMPLES SERVING FOR WOUNDS.

To heale Wounds.

CYprus leaves bruised.

Elme leaves, especially the rinde or skin of the Barke, used instead of a swath.

Gum of Sycamore applied.

Liniment made of the lees of oyle, boyled in a copper vessell.

Greene Dates applied.

Leaves and seed of *Agnus Castus* applied.

Pomegranate flowers applied.

Frankinsence sprinkled on the Wounds.

Ashes of burned wooll applied.

Leaves of wild Cole-worts applied.

Bastard wild poppy[376] applied.

Juyce of Licorice layed to.

Fresh rootes of great Centaury applied.

Leaves of small Centaurie bruised, and applied.

Yarrow applied.

Rootes of Burnet bruised, applied.

Roots of Candie Alexanders applied.

Aloes in powder sprinkled.

Sarcocalla[377] applied.

Policnemon applied with water.

Poley used as a poultis.

Water Germander applied.

Horse-tayle leaves layed to.

Leaves of Spleen-wort applied.

Marsh Mallowes boyled in wine, or in water and hony, applied.

Leaves of Iron-wort[378] aplied.

---

[376]Argemone.

[377]A bitter Gum brought from *Persia.*

[378]Sideritis.

Ground Pine layed to with hony.
Second kinde of Iron-wort applied.
Knot-grasse used in a poultis.
Solomons Seale used as a poultis.
Wall-wort applied.
A poultis made of Comfrey.
Juyce of Clymenum applied.
All sorts of Iron-worts applied.
Roots of wild [379] Buglosse applied in a poultis.
Seed of Basill applied.
Roots of Couch-grasse bruised, and applied.
Flea-wort applied.
Cinkfoile applied.
Scarlet graine powdered, and sprinkled on the wounds.
Verveine applied.
Leaves and flowers of Groundsell, applied with crums of frankinsence.
Leaves of Mullein applied with vinegar.
Fresh Sponges applied with water, and vinegar, without any grease.
Unwashed wooll steeped in vinegar, and in oyle.
Leaves of Dragons boyled in wine.
Leaves of Garden-woad applyed.
Yarrow applied.
Powder of the stone Morochthus, sprinkled.

To stench bleeding of a Wound.

IUyce of wild Olive-tree leaves applied.
    Galls burned, and quenched in vinegar, or in brine, sprinkled.
    Pomegranate flowers applied.
      Dry leaves of Persea[380] applied.
    Cyprus leaves and nuts bruised, and applied.
    Frankinsence sprinkled.
    Ashes of burned Froggs applyed.
    Cobwebs applyed.
    Dung of wild she Goates applied with vinegar.
    Asses dung crude, or burned, and applyed with vinegar.
    Leaves of Scabions applied.
    Purslaine applied.

[379]Lycopsis.
[380]Called Persian Plum-tree.

Plantaine applied.
Roots of Idea applied.
Leaves of Garden-woad applied.
Sage applied.
Flowers of Ladies Bed-straw,[381] put in the wound.
Leaves of Tutsan St. Johns-wort layed to.
Cinkfoile applied.
Wild Darnell fastned to the body with red wooll.
Liverwort applied.
Roots of milke vetch put in the wound.
Henbane seed the weight of an obol drunk in honied water.
Yarrow applied.
Cinnaber, and Dragons bloud put in the wound.
Allome applied.
Brimstone applied.
Plaster applied.
Fresh Spunges applied alone, without any other thing.
Ashes of burned spunges applied with Pitch.
Eretrian earth sprinkled.
Powder of Antimonie sprinkled.

To stench bloud descending from the Braine.

CHickens braines drunk in wine.
    Antimonie powdered, and sprinkled.

To resolve clotted Bloud.

TIme put in the wound.
    Summer Savoury applied.

To heale wounds caused by venemous shot.

IUyce of Dittanie drunk, and dropped into the wound.

To re-incarnate Bones destitute of Flesh.

Illyrian Flower-de-luce applied.
Roots of Hercules All-heale applied.
Liniment made of Myrrhe, and Snayles without their shels.

---

[381]Gallium.

To heale Wounds in the pellicles of the Braine.

BUtter applyed.

Against the inflammations of Wounds.

NEw dung of Oxen at grasse, enveloped in leaves, heated upon embers, and
often applyed and changed.
      Liniment made of the leaves of Pine, and of pitch tree, bruised.
      Beane flower used in a poultis.
      Meale of Lupines applied.
      Yarrow applied.
      Flowers of Labruske put in Cataplasmes.
      Verdigrease applied.

To draw out Splinters, or other things which stick in wounds.

SNailes with their shels, bruised and applied.
      Flesh of a salted Silurus applied.
      A Lizards head cleft, and applied.
      Scalions used in Cataplasmes.
      Clarie applied with water.
      Pimpernell applied.
      Daffodill roots applied with meale of Darnell.
      Round Aristolochia applied.
      Dittany applied.
      The first root of Corn-flag applyed with wine and frankincense.
      Roots of stinking Gladdon applyed.
      Leaves, seed, and juyce of small Saxifrage[382] applyed.
      Seed of Devils bit[383] layed to with polenta.
      Root of Hawthorne applyed.
      Roots of Reed-cane applyed.
      Mustard-seed layed to.

To take away all superfluous flesh.

GAlles bruised and sprinkled.
      Date stones burned, washed, and applied.
      Ashes of a sea Hedge-hoggs skin, applied.

---

[382]Tragium.
[383]Pycnocomum.

Ashes of burned Purple shel-fish, applied.

Liniment made of the Ashes of *Unguis odoratus*, applied.

Head of a Cackerell fish burned, applied.

Ashes of burned wooll applied.

Powder of water Germander.

Burned brasse or Verdigrease applied.

Washed Lead, Antimonie, Lithargy, Ceruse, Borax, Oker, drosse of Brasse, Arsenick, Pumice stone, Corall, flower of the Asian stone, dryed powdered, and put upon the excressence in any sort whatsoever.

Marcasite stone applyed with Rosin.

To Cicatrise a Wound.

CAdmia washed, and applyed.

Washed lead applyed.

SIMPLES SERVING AGAINST VLCERS.

Against corrosive Ulcers.

BArk of Pine, or of pitch-tree bruised, and applied in a liniment with beaten Vitrioll.

Decoction of Mastick tree fomented.

Cyprus leaves bruised, and applyed.

Leaves of both kinds of Savine bruised, and applyed.

Leaves of all sorts of Ramne-thorne applyed.

Flowers of Holly-rose[384] applyed.

Leaves of wild Olive-tree, bruised and applyed.

Rotten wood layed to.

Ripe Olives burned, and layed to.

Date skins in powder applyed.

Mirtle leaves bruised, and applyed with oyle of green Olives, or with a little oyle of roses, and wine.

Bitter Almonds applied with wine.

Head of a Cackerell fish burned, bruised, and layed to.

Pickle of fish applyed.

Gall of a Tortoise layed to.

Liniment made of Darnell meale, Radishes, and salt.

Lin-seed boyled in wine.

Meale of bitter vetch applyed.

Radishes bruised, and applied.

[384]Cistus.

Leaves of Beets applied.

Plantaine applied in any sort.

Roots of great Dragons bruised, and applied with hony, and brionie.

Leaves and roots of Asphodill applyed with wine.

Pimpernell bruised, and applied.

Ivie leaves boyled in wine applyed.

Roots of Celandine applied with wine.

Leaves of Garden woad applied.

Round Aristolochia applied.

Root of black Chamelian thistle used in a poultis.

Green Penni-royall applyed.

Herbe Mastick[385] applied.

Seed and flowers of Esculapius All-heale applied.

Leaves of All-heale bruised, and applied with hony.

Liniment made of Coriander, bread, and Polenta.

Leaves of Hore-hound applied with hony.

Milk of male spurge applied.

Verjuyce applyed with vinegar.

Juyce of Hemlock applied.

Housleek applied.

Meddow Parsnep applied with Rue.

Knotgrasse applied.

Verveine applied with vinegar.

Leaves of Morell applyed with Polenta.

Vinegar fomented.

Sharp brine fomented.

Butter burre[386] sprinkled.

Scailes of brasse sprinkled.

Verdigrease applied.

Burned salt applied with Polenta.

Chalcitis applied.

Drosse of Brasse applied.

Powder of Asian stone applied with vinegar.

Liniment made of Allome, with the like quantity of galls, and lees of vinegar.

Against old inveterate Ulcers.

FLowers of Holly Rose applied.

Smal Centaury applied.

[385]Marum.
[386]Petasitis.

A Tent made of the root of Esculapius All-heal.

Liniment made of Misletoe and Frankinsence.

Germander applyed with hony.

Juice of the leaves of Lillies; boiled in a brasse pot, applyed with hony, and vinegar.

Water Germander bruised, and applied with hony.

Root of Milk vetch[387] applied.

Root of Silver weed[388] applied.

Leaves of Clot bur applied.

Vernish laid to with vinegar.

Fresh Spunges laid to without any other thing.

Flower of Asian stone applied.

Against maligne Ulcers.

PLantain applyed in any sort.

Rootes of Dragons, chopped small, applyed with hony and Briony.

Butter Bur applyed.

Fleawort bruised and applyed with hony.

Leaves, berries, and roots of Briony applyed with salt.

Roots of Brakes bruised and applyed.

Powder of Cadmia sprinkled.

Flos salis applyed.

Flower of Asian stone applyed with hony.

Powder of the stone Ostracites, applyed with hony.

Against hollow Fistulaes and Ulcers.

DEcoction of Illyrian Flower-de-luce surringed.

Hogs grease surringed.

Hony dropped into them.

Juyce of Plantaine dropped into the Ulcers.

Juyce of the roots of great dragons, applyed with hony.

Round Aristolochia, applyed with hony, and roots of Flower-de-luce.

Parings of meddow Parseneps, applyed and fastned about Fistulaes, consumes their hardnesses, and callocities.

Cinkefoile applyed with salt and hony.

Yarrow surringed.

---

[387]Astragalus.
[388]Talichium.

Milk of male Spurge, dropped into the Ulcers.
Vinegar and verjuyce surringed.
Chalcitis surringed.
Cadmia applyed, being first made liquid.
Fresh Spunges soaked in hony applied.
Gentian applyed in any sort.

Against the hardnesse and Callocities of Ulcers.

DRyed rootes of Caper bush, applyed.
Verdigrease applyed with Gum ammoniacum, as a Collyrie.
Dry Spunges tyed with thread, and used as a Tent.

Against Ulcers caused by corrosive things.

LIniment made of all sorts of milk, especially of Cowes milk.

Against the Scurfe, and to kill Lice.

STaphis acre, bruised and applied with oyle.

Against filthy salt Ulcers.

LEaves of wild olive tree, bruised and applied with hony.
Illyrian flower-de-luce applied with hony.
Pickled Olives bruised and applyed.
Turpentine applied.
Tar applyed with hony.
Skin of a Sea Urchin, burned and applyed.
Ashes of purple shell fish burned, applied.
Ashes of *Unguis odoratus*, sprinkled on the Ulcers.
Meale of red vetch applyed.
Liniment made of Coleworts, Fenugreek, and vinegar.
Roots and leaves of Asphodills applied.
Barke of the Caper bush, dryed and applied.
Root of Passe-flower applyed.
Ivy leaves boyled in wine.
Celandine applied with grease.
Round Aristolochia applyed.
Dry roots of Rosemary, applied with honie.
Stinking Horehound applyed with honie.
Leaves of white Hore-hound applied with hony.

Leaves of female Verveine applyed.

Daffodill roots applyed with hony, and meal of bitter vetch.

Roots and berries of Briony applied with salt.

Verdigrease boiled in hony, applyed.

Burned brasse sprinkled on the Ulcers.

All sorts of Nettles, bruised and applied.

Root of Sowfennel bruised.

Cadmia applied.

Hony applied.

True Tuty applied.

Brine applied.

Allome used in any sort.

Flower of Asian stone, dried and applyed.

Against Burnings.

BErries of Sycamore, incorporated in grease, applied.

Decoction of the leaves of Privet fomented.

Flowers of Holly rose applyed with waxe.

Gum of Acacia dissolved in an egge, preventeth bladdering.

Mirtle leaves, crude, or burned, incorporated in wax.

Mulberry leaves, bruised and applyed with vinegar.

Frankincense incorporated in the grease of a Hog, or of a Goose.

Ashes of Cutle fish applied.

Ashes of burned Musles applied.

Ashes of *Unguis odoratus* applied.

Ashed of burned old shoes applyed.

Hogs grease applyed.

Sheeps dung incorporated in wax, and oile of roses.

Dung of Pidgeons, or of Hens, incorporated in oile with Lin-seed.

Sesamum with oile of roses.

Mallowes boiled in oile.

Green leaves of Beets applied.

Ashes of Coleworts incorporated in the white of an egge.

Milke of wild Lettice applied with womans milk.

Flowers of Ivy incorporated in wax, and the leaves boiled in wine.

Roots of Brank Ursine applied.

Seed and leaves of wild Rue applied.

Birdlime dissolved in hot water, and applyed, preventeth bladdering.

Flower of Tiph-wheat incorporated in old Hogs Lard wel washed.

Roots of Lyriconfancy,[389] applied.

---

[389]Hemerocallis.

Leaves of marsh Mallowes applyed with a little oyle.

Leaves and seed of St. *Johns* wort applied.

Leaves and seed of St. *Peters* wort,[390] applyed.

Leaves of Tutsan St. *Johns* wort, applyed.

Roots of Orkanet, boiled in oile, and incorporated in wax.

Wall Pellitory aplyed.

Leaves of horned Poppy, applyed with oile.

Leaves of wild Mullein applyed in a poultis.

Powder of Antimony incorporated in fresh grease, applied; preventeth bladdering.

Allome applyed with water.

Salt with oyle, or Fullers earth alone, preventeth bladdering.

Phrigian stone incorporated in wax, applyed.

Inke applyed with water.

Cinnaber and Dragons bloud applyed.

Flowers of Ladies Bed-straw,[391] applyed.

Burned roots of Lillies incorporated in oyle of roses, or the leaves, applyed.

Leaves of Hounds-tongue incorporated in old Hoggs-grease.

Young Elder leaves applied.

Daffodill roots applied with a little hony.

Oyle boyled in the hollowed roote of an Ashphodil, applyed.

Against Ulcers dropping matter like Hony.

ROots of Pompions applyed with hony.

Garden cresses applyed.

Against Scabs, or red Sores growing in the Fundament.

SCalions rosted in embers applied with the ashes of a Cackarell-fish, head burned.

Against gallings which happen by chafing betweene the Thighes, or else-where.

POwder of old Shooes burned, applied.

Against inflammations of Ulcers.

CObwebs applyed.

---

[390]Ascyron.
[391]*Gallium.*

To incarnate hollow Ulcers.

FRankincense put in them.
>Tarre applyed with hony.
>Pitch applyed.
>Marrow of the bones of all foure-footed beasts applied.
>Hony dropped into them.
>Cadmia sprinkled.
>Corrall put in them.
>Flower of the Asian stone applyed with hony.
>Eretrian earth applied.
>Pumice-stone sprinkled.

To cicatrise Ulcers.

AShes of burned Purple-fish.
>Ashes of Muskles, and of *Unguis odoratus* applyed.
>Aloes applyed.
>Leaves of Agrimonie chopped smal, and incorporated in Hoggs-grease, applyed.
>Powder of the rootes of Brakes sprinkled on them.
>Cadmia applyed.
>Burned brasse applied.
>Scailes of Brasse sprinkled.
>Verdigrease incorporated in oyle and wax.
>Antimonie, Lead Ore, Lithargie, Ceruse, Chalcitis, Pumice stone, wine-lees burned, lime washed, corrall, flower of the Asian stone, or Tiles well baked, applied in any sort whatsoever.

SIMPLES SERVING FOR RUPTURES, AND DISLOCATIONS.

For members out of joynt.

ROots of Rose-bushes applied with vinegar.
>Rootes of Clote burre, bruised and applyed, to ease the paines of the wrinch.
>Decoction of Acacia fomented.
>Leaves and seed of *Agnus Castus* used as a poultis.
>She Goates dung incorporated in wax, and oyle of roses applyed.
>Sparagus roots applyed with wine, or vinegar.
>Decoction of Sow-bread fomented.
>Decoction of Scalions fomented.
>Roots of brank Ursine applied.
>Leaves of sweet Marjerome incorporated in wax, applyed.

A poultis made of the leaves of Orkanet, hony, and meale.

All sorts of nettles applyed.

Daffodill roots bruised, and incorporated with hony layed to.

Leaves of black Brionie applied with wine.

Polipodie applied.

Liniment made of Turnsole leaves.

Liniment made of the ashes of Vine branches, and Grapeskins burned, incorporated in vinegar.

Salt, meale, and hony applied.

For broken Bones.

DEcoction of Mirtill leaves used in fomentation.

Unwashed wooll dipped in oyle, wine, and rose vinegar applied.

Decoction of Mullein drunk.

Painters soote incorporated in wax, applied.

Liniment made of the decoction of Elme leaves, or of the decoction of the barke of the roots.

To draw out broken Bones.

ROund Aristolochia used in a poultis.

Powder of the root of Sow-fennell, put in the wound.

Euphorbium put in the wound.

Roots of stinking Gladon, applied with Verdigrease.

Brionie bruised, and applied.

Root of black Brionie.

For persons which have had a great fall.

IUuyce of Gentian roots, the weight of a dram drunk.

Decoction of the roote of Plowmans Spikenard drunk.

Yarrow drunk with water and salt.

A Lexive made of the ashes of Vine branches, with vinegar, salt, and hony.

For persons which are bursten.

DEcoction of Common sweet Cane drunk.

Graines of Paradise drunk in water.

Decoction of true sweet Cane drunk, with seed of Couch-grasse, or of Parsley.

Electuary made of Elicampane root and hony.

Bdellium drunk.

Juniper berries drunk.

Cedar berries eaten.

Root of Sea Purslaine,[392] the weight of a dram taken in honied water.

Root of great Dragons rosted in embers, or boyled, taken with hony.

Asphodill roots the weight of a dram taken in wine.

Scalions boyled in vinegar eaten.

Pills of Agarick, the weight of three obols taken with honied wine.

Juyce of Gentian roots, the weight of a dram drunk.

Round Aristolochia drunk.

Wild Time drunk.

Roote of great Centaury taken in wine.

Roots of brank Ursine drunk.

Roots of Candie Alexanders eaten, or drunk.

Decoction of our Lady-thistle roots boyled in wine, drunk.

Seed of Southernwood taken in water.

Organie eaten with figgs.

Leaves and roots of Horse-tayle drunk.

Decoction of Calaminte drunk.

Decoction of the rootes of Plowmans Spikenard drunk.

Rosemary roots drunk.

Gum sagapene drunk.

Benzoin taken with some lye.

Galbanum taken in pills.

Polycnemon drunk in wine.

Water Germander eaten with Garden cresses, hony, and rosin.

Decoction of marsh Mallows drunk.

Roots of marsh Mallowes drunk in wine, or in water.

Bettony leaves the weight of a dram drunk in cleare water.

Wall-wort drunk in honied vinegar.

Comfry roots drunk.

Roote of stinking Gladdon drunk in honied wine.

Tops of golden Moth-weed[393] drunk in wine.

Decoction of Mullein drunk.

Electuary made of Briony roots and hony.

Powder of the stone Schistos drunk.

[392]Halymus.
[393]Helychrisum.

SIMPLES SERVING AGAINST VENOME AND POYSONS, AND ALSO AGAINST THE BITING AND STINGING OF VENEMOUS BEASTS.

Against the stinging and biting of venemous Beasts.

ROots of Illyrian Flower-de-luce taken in vinegar.

Graines of Paradise taken in wine.

Celtick Spikenard, taken with decoction of Wormwood.

Valerian put in preservatives prescribed against venemous bitings.

Cinnamomum drunk.

Cinamon drunk.

Decoction of Elicampane rootes drunk.

Bdellium drunk.

Sycomore berries drunk.

Leaves and flowers of Heath drunk.

Seed of *Agnus Castus* drunk.

Acornes eaten.

Wall-nuts eaten.

Rosin of Sycomore applied.

Milk of Fig-tree-put in the wound.

Liniment made of Tarre, and of salt.

Decoction of the leaves and rootes of Christs-thorne drunk.

Chickens braines taken in wine.

Caterpillars applyed with oyle.

Curd of Hares, of Lambs, of Calves, of Hindes, of Bores, of Harts, of Buffles, of Kids, or of fallow Deere, the weight of three obols taken in wine.

Bloud of a sea Tortoise drunk with Cummin, and the curd of a Hare.

Hony drunk with oyle of roses made hot.

Wheat meale applied with wine, and vinegar.

Juyce of Leeks taken with hony, or a liniment made of the leaves.

Wild Leekes eaten.

Pepper taken in any sort.

Sea holly taken in wine.

Great Germander[394] applyed with vinegar.

Bastard wild Poppy taken in wine.

Agarick the weight of three obols taken in wine.

Rhapontick drunk.

Germander drunk.

Gentian roote the weight of a dram taken in wine with Rue, and Pepper.

Long Aristolochia, the weight of a dram drunk, or applied on the wound.

---

[394]Teu[c]rium.

Decoction of Organie drunk.

Poley mountaine[395] drunk in wine, or used in a poultis.

Penni-royall taken in wine.

Juyce of Dittany taken in wine.

Roots of Plow-mans Spikenard taken in wine.

Seed of Hercules All-heale taken with Aristolochia.

Seeds and roots of Lovage drunk.

Seed of All-heale drunk.

Annise drunk.

Roots of Swallow-wort drunke in wine.

Cummin taken in wine.

Ammeos drunk in wine.

Delphinium[396] applied on the wound.

Benzoin drunk and applyed.

Galbanum applyed is very good.

Wild Basill drunk.

Leaves of stinking Trefoile taken with Oximel.

Decoction of Poley drunk.

Bettony leaves the weight of three drams taken in nine ounces of wine, or applyed on the wound.

Juyce of Knot-grasse drunk.

Liniment made of Periwinckle.

Root of Burre reed[397] taken in wine.

Strong brine dropped into the wound.

Lemnian earth drunk.

Liniment made of Organie, salt, hony, and hisope.

Against the bitings of Vipers.

COstus the weight of halfe an ounce drunk.

Cinamon drunk.

Tarre applyed.

Leaves of Juniper, and juyce of the said leaves drunk.

Leaves of Ash, or the juyce of the leaves drunk.

Bay leaves applyed.

Southernwood applyed.

Galbanum applyed instead of the linnen folds usually laid next above the plaister.

Green Organie put in the wound.

[395]Leuc[a]s.
[396]Thought to be wild Larkes spur.
[397]Sparganium.

Chickens cleft alive, and applyed on the wound.

A poultis made of bruised Cammomill, barley meale, and honied vinegar, before you lay it to, foment the Wound often with hot honied vinegar.

Bramble leaves applyed with wine.

Juyce of Leekes drunk in a hemine of pure wine.

Juyce of Baulme drunk in wine.

Curd of a Hare drunk.

The salted flesh of a Tunie[398] eaten, but you must drink presently after, or you may apply it on the wound.

Powder of Harts-horne taken in wine.

The Patients owne urine drunk.

Wheat bran boyled in the decoction of Rue, applyed.

Liniment made of the meale of bitter vetch, steeped in wine.

Raddish applyed.

Juyce of Cole-worts drunke with niter, and the root of Flower-de-luce.

Gum Succory eaten.

Garlick taken in wine, or applied.

Squil boyled in vinegar applied.

Juyce of Pimpernell taken in wine.

Pith of Fennell Gyant taken in wine.

Juyce of Clote burre taken in wine.

Juyce of the roots of Madir drunk, with the leaves.

Juyce of Land Caltraps the weight of a dram taken, or applyed on the wound.

Leaves and roots of the first kinde of Orkanet eaten, drunk, or worne about the neck.

Seed of wild Basill drunk in wine.

Roots of Elder, or of Wall-wort, boyled in wine, drunk.

Brionie roote the weight of two drams drunk.

Ashes of Vine branches applied with vinegar.

Against the bitings of Serpents, and Aspes.

RIver Crabbs bruised, and drunke with Asses milk.

The stones of River Horses[399] drunk.

Castorium drunk.

Powder of Weesils salted, and dryed in the shadow, the weight of two drams taken in wine.

Froggs boyled in oyle, eaten with salt.

---

[398]Omotarichus.

[399]A beast living in *Nilus*.

Gudgeons eaten.

Seven punies taken in any sort.

A Bores liver dryed, and taken in wine.

Hens cleft alive and laid upon the wound, letting them remaine so long as they are hot, then laying to others.

Butter applied.

Wild Goates dung boyled in wine, or in vinegar, and applyed.

Hony drunk with oyle of roses.

Asphodill rootes the weight of three drams drunk, or used with the leaves and flowers in a poultis.

Garden cresses drunk.

Seed of white Thistle drunk.

Southernwood taken in wine.

A poultis made of Hisope bruised with hony, salt, and cummin.

Feild Calaminte[400] drunk, or used in a poultis.

Seed and flowers of Esculapius All-heale drunk, or applyed.

Panaces de Chiron[401] drunk, or applyed.

Juyce of Hawk-weed taken in wine.

Seed of Wild Parsnep[402] drunk.

Incision made in the Patients head unto the bone, Euphorbium put therein, and the wound re-closed.

Lions leafe[403] drunk, taketh away the paine.

Lilly leaves applyed.

Baulme drunk in wine, and applied on the wound.

Leaves of Hore-hound drunk.

Wild Time drunk, and applyed.

Rue eaten with Wall-nuts, and dry Figgs.

Dry water Germander taken in wine.

Harts-tongue taken in wine.

Roots of Candie Alexanders applyed.

Fennell taken in wine.

Gum Sagapene taken in wine.

Rosemary roots taken in wine.

Fleawort applyed.

Periwinckle taken in vinegar.

Roote of Vipers Buglosse[404] taken in wine, also whosoever drinketh the roots, leaves, or seed of Vipers Buglosse, shall be preserved from being bitten by Serpents.

---

[400]Nepeta.

[401]It beares a leaf like sweet Marjerome, a yellow flower, and hath a small roote.

[402]Elapphoboscum.

[403]Leontopetalon.

[404]Echium.

Seed of wild Basill drunk.

Seed and leaves of Agrimonie taken in wine.

Sprigs of golden Moth-weed taken in wine.

Roots and leaves of female Verveine taken in wine, or applyed.

Mandragore roots applied with hony, or oyle.

Roots of Oleander taken in wine.

Fomentation with hot vinegar, if the poyson be cold, otherwise if the poyson be hot, use cold vinegar.

Decoction of Maiden-haire drunk.

Sea water fomented.

Liniment made of salt, organie, hony, and hisope.

Ashes of Vine branches applyed with vinegar.

Samian earth drunk in water.

Serpentine marble worne about the neck.

Against the bitings of the Serpents called Emourrous.

GArlick drunk, and applyed.

Pure wine drunk abundantly.

A poultis made of Vine leaves, boyled, and incorporated in hony.

Against the bitings of horned Serpents, called Cerastes.

SEsamum applyed with oyle of roses.

Seed of Radishes drunk in wine.

Liniment made of salt, incorporated in rosin of Cedar, or in pitch, or in hony.

Against the bitings of Scolopendra.[405]

SEEd and rootes of Asphodill taken in wine.

Salt with hony, and vinegar.

Wild Rue applyed, or drunk in wine.

Strong brine fomented.

Aristolochia taken in wine.

Wild Time taken in wine.

Calaminte taken in pure wine.

Against the bitings of the Serpent called Dryinus.[406]

ARistolochia taken in wine.

Leaves of stinking Trefoile drunk.

---

[405] A venemous worme having many leggs.

[406] A most venomous stinking scailie Snake, broad headed, and of a darke tawny colour.

Asphodill roots drunk.

Acornes drunk.

Roots of Holme Oake bruised, and applyed on the wound.

Against the bitings of a water Adder.

ORganie bruised, incorporated in water, and applyed with oyle, or lye.

Liniment made of the rinde of Aristolochia chopped small, with roots of oake, barley meale, and hony.

Aristolochia the weight of two drams taken in water, and vinegar.

Juyce of Hore-hound taken in wine.

New Hony-combe taken with vinegar.

Against the bitings of the Serpent called Cenchrus.[407]

LIniment made of the seeds of Lettice, and wine.

Summer Savoury taken in wine, with wild Rue, wild Time, and Asphodill roots.

Gentian drunk.

Graines of paradise eaten.

Against the bitings of shrew Mice.

THe shrew Mice themselves cut in peeces, and applyed on the wound.

Liniment made of Garlick, Fig-tree leaves, and Cummin.

Worm-wood taken in wine.

Roots of Tormentill[408] chopped smal, and applyed with vinegar.

Galbanum applyed on soft linnen folds.

Liniment made of barley meale, and honied vinegar.

Kernels of sweet Pomegranats boyled, and applyed.

Bruised leekes applyed.

Decoction of Southernwood drunk in wine.

Wild Time taken in wine.

Rocket taken in wine.

Cyprus apples taken with vinegar.

Sow-bread taken in honied vinegar.

Pellitory of Spaine drunke in wine.

Roote of Carline Thistle drunk.

---

[407]A Serpent covered with greene scailes, and spots resembling Millet-seed.
[408]Chrisogonum.

Against the stinging of the Fork-fish, sea Scorpion, and sea Dragon.

DEcoction of Sage drunk.

    All simples good against the bitings of Vipers.

    Decoction of Wormwood, or of Brimstone boyled in vinegar.

    The Beasts themselves which stung the Party, cut in peeces, and applied on the wound.

    Great sea Barbell cleft, and applied.

    Basil applyed with polenta, and vinegar.

    Lead rubbed on the wound.

    Brimstone applyed.

Against the bitings of Weesils.

ROcket eaten, but you must drinke good wine presently after.

Against the bitings of Cockatrices.

CAstorium the weight of a dram taken in wine.

    Opium drunk.

Against the biting of Lizards.[409]

PUrslain well boiled.

Against the bitings of mad Dogs.

IUice of Box thorn[410] taken in pills, or drunk in water.

    Ashes of river Crabs drunk the weight of two drams in wine of Gentian roots, three dayes together.

    Salted Cackarell fish eaten.

    The salted flesh of a Tuny[411] applied.

    Pickle of all fish fomented.

    The Liver of a mad dog rosted and eaten taketh away all feare of water.

    Blood of a dog drunk.

    Urine of a dog drunk.

    Hony drunk with hot oyle of roses.

    Wheat chewed and applied.

---

[409] A broad headed sharp mouthed Serpent of many coulors.

[410] *Lycium.*

[411] *Omotarichus.*

Onyons incorporated in rue, salt, and hony applyed.

Garlick drunk in wine, or used in a poultis.

Hercules All-heal incorporated in pitch, used as a poultis.

Fennell roots chopped small applied with hony.

Asa fetida applied.

Stinking Hore-hound applied with salt.

Mad-wort eaten.

Crow Garlick eaten and applied.

Salt things applied.

Benzoin.

Against bitings of Dogs.

BItter Almonds incorporated in hony applied.

Muskles flesh eaten.

Gudgeons applied.

Meale of bitter Vetch steeped in wine applied.

Plantain used as a poultis.

Cowcumber leaves applied.

A poultis made of Scallions, hony, and powder of Pepper.

Minte applied.

All sorts of Nettles applyed with salt.

Leaves and roots of Hounds tongue incorporated in old Hogs grease, applyed.

Liniment made of the leavs of Elder and of Wall-wort.

Ashes of vine branches applyed with vinegar.

Againts the stinging of the Spider called Phalangium.[412]

BErries of Tamarisk, drunk.

Mirtill drunk in pure wine.

Juyce of Mulberry leaves, the weight of a Cyath, drunk.

Lexive of the ashes of figtree drunk with wine and white salt.

River Crabs, bruised, boiled, and drunk with Asses milk.

Great Sea Barbell, cleft and applyed.

Decoction of mallowes applied.

Sweet Chervil taken in wine.

Decoction of Sparagus roots drunk in wine.

Wild Lettice drunk.

---

[412]A most venemous Spider, having a perilous and deadly sting.

Seed of bastard St *Johns*wort[413] drunk in wine.

Juyce of Ivy taken in vinegar.

Southern wood drunk in wine.

Seed of Yellow Carrot taken in wine.

Gith the weight of a dram drunk in water.

Clavers drunk in wine.

Baulme drunk in wine or applyed in a poultis.

Leaves, flowers and seed of Spider-wort[414] drunk.

Tender leavesgrowing near the bottom of Sea Rushes, applyed.

Roots of Jacynth applyed.

Housleek drunk.

Sea water fomented.

Rootes of wilde Pomegranat tree powdered very small, or Aristolochia
  incorporated in Barly flower; and vinegar, applyed.

Decoction of Baulm, or of the leaves fomented.

Seeds of Southernwood, of Annise, of Ethiopian Cummin, and of wild
  Ciches, the weight of two drams of any of them taken in anHemin of
  wine.

Fruit of the Cedar bruised, applyed on the wound, or drunk.

Bark of Sycomore drunk.

Decoction of green Cyprus apples drunk with wine.

Decoction of ground Pine drunk.

Seed of Trefoile drunk.

Against the bitings of the Lizard called Stellio.

SEsamum applyed with oile of roses.

Against the bitings of Crocodiles.

SAlt applyed on the wound.

Against the bitings of all four footed beasts.

A Boares Liver fresh or dry drunk.

Against the stinging of Scorpions.

GAlingall applyed.
  Graines of Paradise taken in wine.

---

[413]*Coris,*
[414]*Phalangium.*

Amomum applyed with Basill.

Bay berries drunk in wine.

Juyce of Mirtill taken in pure wine.

Milk of domesticall fig-tree dropped into the wound.

River Crabs bruised, boyled, and drunk with Asses milk.

Scorpions bruised, and applyed, or rosted and eaten.

Wild Larks spur[415] applyed.

Great Sea Barbell opened and applyed.

Salted Cackarell fish applyed.

Lizards opened, and applyed take away the paine.

Mice opened, and applyed.

Dung of Asses, or of Horses at grasse mingled with wine, drunk.

Mans urine, drunk

Wheat meal applyed with wine and vinegar,

Seed of Rose Campion[416] drunk in wine.

Seed of sharp pointed dock, or of Sorell drunk in win[e], or in water.

Juyce of Sow-thistles eaten, or applyed in a poultis.

Succory laid to as a poultis.

Spider wort drunk.

Wild Lettice drunk.

Basill applyed with Polenta

Seed and flowers of Asphodills drunk in wine.

Southern-wood taken in wine.

Sweet Marjerome applyed with salt and vinegar.

Both kinds of Hawkweed applyed in a poultis.

Benzoin dissolved in oyle applyed.

Wild bastard thistle[417] drunk in wine with Pepper, or carryed in the hand, asswageth the pain.

Leaves of Baulme applied.

Roots of spatling Poppy woorne about the neck.

Black-berries, and their flowers.

Leaves of Mullein bearing yellow flowers applied.

Juyce of Spurge Time applied.

Scorpions grasse applyed.

Turnesole drunke in wine, and applyed.

Sea water fomented.

Naturall Brimstone[418] incorporated in Turpentine applyed.

[415]*Delphinium.*
[416]*Lychnis.*
[417]*Colus agrestis.*
[418]Sulpher viv.

Bruised Calaminte applyed, or fomented with water and vinegar.
Galbanum applyed as a bolster.
Barley meale mingled with wine.
Decoction of Rue fomented.
Bruised Trefoile put in the wound.
Cyprus applyed with wine, and Rue.
Juyce of Sow-fennell drunk.
Decoction of Penni-royall, or of Gentian drunk.
Rinde of Aristolochia the weight of two drams taken.
Salt with Lin-seed.
Saphire stone applyed.

Against the stinging of Waspes, and Bees.

BAy leaves bruised, and applyed.
Mallowes chopped small, applied with oyle.
Leaves of Water-cresses.
Decoction of marsh Mallowes drunk in water and vinegar.
Salt applyed with Calves grease.

To drive away all venomous Beasts.

PErfume of the Juniper plant.
Cedar berries incorporated in the fat of Venison, or in Deeres marrow; anoynt all the body over with this composition.
Perfume of the leaves of *Agnus Castus*, or strew them in the place whence you would drive the venomous Beasts.
River Crabbs bruised, boyled with Basill, and given to Scorpions.
Perfume of Harts-horne.
Liniment made of the suet of red Deere, and of Elephants, to anoynt the body.
Deeres marrow to annoynt the body.
Perfume of Garden Cresses.
Southernwood strewed, or perfumed.
Leaves of Organie put under the Pillowes and Matteresses where men lye.
The savour of Dittanie killeth all venemous beasts.
Perfume of Calaminte.
Perfume of Sow-fennell.
Perfume of Willow-herb chaseth away all serpents and flies.
Perfume of Gith.
Perfume of Galbanum.
Perfume of both kinds of Poley, or strew them about the place.
Perfume of Fleabane.
Perfume of Jet.

Against all sorts of Poysons.

VAlerian put in preservatives.

Cinamon drunk.

Tarre made into a Lohoch with hony, the weight of cyath taken.

Cedar berries put in preservatives.

Wall-nuts eaten fasting with Rue, and dry Figs.

Juyce of Cinkfoile roots drunk.

Curd of a Hare drunk.

Wild white Hellebore[419] drunk.

Castorium drunk.

Calamint drunk as a defensative.

Powder of Weesils salted, and dryed in the shadow taken in wine.

The cod-skin, or ventricle of a Weesill stuffed with Corianders, dryed,
  and taken in wine.

Milke of a Bitches first Litter drunke.

Sea Holly taken in wine.

Oyle of olives, or butter, drunk.

Bloud of Geese, Drakes, and Kids, put in preservatives.

The Patients urine drunk.

Turnep-seed drunk.

Rue-seed the weight of five drams drunk in wine.

Seed of Navew gentle drunk.

Decoction of Mallowes, and the roots, often drunk and vomited.

Cole-wort seed put in preservatives.

Seed of bank Cresses drunk.

Laser-wort[420] drunk.

Agarick the weight of a dram taken with wine and water.

Roots of Carline thistle drunk in wine.

White Thistle[421] worne about the neck.

Seed of Southerne-wood drunk in wine.

Decoction of Parsley drunk.

Leaves of Hore-hound drunk.

Bettony leaves the weight of a dram taken in wine.

Roots of spatling Poppie taken in wine.

Juyce of Land Caltraps drunke in wine.

Berries of Sharp pricking Ivie[422] taken as a preservative.

---

[419]*Epipactis.*
[420]Laser pitium.
[421]Bedeguar.
[422]Hedera-spinosa.

Luke warm vinegar drunk.

Lemnian earth drunk in water.

Samian earth taken in water.

Against the poyson of the Sea Hare.

ROsin of Cedar dissolved in wine, drunk.

River Crabs boyled, and eaten with their broth.

Asses milk, or sod wine, drunk continually.

Decoction of the rootes of Mallows drunk.

  Roote of Sow-bread drunke in wine.

Black Hellebore, or juyce of Scammonie, the weight of a dram taken with honied water, and kernels of Pomegranats.

Warme Goose bloud supped.

Beares eare,[423] the weight of one or two drams drunk in wine.

Against the Venomes and Poysons of Toades and greene Froggs.

BLoud of a sea Tortoise drunke, with the curd of a Hare, and Cummin.

Roote of Beares eare the weight of one or two drams taken in wine.

Wine abundantly drunke, and vomited.

Roots of Rose bushes, or of Galingall, the weight of two drams drunk.

Against Long-leggs,[424] and Caterpillars that breed upon Pine Trees.

OYle of Flower-de-luce, or of Quinces drunk.

Dry Figgs eaten, or the decoction of them boyled in wine, drunk.

Thebane Dates eaten, or bruised and drunk in honied wine, or in milk.

All sorts of Peares eaten.

Womans milk drunk abundantly.

All Simples good against Cantharides, are good against these.

For persons which have swallowed Horse-Leeches.

BRine drunk.

Benzoin drunk.

Leaves of Laser-wort taken in vinegar, or their juyce gargarized with vinegar.

Leaves of Beets taken with vinegar.

---

[423]Alisma.

[424]A venemous black fly.

Snow taken with water and vinegar.
Punies drunk in wine, or in vinegar.
Vinegar with salt drunk.
Niter and water gargarized.
Vitriol dissolved in water, gargarized.

For those which have drunk Cantharides.[425]

Decoction of Furmentie, of Rice, of small Saxifrage, of Mallowes, of Lin-seed,
of Fenugreek, or of marsh Mallowes given in a Glister.
Niter drunk in honied water.
Kernells of Pine-apples taken in wine.
Seed of Cowcumbers bruised, and taken in honied wine, or in milk.
Goose-grease drunk in sod wine.
Milk supped.
Sweet wine drunk plentifully.
Bark of the Frankincense-tree taken in sod wine.
Samian earth drunk in sod wine.
Penni-royall bruised, and drunk in water.
Oyle of roses, and of Flower-de-luce taken in decoction of Rue.
Tendrells of Vine bruised, and taken in sod wine.
Broth of all fat things.

For Persons which have drunke Salamander.

ROsin of Pine-tree taken in an Electuary.
Galbanum taken with hony.
Pine-apple kernels bruised, and drunk in decoction of ground pine.
Nettles boyled with Lillies in oyle, drunk.
Eggs of Land and Sea Tortoises eaten.
Decoction of Froggs, and Sea Holly drunk.

To dissolve milke and bloud clottered and co-agulated in the stomach.

CUrd of a Hare drunk.
Warme vinegar drunk and vomitted.
Early Figgs having their milke in them, taken in water and vinegar.
Niter drunk.
All kinde of Curds taken with vinegar, and roote of Laserwort, or with
  Benzoin.

---

[425]Venemous green flyes, breeding in the tops of Ash, and olive-trees.

Seed of Coleworts drunk in Lye, made of the ashes of Fig-tree.

Seeds of Flea-wort drunk with pepper and vinegar.

Juyce of bramble drunk in vinegar.

Liniment made of Barly-meale, and of honied water, to annoynt the mouth of the stomach, and the belly.

Time drunk in wine.

Dry leaves of Calaminte drunk.

Against the malignity of Meddow Saffron.[426]

ORganie drunk in sod wine, or in oximel.

Cowes milke drunk, or Asses milke taken in great quantity,

Decoction of Acornes, or of Oake-leaves drunk.

Pomegranate shell drunk.

Wild Time boyled in milk drunk.

Juyce of Bucks-horne[427] drunk.

Juyce of the Tendrels of Vine drunk.

Juyce of bramble drunk.

Pith of Fennell gyant taken in wine.

Myrtill-berries drunk in water.

The inward skin of Chesnuts powdered, and drunk with juyce of Bucks-horne.

Organie drunk with Lye.

All Simples good against Tad-stooles, are proper against this.

Against sleepy Night-shade.

HOnied water much drunk.

Milke of Goates, or of Asses drunke.

Sweet wine drunk warme with Annise.

Bitter Almonds eaten.

All beasts having shels, eaten raw, or rosted.

Sea Crevices, Lobsters,[428] and river Crevices eaten, and their broth supped.

Against Henbane.

BArke of Mulberry-tree drunk.

Honied Water drunke abundantly.

Any kinde of milke drunke, especially Asses milke.

[426]Colchicum the Apothecaries Hermodactylus.
[427]Coronopus.
[428]Those which have undivided cleyes, and prickles on their backs.

Decoction of dry Figgs drunk.

Pine-apple kernels eaten.

Seeds of Cowcumber drunke in sod wine.

Brackish wine drunk with sod wine, and fresh Hogs-grease.

Nettle-seeds drunk in water.

Niter drunk in water.

Succorie eaten.

Mustard taken in any sort.

Garden-cresses, Radishes, Garlick, or Onions taken in wine.

Against Aconitum.[429]

CUrds of Hares, of Kids, or of Calves drunk in wine.

Decoction of Ground pine drunk.

Drosse of Iron taken in honied vinegar.

Decoction of Organie, of Rue, of Hore-hound, and of worme-wood, taken with wormwood wine.

Housleek, southernwood, Ground-pine, and widdow-waile,[430] taken in wormwood wine.

Baulme the weight of a dram, milke or hony, castorium, pepper, and rue, of each a like quantity; the whole to be taken in wine.

Wine wherein gold or silver, or iron, red hot hath been quenched drunk.

Broth of Hens mingled with lye, and wine, drunk.

Decoction of fat things taken with wine.

Against Yew.

HOt vinegar drunk, and vomited.

All Simples serving against Hemlock are proper against this.

An addition to the Simples serving against poysons.

BLoud of Hee Goates, She Goates, of Hares, of Harts, or of Doggs, fryed and eaten.

Galbanum drunk with myrrhe.

Cinkfoile roots drunk.

Roots of oake, of beech, or of holme oake powdered and taken in milke.

Quinces eaten, or drunk with penni-royall and water.

Amomum, or fruite of the Balsam-tree[431] taken in wine.

---

[429]Of which there is two sorts, Libbards bane, and Wolfes bane.

[430]*Chamelea.*

[431]*Carpobalsamum.*

Against the juyce of black Poppy,[432] and of horned Poppy.

HOny drunke with hot oyle of roses.

    Organie drunk with sod wine, or with oximel.

    Root of Beares-eare, the weight of two drams taken in wine.

    Vinegar drunk and vomited.

    Salt taken in Oximel.

    Pure wine drunk with wormwood, and cinamon.

    Niter drunk in water.

    Organie drunk with Lye, or sod wine.

    Seed of wilde Rue taken in wine, with pepper, and All-heale.

    Pepper with Castorium drunke in wine, and honied vinegar, or decoction
of Summer savoury, or of organie.

    Decoction of fat things supped in wine, or in sod wine.

    Marrow of bones drunk with oyle.

Against Hemlock.

VVOrmwood drunk in wine.

    Organy drunk in sod wine, or in oximel.

    Vinegar drunk and vomited.

    Pure wine a great quantity drunk at times.

    Milk of Cows, or of Asses drunk.

    Castorium taken in wine with rue, and minte.

    Amomum, graines of Paradise, or storax drunk respectively the weight of
    an ounce.

    Pepper taken in wine with seeds of nettles.

    Bay leaves drunk.

    Benzoin taken in oyle, or in sod wine.

    Sod wine drunk abundantly.

Against the Gum of Carline Thistle.

WOrmwood drunk in wine.

    Organie taken in wine.

    Vinegar drunk and vomited,

    Seeds of wilde rue drunk.

    Roots of Laserwort drunk.

    Decoction of Goates organie drunk.

    Turpentine swallowed.

---

[432]*Opium.*

Spikenard drunk.

Castorium and Laserwort the weight of an obol taken.

Wall-nuts, rue, rosin, and castorium, of each a dram; bruise all
  together, and drink them in wine.

Juyce of widdow-waile, of stinking deadly Carrot, or of worm-wood, the
  weight of a quarter of an ounce of any of them, taken in honied water.

Against Coriander.

PVre wine drunke, alone, or with wormwood.

Oyle swallowed.

Eggs dressed with oyle, eaten, or drunk in brine.

Decoction of Hens, and of Geese, drunk with good store of salt.

Sod wine drunk with Lye.

Against Flea-bane.[433]

ALL Simples prescribed against coriander, are proper for this.

Against Apium risus.[434]

Honied water drunk much.

Milk drunk in great quantity.

Fomentation with hot water.

Against Mandragore.

HOnied water drunk largely.

Niter taken in sweet wine, or in sod wine with wormwood.

Vinegar and oyle of roses, sprinkled on the head.

Agrimony, pepper, mustard, castorium, or rue; any of them bruised with
  vinegar, and applyed to the nose to smell to.

The odour of Lamps extinguished.

Against Tad-stooles.

HEns dung drunk in vinegar.

Hony drunk in hot oyle of roses.

Radishes eaten, or drunk.

Wormwood taken with vinegar.

[433]*Psyllium.*
[434]Some think it to be a kind of Crow-foot.

Leaves of baulme drunk with niter.
Lexive made of the ashes of vine branches drunk.
Decoction of Summer savory drunk.
Decoction of Organy drunk.
Hot Vinegar drunk and vomited.
Vitrioll drunk with water.
Salt drunk with Oximel.
Leaves of wild pear-tree, drunk and eaten.
Hens eggs eaten in water and vinegar with a dram of Aristolochia.
Seed and roots of All-heal drunk in wine.
Wine Lees burned, and drunk in water.
Mustard drunk.
Garden Cresses eaten.

Against Plaster.

ORgany drunk with sod wine, or Oximell.
Decoction of Mallowes drunk, also wash all the body therewith.
Oyle drunk.
Honyed water drunk.
Decoction of dry figs, drunk.
Lie made of the ashes of vine branches or of fig tree, taken with a good quantity of wine.
Organy taken in lye, or vinegar, or sod wine.
Time taken as aforesaid.
All Simples serving against Tad-stools, used for this.

Against Ceruse.

OYle of great Marjerome, or of flower-de-luce, drunk.
Juyce of Elme leaves drunk.
Kernells of Peach stones drunk in barly water.
Decoction of dry figs, or of Mallowes drunk.
Milk drunk luke warm.
Sesamum bruised and taken in wine.
Lye of the ashes of vine branches drunk.
Pidgeons eggs supped with Frankensence.

Against Lithargy.

SEEds of wild Clary drunk.
Myrrhe, Wormwood, Hysope, Parsely seed, Pepper and flowers of Privet, any of them taken with wine.
Dryed dung of Stock Doves drunk in wine with Spicknard.

Against Quick-silver.

MIlk drunk in great quantity and vomited.
>Also all Simples serving against Lithargy.

Against unslecked Lime, red Arsenicke, and Orpine.

MIlk with honied water drunk and vomited.
>Decoction of fat things supped.
>Decoction of Mallowes, and of marsh Mallowes boiled till it be very
thick, drunk.
>Seedes of small Sea Grapes[435] drunke.
>Decoction of Linseed drunk.
>Decoction of Rice supped.

SIMPLES SERVING TO EMBELLISH THE BODY.

Against the shedding of Haire.

LIniment made of Myrrhe, Labdanum, and Myrtill wine.
>Ashes of the rind of Canes applyed with vinegar.
>A Poultis made of Labdanum, wine, Myrrhe, and oyle of Myrtill.
>Juyce of Myrtil berryes applyed.
>Ashes of Wallnut-shells powdered, and applyed.
>Liniment made of the ashes of burned Filbeards incorporated in grease of
Bears.
>Ashes of a land Hedge-hog skin applyed with Tarre.
>Ashes of a burned Hares head, incorporated in Bears grease.
>Ashes of burned Frogs incorporated in Tar.
>Ashes of Rats dung applyed with vinegar.
>Bears grease applyed.
>Dung of she Goats applied with vinegar.
>Raddishes bruised and applyed with Darnell meale.
>Coleworts used in frication with salt.
>Fresh leaves of Beets applyed raw.
>Ashes of Asphodill roots applyed.
>Onions used in frication.
>Ashes of Garlicke applyed with hony.
>Mustard applyed.
>Rub the place with Garden Cresses.
>Juyce of Sow-bread applyed.

[435]*Tragos.*

Leaves and roots of Crowfoot applied: but it must be soon removed.

Alloes and wine applyed.

Ashes of Southernwood incorporated in juyce of Raddishes, or in oyle of
   Palma Christi.

Juyce of Laserwort applyed with pepper, and vinegar.

Roots of water-Lilly applyed with pitch.

Leaves of Hounds-Tongue incorporated in old Hogs grease.

Maiden-haire applyed with oyle of Lillyes, or oyle of Myrtill, or with
   wine, or Hysope.

Juyce of stinking deadly carrot applyed.

Rust of Iron applyed.

Red Arsenicke applyed with Rosin.

Third kind of *Spuma Maris*, burned and applyed.

Naxian stone applyed.

Ashes of burned Sea horses, incorporated in pitch, in grease, or in oyle
of great Marjerome.

Ashes of she Goates hoofes, applyed with vinegar

To cause shedding of the Hair.

TUrmerick applyed.

Oyle wherein a Scolopendra hath been boyled, anointed.

   Sea Hare applyed alone, or with Sea-Nettle, having first bruised it.

Ashes of a Salamander with oyle.

Gum of Ivy Tree applyed.

Roots of Oake fearn bruised, and applyed, after the person hath been
made to sweat.

Water which issueth out of green vine branches, when they are burned,
   applyed.

Arsenick applyed.

Babilonish Galingall, applyed.

To cleanse the head from Dandriffe and Scurfe.

DEcoction of the leaves and Bark of Willow, to wash the head,

Juyce of Myrtill berries applyed.

Liniment made of Oxe gall, Niter, and Fullers earth.

Stale mans urine used in Lotion.

Maiden hair put in Lye.

Fenugreek put in Lye, then wash the head therein.

Mallowes with mans urine.

Decoction of Beets applyed.

Ashes of Garlick with hony.
Burned Lilly roots with hony.
Liniment made of Scallions, and burned Niter.
Allome with bitter Vetches and pitch.

To colour haire yellow.

PRivet leaves bruised and infused in juyce of Sopewort, to reduce them to a Liniment.
Juyce of Boxthorn[436] applyed.
Wash the head in the decoction of Lote Tree.
Burned Lees of wine incorporated in oyle of Mastick, applyed on the head the space of one night.

To colour hair black.

CYprus leaves bruised and applyed with vinegar.
Decoction of Sumack aplyed.
Mulberry leaves bruised and applyed with vinegar.
Galls infused in vinegar, or in water applyed.
Decoction of the bark of Date trees often applyed.
Decoction of Myrtill leaves, put to some lye.
Juyce of Acacia applyed.
Rinde of the roots of Holme oake, boyled in water till it become soft, applyed a whole night.
Ivy berries applyed.
Decoction of Sage often used.
Bramble leaves applyed.
Sory applyed.

To kill Lice and Nits.

ROsin of Cedar applyed.
Wash the head with the decoction of Tamarisk.
Hony applyed on the head.
Decoction of Beets used.
Garlick drunk in the decoction of Organy.
Gum of Ivy tree applyed.
Staphis acre applyed.

---

[436]*Lycium.*

Red Arsenick applyed with oyle.
Allome applyed with water.

Against Sun-burne.

WHites of Egges, applyed.
    Juyce of Sow-bread, applyed.

To make the Face smooth, and to give it a luster.

LIquor growing in certaine purses upon Elmes.
    Mastick applyed.
    Meal of Lupines applyed.
    Seeds of wild Turnips applyed.
    Liniment made of juyce of Pompions dryed in the sun, with their seeds,
      and flower.
    Solomons seale applyed.
    Ben applyed with urine.
    Seed of *Palma Christi* applyed.
    Berries of wild vine applyed.
    Lithargy washed and applyed.
    First and second kind of *Spuma Maris* applyed.
    Earth of Chio applyed.
    Dung of Land Crocadiles applyed.

To cause a good colour.

CIch pease much eaten.
    Agarick the weight of a dram drunk.
    Hysope drunk and eaten.
    Earth of Chio applyed.
    Gum of Cherry-trees applyed.
    Dry figs eaten.

To take wrinckles out of the Face.

BErries of Mountain Horse-foote[437] incorporated in wax used as a Liniment.
    Liniment made of Briony roots, of bitter Vetches, of earth of Chio, and
of Fenugreek.
    Earth of Chio applyed.

---

[437]*Caealia.*

To take Moles out of the face.

THe face washed in the decoction of Savine.
    Ashes of *Unguis odoratus* applyed.
    Ben bruised and incorporated in urine.
    Ashes of River Crabs.
    Daffodill roots with nettle seeds and vinegar.
    Berrys of wild vine applyed.
    Cinamon with hony.
    Roots of Costus applyed with water, or hony.
    Briony roots applyed alone, or with bitter Vetches, earth of Chio, and
      Fenugreek.
    First and second kind of *Spuma Maris*, applyed.

To rase Pocke-holes and Scars out of the Face.

MYrrhe applyed with hony, and Cinamon.
    Leaves of Leeks, and seed of Sumack applyed.
    Juyce of Onyons applyed with salt.
    Scallyons applyed alone, or with the yolk of an egge.
    Penniroyall incorporated in wax.
    Sory applyed with water.
    First and second kind of *Spuma Maris* applyed.

To take blemishes and red pimples (caused by the Sun) out of the face.

ROOts of Illyrian flower-de-luce applyed with Hellebore.
    Cinnamon with hony.
    Roots of Costus applyed with water or hony.
    Decoction of the bruised roots of bitter Almond tree, applyed.
    Milk of fig-tree applyed.
    Snails and their shells burned to ashes, and applied with hony.
    Blood of Hares applyed.
    Ashes of burned Cuttle fishes applyed.
    Linseed applyed.
    Meale of bitter vetches applyed.
    Water-Cresses applyed.
    Burned Scallions applyed with *Spuma Maris*.
    Decoction of Ivy leaves boiled in wine.
    Roots of black Chameleon thistle applyed.
    Madwort chopped small, and applied with hony.

Melian earth[438] applied.

Juyce of Sow-bread, applyed.

To take away Freckles.

ILlyrian Flower-de-luce applied with white Hellebore.

    Liniment of Cinamon and Hony.

    Costus applied with water and hony.

    Blood of Hares applyed hot.

    Wheat flower applyed with honyed vinegar.

    Radishes applyed with Darnel meal.

    Seeds of Coleworts powdered, and sprinkled on them.

    Water Cresses bruised and applyed.

    Ashes of Garlick applyed with hony.

    Roots of great Dragons applied with hony.

    Scallions applyed with hony and vinegar.

    Gith rubbed on them.

    Galbanum with vinegar.

    Madwort chopped small and applyed with hony.

    Daffodill roots applyed with nettle seed and vinegar.

    Seeds of *Palma Christi* applyed.

    Liniment made of the berryes of wild vine.

    Briony roots applyed with bitter vetches, fenugreek and earth of Chio.

    Adarca applyed.

To rase out Moles naturally printed in the Body.

Spuma Maris applyed.

To keep the body faire.

MAstick sprinkled.

    Liquor growing in purses upon Elms, applyed.

    Butter applyed.

    Dung of Land Crocodiles applied.

    Juyce of Pompions dryed in the Sun, applyed with their seeds, and water.

    Briony roots applyed.

    Juyce of Sow-bread applyed.

---

[438]The earth of an Isle called *Melia*, it is of like vertue as Allome.

To take away Scarres.

ASses grease applyed.

Beane-flower used in a poultis.

Leaves and rootes of Crowfoot applyed.

Calaminte boyled in wine applied.

Roots of wilde Cowcumber bruised, and applyed.

Ben boyled in vinegar, and applyed with niter.

A Poultis made of briony rootes, bitter vetches, earth of chio, and fenugreeke.

Borax applyed.

First and second kinde of Spuma maris applyed.

Against the Leprosie, and St. Anthonies fire.

SNayle shels burned, and applied.

Bloud of Hares applied.

Ashes of burned Cuttle-fishes applied.

Beane flower applied.

Meale of Lupines applied.

Raw leaves of Beets applied.

Leaves and rootes of Gum succory, bruised, and incorporated in hony, niter, and water.

Rootes of great Dragons applied with hony.

Juyce of Asphodill rootes applyed, first well chafing the skin of the offended part in the Sun.

Juyce of Onions applyed in the Sunne.

Ashes of Garlick with hony.

Pepper applyed with niter.

Roots of Caper-bush bruised, and applyed with niter, wine, and brimstone.

Bastard wild Poppie dried, bruised, and applied with nitre, wine, and brimstone.

Leaves of Spanish Orpine[439] applyed with Barley meale, oyle, and water, but it must remaine but six houres.

Juyce of Gentian roots applyed.

Roote of black Chameleon-thistle applyed with brimstone.

Rue used in frication with wine, pepper, and niter.

Seeds of Rosemary with strong vinegar.

Burned Lilly-roots applyed with hony.

Rootes of water Lillies applied with water.

Roots of madir with vinegar.

---

[439]*Telephium.*

Seeds of marsh mallowes, fresh or dry, bruised, and applied in the Sun.
Roots of Orkanet with vinegar.
Daffodill roots, and nettle-seeds applied with vinegar.
Liniment made of briony, bitter vetches, earth of chio, and fenugreek.
Ben boyled in vinegar, applied with niter.
Roots of wilde Cowcumbers bruised, and applied.
Seeds of *Palma Christi* applied.
Black Hellebore applied with vinegar.
Brimstone applied in any sort whatsoever.
First and second kind of Spuma maris applied.

Against Tetters, and Ring-worms.

BArke of the Pine, and of the Pitch-trees applyed.
Decoction of the leaves of mastick tree fomented.
Liniment made of Cyprus leaves, and dry polenta.
Leaves of Rhamne-thorne applied.
Rotten wood sprinkled.
Seeds of Garden-cresses applied.
Rhapontick applied with vinegar.
Black Hellebore applied with vinegar.
Ben applied with urine.
Gum of vine-stocks applied with niter, having first well chafed the
   place.
Brimstone with Turpentine.
The place rubbed with salt, oyle, and vinegar.
First and second kinde of *Spuma maris* applied.
Adarca applied.
Tarre applied.
Frankincense sprinkled.
Gum of Aethiopian Olive-tree applied.
Plum-tree gum applyed.
Milk of Fig-tree applied with Polenta.
Liniment made of hony, boyled with allome.
Virgins wax applyed.
New wheaten bread applyed with brine.
Ciches and barly with hony.
Roots of sharp-pointed Docks boyled in vinegar, applyed; having first
   well chafed the place, and rubbed it with niter.
Garden-cresses applyed with hony.
Liniment made of the ashes of Garlick, and hony.
Liniment made of mustard and vinegar.
Roote of black Chameleon-thistle boyled in vinegar, applyed.

Rue with allome and hony.

Benzoin, or *Asa fetida* applyed with vinegar.

Birdlime dissolved in vinegar, applyed.

Roots of wilde Cowcumbers, bruised, and applyed.

Milk of male spurge applied.

Liniment made of briony roots, of bitter vetches, earth of chio, and fenugreek.

Sea-water fomented.

Against Blisters, Wheales, and Heat Pushes.

ANy kinde of raw milke, drunke with hony, water, and a little salt.

Whey drunk.

Vinegar applied.

Butter applyed.

Stale mans urine.

Meale of Lupines applyed.

Juyce of Sow-bread applyed.

Lotion with the decoction of Penniroyall.

A poultis made of rue, wax, and oyle of myrtil.

Staphis-acre applyed.

Liniment made of Ben and urine.

Rust of Iron applyed.

Allome with hony.

Cinnaber, or Dragons bloud applied.

Tiles calcined in a Furnace applyed.

Against Morphew,[440] and other blemishes of the face.

LIniment made of the juyce of stinking deadly Carrot.

Liniment made of Ben, and urine.

Daffodill rootes applyed with nettleseeds, and vinegar.

Lote-tree applyed with hony.

Powder of wilde cowcumber rootes applyed.

Seeds of Palma Christi applyed.

Liniment made of the berries of wilde vine.

Liniment made of briony, bitter vetches, earth of chio, and fenugreek.

Against the wilde Scab.[441]

LIniment made of Staphis-acre bruised, and oyle.

Seeds of briony applyed.

[440]*Alphos.*
[441]*Psora.*

Sea water fomented.
Ben boyled in vinegar.
Salt applyed.

Against the Scurfe.

LIniment made of Cardamomes and vinegar.
   Liniment made of the sap, or liquor issuing out of green olive-trees
when they are burned.
   Milk of figge-tree applyed.
   Skin of a Sea Hedge-hogge raw, or burned, applyed among other medicines,
prescribed to mundifie the scurfe.
   The head annointed with liniments made of the ashes of burned
Sea-Horses, incorporated in Tarre, or grease, or in oyntment of great
Marjerome.
   Stale urine applyed.
   Whey drunk.
   Ciches with barley and hony.
   Meale of Lupines.
   Bastard wild Poppy dryed, bruised, and used in frication with niter in a
bath.
   The lesser Celandine rubbed on the scurfe.
   Liniment made of the roots of black Chameleon-thistle, with a little
      vitriol, rosin, cedar, grease, brimstone, and allome.
   Liniment made of ben, and urine.
   Lotion with the decoction of Organy
   Liniment made of boyled Cinkfoile roots.
   Pondweed[442] applied for the Itch.
   Lote-tree applied with hony.
   Liniment made of black hellibore, wax, pitch, and oyle of cedar.
   Antimony incorporated in wax, with a little ceruse.
   Allome sprinckled, or dissolved in water, is good for the Itch.

Against the Scurfe, and scabbinesse, tending to the wild scab.

OXe Gall, with niter, and fullers earth.
   Mans urine and niter fomented.
   Barke of the Juniper plant burned, and applyed with water.
   Bark of the Ash-tree burned, and applyed with water.
   Elme leaves chopped small, and applyed with vinegar.
   Gum of Ethiopian Olive-tree applyed.

---

[442]*Potamogeiton.*

Liniment made of turpentine, or of the rosins of Larch-tree, or of Firre-tree, with verdigrease, vitriol, and niter.

Milk of Figge-tree applyed with dry polenta.

Wheat bran boyled, and incorporated in strong vinegar.

Barly meale applyed with strong vinegar, oyle, and water.

Darnell meale, brimstone, vinegar, and wine applyed.

Roots of sharp-pointed Docks applyed, having first chafed the place, and rubbed it with niter.

Coleworts chopped small, and applyed with polenta.

Black Hellebore with vinegar.

Ashes of Garlick with hony.

Mustard with vinegar.

Briony seeds applyed.

Garden-cresses with hony.

Roots of orkanet with vinegar.

Roots and leaves of Crow-foot applyed.

Gith applyed.

Roots of Cowcumber powdered, and applyed.

Ben boyled in vinegar, applyed with niter.

Juyce of stinking deadly Carrot applyed.

Liniment made of Scammony boyled in vinegar.

Gum of Vine-stocks applyed, rubbing the place first with niter.

Verdigrease and niter incorporated in turpentine.

Allome boyled with Cole-worts and hony applyed.

Brimstone incorporated in turpentine and vinegar.

Salt, oyle, and vinegar boyled together.

First and second kind of *Spuma maris* applyed.

Adarca applyed.

Melian earth applyed.

Against the Itch.

MIlk of Fig-tree applyed with polenta.

Brimstone and niter.

Frication with salt, oyle, and vinegar.

Allome applyed with water.

Against the Leprosie.

LAnd Hedge-hoggs dryed, and frequently eaten.

Rosin of Cedar applyed.

Liniment made of the ashes of snailes.

Salamander put among other medicines prescribed for the same effect.

Whey drunk.

Liniment made of the galls of Hee or Shee Goates.

Calaminte eaten with Whey.

Tamariske much eaten.

Against hardnesse of the skinne, and Warts.

LIniment made of ashes of the barke of willow, and vinegar.

    The salt head of the Cackarell-fish burned, applyed.

    A Lizards head cleft and applyed.

    Sheeps dung applyed with vinegar.

    Hony boyled with allome.

    At the new of the Moone, take as many cich pease as you have warts, and with every pease touch one wart, then binde the said pease in a linnen cloth, and cast them behinde you.

    Seeds of Turnesole applyed.

    Burned squill applyed.

    Leaves and roots of Crow-foot.

    Roots of Teasell boyled in wine, bruised and applyed.

    Gith applyed with stale urine, having first chafed the place.

    Benzoin or *Asa fetida* mingled with wax applyed, having first scarified the place.

    Wild basill drunke certaine dayes together.

    Branches of spurge time bruised, and applyed.

    Water issuing out of green vine branches, when they are burned, applyed.

    Verdigrease applyed.

Against Cornes.

WIne of Pomegranats applyed.

    Milk of figge-tree incorporated in grease, applyed all about the place where the Corne is.

    Liniment made of frankincense, vinegar, and pitch.

    Frication with rue, pepper, wine, and niter.

    Ciches with barly and hony.

    Leaves and roots of crow-foot.

    Rootes of Teasell boyled in wine, bruised and applyed.

    Liniment made of the juyce and milk of male spurge.

    Branches of spurge time bruised and applyed.

    Seeds of Turnesole applyed.

    Small Turnesole applyed.

    Water issuing out of greene vine branches burned, applyed.

    Oyntment made of Calves grease, and salt.

Against the stench of the Arme-holes.

LIniment made of myrrhe, and liquid allome.
> Powder of dry myrtill leaves cast into the Arme-pits.
> A poultis made of the roots of cardoones.
> Allome applyed.

Against clefts and chaps in the Lips.

OYntment made of Hens-grease, or of Goose-grease.
> Juyce of boxe-thorne applyed.

To provoke sweat.

SEedes of fennell giant applyed with oyle.
> Red fetchlin applied with oyle.
> Heraclian hony eaten.
> Ripe figges eaten.
> Mustard eaten.

To hinder sweating.

SCalions eaten.
> Frication with sulpher.
> Plaster, the Stone Morochthus, or samian earth applyed.

To made the skinne thin.

LIniment made of the rootes of Sow-bread.

SIMPLES SERVING TO EVACUATE HUMOURS, EITHER UPWARD, OR DOWNWARD.

To purge Choller.

ILlyrian flower-de-luce, the weight of seven drams taken in honied water.
> Seed of Triacle mustard[443] drunke.
> Aloes drunk.
> Wormwood drunk.
> Decoction of Goates organy drunk.
> Seed of wild rose campion, the weight of two drams drunk.
> Seed of Tutsan St. *Johns*-wort, the weight of two drams drunk.

---

[443]*Thlaspi.*

Black Hellebore taken alone, or with scammonie, and one dram of salt.

Roots of Devils-bit,[444] the weight of two drams taken in honied water.

Small Centaury eaten.

Dry fever-few taken with salt, or in honied vinegar.

Milke of stinking deadly Carrot[445] taken in honied water.

Seed of withiwind bruised and drunk.

Bastard-woad bruised and drunk.

Juyce of wild Cowcumber roots, and their rinde, the weight of one obol
  and a halfe drunk.

Juyce of Teasell, the weight of an obol taken.

Thirty graines of *Palma Christi* bruised, and drunk.

Juyce of all sorts of spurge, the weight of two obols taken in water and vinegar.

Juyce of mercury supped.

Sixe or seven graines of spurge, taken in pills, with figgs, or dates.

Petty spurge[446] taken in a cyath of honied water.

Juyce of scammonie the weight of a dram, or of foure obols taken in
faire water, or in honied water.

One part of the leaves of widdow-waile[447] incorporated in two parts of
wormwood, and made into pills with honied water.

The inward part of spurge flax,[448] the weight of twenty graines drunk.

Leaves of elder, and of wall-wort, eaten in pottage.

The lowest part of the root of Apios eaten.

Samphire[449] taken in honied water, or in some broth.

Powder of dry Polipodie taken in honied water.

Decoction of Dogs mercury[450] drunk.

Decoction of Turne-sole taken with water.

One or two drams of Agarick drunk in honied water.

Roots of spurge the weight of two drams taken in honied water, or a dram
  of the seeds taken, or the juyce thereof made into pills, with meale,
  the weight of a dram taken.

To purge Phlegme.

ILlyrian Flower-de-luce, the weight of seven drams taken in honied water.

  Juyce of mandragore the weight of two obols taken.

  Black Hellebore taken alone or with Scammony and a dram of salt.

---

[444]*Pycnocnmum.*
[445]*Thapsia.*
[446]*Esula rotunda.*
[447]*Chamelaea.*
[448]*Thymelea.*
[449]*Empetrum.*
[450]*Cynocramhe.*

Seed of box-thorn, the weight of a cyath taken.

Elme bark the weight of an ounce taken in wine, or in clear water.

Broth of old Capons, prepared after *Dioscorides* his manner.

Roots of Sow-bread taken in honied water.

Squil boiled in hony drunk.

Hysope boiled in water with hony and Rue, drunk.

Time drunk with salt, and vinegar.

Seeds of meddow Parsenep drunk.

Gum Armoniack, the weight of a dram drunk.

Dry or green leaves of spurge Laurell drunk.

Juyce of Hyppophastus, the weight of three obols, taken.

Dodder growing about Time, drunk with hony.

Juyce of Briony taken in honyed water.

Juyce of the seed of bastard Saffron[451] taken in Capons broth, or in honyed wine.

Powder of Load stones, the weight of three obols, taken in honyed water.

Decoction of small Centaury drunk.

Dry Feverfew taken in honied vinegar, or with salt.

Seeds of Withiwind bruised, and drunk.

Bastard woad bruised and taken.

Juyce of wild Cowcomber roots, and their bark the weight of an oboll and a halfe, taken.

Juyce of Teasell the weight of an obol taken.

Thirty graines of Palma Christi, drunk.

Juyce of all kinds of Spurge, the weight of two obols, taken in water, and vinegar.

Six or seven graines of Spurge taken in pills with figs, or dates.

Petty Spurge taken in a cyath of honied water.

Juyce of Scammony, the weight of a dram, or of four obols, taken in clear water, or honyed water.

One part of the leaves of Widdow-waile incorporated in two parts of Wormewood, and made into pills with honyed water.

Pith of Spurge flaxe, the weight of twenty grains, drunk.

Leaves af Elder, and Walwort eaten as other pot hearbs.

The lowest part of the root of Apios eaten.

Samphiere taken in broth, or in honied water.

Powder of dry Polipodi, taken in honied water.

Decoction of wild Mercury drunk.

Decoction of Turnsole, boyled in water, drunk.

One or two drams of agarick, taken in honyed water.

---

[451] *Carthamu.*

Roots of Spurge, two drams taken in honyed water, or a dram of the seeds taken, or the juyce thereof made into Pills with meale, the weight of a dram, taken.

To Purge Melancholy.

IUyce of Mandragore, the weight of two obols, taken in honied wine.
Broth of old Capons, prepared after *Dioscorides* his order.
Dodder growing about Time, taken with hony.
Whey drunk.
Dry Organy the weight of an acetabule, taken in honied water.
Penniroyall drunk.
Black Hellebore, drunk.
Broom, drunk.
White Turbith, Epithyme, Salt, and Vinegar, of each a like quantity, taken.

To cause vomiting.

TRiacle Mustard seed drunk, expelleth red choller.
Mandragore drunk expelleth Melancholy.
Milk of stinking deadly Carrot drunk in honied water.
Juyce of Spurge the weight of two obols taken in honied water.
The uppermost part of the root of Apios eaten.
Flowers and seeds of *Spanish* Broom drunk in honyed water.
Seeds of stinking bean Trefoile, chewed.
Bettony roots taken in honied water expell Flegme.
Seeds of Spatling Poppy, the weight of an Acetabule, taken in honied water.
Five grains of Staphis acre, taken in honied water.
Roots of Sylibum a dram drunk.
Ben taken in honied water.
Boyled Daffodil roots, either eaten, or drunk.
Thirty grains of *Palma Christi*, drunk.
Rind of Radish, drunk in honied water.
Juyce of all kind of Spurge drunk,
Burned brasse taken in honied water.

For the Dropsie, and to expell water being between the skin and the flesh.

ROOts of Sow-bread taken in honied water.
Decoction of Poley drunk.
Juyce of Hyppophestus, the weight of three obols, taken.
Juyce of Hyppophae the weight of an obol taken.
Thirty grains of *Palma Christi*, drunk.

Six or seven grains of any kind of Spurges, taken in pills, with figs or Dates.

Leaves of elder, and of wall-wort eaten in Pottage.

Samphire taken in broth, or in honied water.

Decoction of wilde mercury drunk.

Asarabacca drunk.

Juyce of wild Lettice taken in honied vinegar.

Roots of Trefoile, the weight of two drams taken in wine.

Juyce of spurge drunk.

Pith of spurge flax, the weight of twenty graines drunk.

Roots of wild vine boyled in water, taken in two cyaths of wine, allayed with sea water.

Scailes of brasse taken in honied water.

Decoction of mercury supped.

To loosen the Belly.

CHerries new gathered eaten.

Prunes eaten.

Carob beanes eaten.

Ripe figs eaten.

Milk of fig-tree supped.

Decoction of Cockles, or of great sea muscles.

Unguis Odoratus drunk.

Radish eaten.

White beets eaten.

Blites eaten.

Decoction of sorrell, and also the hearb eaten.

Mallowes eaten,

Orage eaten.

Coleworts lightly boyled eaten.

Decoction of husked lentills.

Sparagus eaten.

Juyce of gourds boyled entire drunk.

Ginger taken in any sort whatsoever.

Sow-fennell drunk.

One or two drams of dry squill taken fasting.

Seeds of Tutsan St. *Johns*-wort bruised, and drunk.

Juyce of wall Pellitory drunk.

Seeds of wild poppy the weight of an *Acetabule* taken in honied water.

Decoction of Hounds-tongue drunk.

Boyled sprigs of spurge time eaten.

Young tender shoots of briony, boyled and eaten.

A note of the VVeights and Measures used in this Book.		
24 Graines		Penny weight
10 Graines		Obol
2 Obols		Scruple
3 Scruples	makes a	Dram
8 Drams		Ounce
1 Ounce and a half		Cyath
2 Ounces and a half		Acetabule
10 Ounces		Hemine

The Contents

*An orphan entry in the original text.

Simples serving for the Armes and Leggs.   87

Simples serving generally against many Maladies, and first of those which serve against Feavers.   94

Simples serving to evacuate Humours, either upward, or downward. 149

A Table of the vertues of the Simples contained in this Booke.

Note the severall kinds of Herbs are expressed in the Page.

Allome, good against Rheumes of the eyes, p. 20. ordure in the eares, 23. to fasten loose teeth, 29. stays watering or rotten gums, 30. against inflammations of the jaws, 31. Rheumes of the throat, 32. Ulcers in the privie parts, 74. heales Kybes, 91. stops bleeding of Wounds, 107. good against all Ulcers, scurfe, and scabbinesse, vid, 26, 83, 92, 110, 113, 147.

Almonds, ease the Head-ach, p. 1. provoke sleepe, 3. helpe a Cough, 35, 36. obstructions of the Liver, 48. Collick, 59. gravell of the Reines, 65. Ulcers, 109. cures the venome of the sleepy Night-shade, 132. takes away red pimples, 141.

Aloes, good against the Head-ach, p.1. provokes sleep, 3. heales the Itch of the Eye-lids, 13. putrified Gums, 30. jaw inflamation, 31. spitting bloud, 33. the Jaundise, 48. Emeroids, 64. Ulcers, 62, 74, 92. shedding of haire, 138. purgeth Choller, 149.

Amber, good to stay vomiting, p. 43.

Amilum, profitable against ulcers and rhumes in the Eyes, 16, 20. sharpnesse of the throat, 32. spitting bloud, 33.

Ammeos, good against the Belly-ach, p. 55. Paine-pisse, 70. provokes womens Courses, 78. healeth the stinging of venemous beasts, 119.

Amomum, provokes sleep, p. 3. cures inflammations of the Eyes, 17. heats the Liver, 51. helpeth the Reines, 64. Gout of the leggs and feet, 87. stinging of Scorpions, 127. and cureth poysons, 133, 134.

Annise and the Seede, against the Head-ach, p. 2. filth in the eares, 23. sweetens breath, 27. increases milke, 42. helps the Dropsie, 50. gravell of the reines, 65. stayes Womans Courses, 80. helps the biting of venemous Beasts, 119.

Anthyllis, cureth the Falling-Sicknesse, p. 6.

Antimony, good against Ulcers, and Fistulaes of the eyes, p. 16, 17. and other parts, 115, 146. Burnings, 114. stayes bleeding of wounds, 107.

Sweet apples, loosen the belly, p. 59.

Arabian-thistle, helpes spitting of bloud, p. 33.

Arbute-berries, mittigates the Head-ach, p. 3.

Aristolochia, or **Birthwort**, round and long, cures the Spasme, p.9. shortnesse of breath, 34. paines of the sides, 38. Hickop, 46. Ulcers, 110. drawes out broken bons, 116. diminishes the Spleen, 52. keepes teeth cleane, 27. heales the stinging of venemous beasts, 118, 122.

Gum-Ammoniacum, cures the Falling Sicknesse, p. 6. hardnesse of the Liver, 51. provoks womens terms, 78. causes abortion, 83.

Arsenicke or **Orpine**, cures *Nole me tangere* and ulcers of the nose, p. 25. old Cough, 35, 37. Apostumes of the Fundament, 63. shedding of haire, 138. kills Lice and Nits, 140. takes off rough nailes, 92. and proud flesh, 109.

Asa-Fetida, takes away Warts on the Fundament, p. 64. cures the Sciatica, 89. Carbuncles, 97. Gangrenaes, 98. Bitings of a mad Dog, 125.

Asarabacca, cures the Dropsie, 50. expells urine, 66. provoks womens Terms, 76. cures the Sciatica, 88.

Ash-leaves cures the biting of Vipers, p. 119.

Aspe-tree, the seed cures the Falling Sicknesse, p. 5. the leaves the Gout of the hands and feet, p. 87.

Asphodills, cures the Spasme, p. 9. filth in the eares, 23. Deafnesse, 23. Tooth-ach, 28. Cough, 36. paines of the sides, 38. Inflammations of womens Dugs, 41. expells Urine, 67. increaseth Venery, 73. cures the Gout of the legs, 87. Kybes on the heels, 91. Inflammations, 96. Ruptures, 117. venemous bitings, 121, 122. and stings, 127. staies shedding of haire, 137. heales Ulcers, 110.

Asse and its parts, the hoofe cures the Falling sicknesse, p. 5. Kybes on the heeles 91. The dung stops bleeding 106. Cures the stings of Scorpions 127. The grease taketh away Scarres 143.

B

Barbell of the sea, good against the stings of venemous beasts, p. 124, 127.

Barly, good for Sinews, p. 11. Throat, 32. Sides, 38. is binding 58. Expells urine 67. Increaseth milk plentifully, 42.

Barrenwort, Drawes forth womens Dugs p. 41. Hinders conception 84.

Basill, Good against Melancholy p. 7. The Spasme, 10. Paines in the eyes, 18, 20. Paines in the eares, 22. causes Sneesing, 26. takes away inflammations of the Lungs, 38. Bindes 58. helps the Strangury, 71. provoks Terms 78. Helpes venemous stings, 119.

Baulme, Good against Vertiginosities, and the Falling sicknesse, p. 4, 5. Spasme, 9. dimnesse of Sight, 16. Tooth-ach, 28. difficulty of Breath, 39. Belly-ach, 54. Bloody-Flux, 57. the Bitings and Stingings of venemous beasts, 120, 121, 126, 127.

Bayes, Profitable against Aches, p. 11. pain of the eares, 21. Tisick and shortnesse of breath, 34. causes vomiting, 44. helps obstructions of the Liver, 48. gravell in the Reines, 65. Expells Urine, 67. provoks the Menstrues, 77. is good against Venome and Poyson, 119, 127, 128, 134.

Bdellium, Good against the Spasme, and Aches, p. 9, 11. Rheumes of the Throat, 32. paines in the Sides, 38. Stone in the Bladder, 72. Ruptures, 117. Stinging and biting of venemous beasts, 118.

Beanes, cause dreadfull dreams, p.4. good for the eyes, 17, 19, 20. Swelling behind the ears, 22. against a Cough, 36. difficulty of Breath, 39. Inflammations of womens dugs, 41. to resolve curdled milk, 42. stayes Vomitting, 43. Bloody Flux, 57. heales Inflammations of the Genitalls, 74. and of Wounds, 108.

Beare, the Gall good against the Falling sicknesse, p. 5. the Grease heales Kybes, 91. and shedding of Haire, 137.

Herbe Beares-eare, good against Belly-ach, p. 55. Loosenesse and Bloody Flux, 56. Stones in the Reines, 65. Suffocation of the Matrix, 76. poysonous things, 130, 134.

Beaver stones causeth Sneesing, p. 26.

Beets purge the Brain, p.3. help pains in the ears, 21. are loosening, 60. heal Kibes, 91. Ulcers, 110. Burnings, 113. those who have swallowed Horse-Leeches, 130. shedding of Hair 137. cleanse the head from Dandriffe, 138. kill Lice and Nits, 139. cures the Leaprosie, 143.

Ben, or **Behen**, diminishes the Spleen, p. 53. cures the Gout of the legs or feet, 88. takes away Scars, 143. Morphew, 145. Scurfe, 146, 147.

Benzoin, Helps the Falling Sicknesse, p. 5. the Spasme, 10. Dimnesse of sight 16. Pimples on the Nose, 25. Tooth-ach, 28. Squinancy, 31. sharpnesse of the throat, 32. Cough, 36. is good against paines in the sides, 38. resolves clotted milke, 47. is good in shaking Feavers, 95. and in Ruptures 117.

Bettonie, good against the Falling sicknesse, p.6. Melancholly, 7. Spasme 10. stanches bleeding at the nose, 24. helps the tooth-ach, 28. spitting blood, 32, 33. the Tisick, 34. spitting Matter, 38. Vomitting, 43. Belching, 46. helpes digestions 47. removes obstructions of the Liver, 48. cures the Dropsie, 51. diminishes the Spleen, 53. expells urine, 68. helps the suffocation of the Matrix, 76. the Sciatica, 89. Ruptures, 117. and poysons, 119, 129. causes vomitting, 152.

Binde-weed, causes horrible dreames, p. 4.

Birdlime, helpes burnes, p. 113. Tetters and Ring-worms, 145.

Birth-wort, vid. **Aristolochia**.

Bitumen, helpes rheumes of the head, p. 7. Spots in the eyes, 13. skaries out of the eyes, 14. Suffocation of the Matrix, 76. provoks terms, 77.

Blites, loosen, p. 153.

Bolearmonicke, restrains falling of hair from the eye-lids, p.12. causes vomiting 45.

Borax, takes away scars, p. 143.

Boxthorne and the **juyce**, takes away sharpnesse of the eyes, p.12. dimnesse of sight, 15. filth of the ears, 23. helps rotten gums, 30. sharpenesse of the throat, 32. Rheumes of the Stomach, 43. the Jaundise, 49. restraines excesse of womens Terms, 80. helps the biting of a mad dog, 124.

Bramble, Heales the Scurfe, p.8. retires eyes which stand too far forth of the head 17. heals Ulcers, 26. staies watering of the gums, 30. helps Inflammations of the Jawes, 31. panting and throbbing of the heart, 40. stayes vomiting, 43. Binds, 59. helps apostumes of the fundament, 62. stops bleeding of Emeroids, 64. is good against the gravell of the Reines, 65. restrains excesse of womens terms, 80. against the bites of Vipers, 120. dissolves clotted milke, 132. helpes the malignity of Meddow-Saffron, 132.

Bran, drawes forth womens dugs, p. 41. helps the Belly-ach; 55. Inflammations, 96. bitings of Vipers, 120.

Brankursine, helps the Tisick, p. 34. Binds, 58. expels urine, 68. helps burns, 113. Members out of joynt, 115. Ruptures, 117.

Brasse, the scales helps sharpnesse of the eyes, p. 13. blemishes out of the eyes, 14. Ulcers and Rheumes of the eyes, 17, 20. Ulcers in other parts, 110, 113. and cicatriseth them 115.

Brimstone, cures bruised eares, p. 23. deafnesse, 24. shortnesse of breath, 35. Cough 37. spitting of putrified matter, 39. Jaundise, 50. causes abortion, 83. cures the Gout of the legs or feet, 88. Leprosie, 144. the Itch, 147.

Bricks, cure the Gout, p. 88.

Brine, heals the Scurfe on the head, p. 8. Bloody Flux, 58. falling of the fundament, 63. pissing of blood, 73. Sciatica, 90, corrosive Ulcers. 110, 113. stinging and biting of venemous beasts 119. and persons who have swallowed Horse-leeches, 130.

Briony white and black, heales vertiginosities, and the appoplexy, p. 4, 5. the Falling sicknesse, 6. Spasme, 10. Palsie, 10. Deafnesse 23, shortnesse of breath, 35. Cough 37. paines
of the sides, 38. increases milk 42. diminishes the spleen, 53. expells urine, 69. cures the
Gout of the legs, 88. Ulcers at the fingers ends, 92. Inflammations, 96. Gangrenaes, 98.
Ulcers which are filthy and salt, 111, 113. members out of joynt, 116, drawes out broken
bones, 116. helps Ruptures, 117. the bitings of Vipers, 120. taketh wrinckles and moles out
of the face, 140, 141. keeps the body faire, 142. kills Tetters, and Ring-wormes, 145. takes
away Morphew, 145 cures scabbines, 145. and purges phlegm 151.

Brooklime, heals the Ich of the Bladder, p. 72.

Broome, cures the Squinancie, p. 31. expells urine, 69. helps the Sciatica, 90. purges
Melancholy, 152.

Bucks-horne, helps Ordure of the ears p. 23. Rheumes of the Stomach, 43. corrects the
malignity of Meddow-Saffron 132.

Buglosse, profits against swoundings of the heart, p. 40. causes abortion, 83. is good
against shaking Feavors, 95. *Anthonies* fire, 99.

Vipers-Buglosse, increases milk, p. 42. takes away pains of the sides, 93. cures the
bitings of Serpents, 121.

Bull, the urine is profitable against paines of the eares, p. 21. his gal cleanseth the eares
from filth, 23. takes away noyses in the ears, 24. cures the Squinancy, 30. and Ulcers of
the Genital members, 75.

Burnet, good for weak or cut sinews p. 11, 12. Inflammations of the eyes, 18. against
rheume of the eyes, 20.

Bur-docke, good against spitting of blood, p. 33. and putrified matter, 38.

Bur-reed, Profits against the bitings and stingings of venemous beasts, p. 119.

Butter, helps cut sinews, p. 12. Ulcers of the eyes, 16. Rheumes, 20. the Collick 54. is
loosening, 60. cures wounds in the bladder, 71. inflammations of the Matrix, 85.
wounds in the pellicles of the braine, 108. bitings of Serpents, 121. blisters, wheales,
and heat-pushes, 145.

Butter-bur, helps corrosive, maligne ulcers, p. 110, 111.

Butter-flower, vid. **Crow-foot**.

C

Cackarell-fish, takes away Warts from the genitall member, p. 75. consumes superfluous
flesh, 109. cures corrosive Vlcers, 109. bitings of mad doggs, 124. stings of Scorpions,
127.

Cadmia, cures and incarnates salt, hollow Ulcers, 111, 112, 113, 115

Calamarie-fish-shell, makes the teeth cleane, p. 27.

Sea-calfe's curd, cures the Falling-Sicknesse, p. 5.

Calamine, heales Ulcers of the eyes, p. 17.

Calaminte, profitable against the Spasme, p. 9. wormes in the eares, 24. difficulty of breath,
39. the Jaundise, 49. Belly-ach, 55. Wormes, 61. to expell Urine, 67. against Feavers, 95.

Ruptures, 117. bitings of venemous beasts, 121, 122, 128. drives away venemous beasts, 128. dissolves milke coagulated in the stomach, 132. takes away scarres, 143.

Caltraps, cure Cancers, p. 26. putrified Gums, 30. inflammations of the jawes, 31. gravell in the reines, 65. inflammation of any diseased part, 96. bitings of Vipers, 120. poyson, 129.

Cammels Hay, vid. **Squinanth**.

Cammock, cures the Tooth-ach, p. 28. viz.Rest-harrow.

Cammomill, heales Fistulaes in the eyes, p. 17. Cancers, 26. obstructions of the Liver, 48. Jaundise, 49. wind in the guts, 60. gravell in the reines, 65. expels urine 68. provokes womens Termes, 79. is good against bitings of Vipers, 120.

Rose-Campions, cures the stinging of Scorpions, p. 127.

Canary-grasse, helps pissing with pain, p. 70.

Capers and the Plant, profitable against the Spasme, p. 9. Palsie, 10. Wormes in the eares, 24. Ulcers in the mouth, 26. Tooth-ach, 28. diminishes the spleen, 52. expels urine, 67. hard lips of ulcers, 112.

Caraway and the Seed, aydes digestion, p. 47. expels urine, 68.

Carline-thistle, cures the Dropsie, p. 50 kils wormes, 61. helps the pain-pisse, 70. the biting of Shrew-mice, 123. is an Antidote against poyson, 129.

Carobs, helps the Bloudy-flux, p. 56.

Stincking deadly Carrot, profitable against shortnesse of breath, p. 35. Cough, 37. Fellons, 97. stayes shedding of Haire, 138. heales morphew, 145. scabbinesse, 147.

Yellow Carrot, good against a cold, p. 36. expels urine, 69. provokes menstrues, 78. causes abortion, 83. is helpfull against venemous bites, 126.

Castorium, cures the Lethargy, p. 3. Spasme. 9. trembling of the Sinewes, 10. aches of the same, 11. filth of the eares, 22. wind in the stomach, 46. kils wormes, 54. expels menstrues, 77. the after-birth, 81. is an Antidote against the biting of Cockatrices, 124, against Hemlock, 134.

Cedar and the Berries, helpes the Spasme, p. 9. skarres out of the eyes, 14. dimnesse of sight, 15. Noise or Wormes in the eares, p. 24. Tooth-ach, 27. cause viciate teeth to fall out, 29. good against a Cold, or Cough, 35. expels urine, 66. provoke Menstrues, 77 cure ruptures, 117. is good against all poyson and venemous beasts, 126, 128, 129, 130. kils Lice and Nits, 139.

Celandine, purges the braine, p. 3. helps dimnesse of sight, 15. the Jaundise, 48. causes rough nayles to fall off, 92. cures ulcers, 110, 112. and the scurfe, 146.

Centaury greater and lesser, profits against the Spasme, p. 9. aches of the sinewes, 11. darknesse of sight, 15. spitting of bloud, 33. shortnesse of breath, 34. Cough, 36. paines of the sides, 38. Wormes, 55. Purges the menstrues, 77. causes abortion, 82. easeth gripings of the Matrix, 87. cures old inveterate ulcers, 110. ruptures, 117. and purges Choller, 150.

Ceterach, helps yexing, p. 46. and the Jaundise, 49.

Chalcitis, cures sharpnesse of the eyes, p. 13. blear-eyednesse, p. 20. stenches bleeding at the nose, 25. cleanseth rotten gums, 30. helps inflammations of the jawes, 31. restraines the menstrues, 81. cures ulcers, 110.

Green minerall Chalk, takes away paine in the eares, p. 21.

Camelian-thistle, causes bleeding, p. 25. helps the tooth-ach, 28. causeth viciate teeth to fall out, 29. diminishes the spleen, 52. expels urine, 68. cures ulcers, 110. takes away red pimples, 141. tetters, and ring-worms, 144.

Cheese, helps inflammations of the eyes, p. 18. bindes 58.

Chelidonie, good against dimnesse of sight, p. 15.

Cherries and the tree, is profitable against darknesse of sight, p. 15. Coughs, 35. loosen, 59 helpe gravell in the reines, 65. expell urine, 67. break the stone in the bladder, 72.

Chervill, cures the Tisick, p. 34. provokes menstrues, 79. causes abortion, 83. usefull in pestilentiall Feavers, 95.

Chesnuts, stay the Bloudy-flux, p. 56. is an Antidote against Meddow-Saffron, 132.

Earth of Chio, gives the face a luster, p. 140. causeth a good colour, 140. takes wrinckles and moles out of the face, 140.

Christs-thorne, cures a Cough, p. 35. Bloudy-flux, 56. expels urine, 67. preserves against venemous beasts, 118.

Ciches, help the scurfe of the head, p. 8. Jaundise, 48. Dropsie, 50. loosen, 60. expels urine, 67. remove inflammations of the genitals, 74. cause abortion, 82. prevent Gangrenas, 98. cause a good colour, 140. cures tetters, and ring-wormes, 144. take away warts, 148.

Cimolian-earth, heales swellings behind the eares, 22. allayes inflammations of the genitals, 74. cure fellons, 97.

Cinnaber, stenches bleeding of wounds, p. 107. helps burnings. 114.

Cinnamon, good against Catharres, p. 7. dimnesse of sight, 15. Cough, 35. Dropsie, 50. expels urine, 66. provokes menstrues, 76. against falling of the Matrix, 86. poysons, and venemous beasts, 118, 119, 129. takes away Sun-spots out of the face, 141. and freckles, 142.

Cinnamomum, helps dimnesse of sight, p. 15. expels urine, 66. provokes menstrues, 76. helps the stings of venemous beasts, 118.

Cinquefoile, or **five-leaved grasse**, good against the Falling-Sicknesse, p. 6. Cancer in the mouth, 26. Tooth-ach, 28. sharpnesse of the throat, 32. maladies of the breast, 40. Jaundies, 49. bindes, 59. cures impostumes of the fundament, 62. Sciatica, 89. Gout in the hands, 90. ulcers on the fingers ends, 92. Falling of the Guts, 93. Quartan Feavers, 94. and others, 95 *Anthonies* fire, 99. bleeding of wounds, 107. Fistulaes, 111. all kind of poysons, 129, 133. Scurfe, 146.

Cyprus and the Apples, allayes inflammations of the eyes, p. 17. is profitable against *Noli me tangere*, 25. expels urine, 66. cause rough nayles to fall off, 92. Carbuncles, 96. Holy Fire, 98. stinging of venemous beasts, 128. Tetters, and Ring-wormes, 144.

Citrons, sweeten the breath, p. 27.

Clarie, takes spots and blemishes out of the eyes, p. 14. causes venery, 73. drawes splinters out of wounds, 108.

Clavers, heale venemous stinging, p. 126.

Clote-burre, good against the Tooth-ach, p. 29. paine-pisse, 70. Sciatica, 90. Kybes, 91. inveterate ulcers, 111. dislocations, 115. bitings of Vipers, 120.

Cobwebs, stanch bleeding, p. 106. allayes inflammations of Ulcers, 114.

Cocks-gizerne, good against Fluxes, p. 61. the broth against the Gout, 90. and old Feavers, 94.

Cockles, loosen, p. 153.

Cole-worts, purge the braine, p. 3. prevent drunkennesse, 7. helpe the trembling of the Sinewes, 10. weaknesse of sight, 19. cleare the voyce, 37. good against hardnesse of the Spleene, 51. both binde and loosen according as they are boyled, 58, 60. kill wormes, 61. expels urine, 67. and menstrues, 77. hinder conception, 84. are profitable against the Gout, 87, 90. Gangrenas, 98. Holy Fire, 98. filthy Ulcers, 112. burnes, 113. biting of Vipers, 120. stayes shedding of hair, 137. take away freckles, 142.

Colts-foot, good against impostumes of the Lungs, p. 34. Cough, 35. difficulty of breath, 39. expels dead Children, 84. helps Paines of the sides, 93. inflammations, 96. Holy fire, 99.

Coloquintida, purges the head, p. 3. is profitable against the Palsie, 10. Tooth-ach, 29. Collick, 54. Sciatica, 90.

Columbine, good for persons which spit bloud, p. 33.

Comfrie, good against the Spasme, p. 10. spitting of bloud, 33. inflamations of the fundament, 63. and persons which are bursten, 117.

Coriander and the Seed, kills Wormes, p. 61. augments Sperme, 73. allayes inflammations of the Genitalls, 79. is good against Carbuncles, 97. Holy fire, 99. and Ulcers, 110.

Corn-flag, causes venery, p. 73. purges the menstrues, 79. drawes splinters out of wounds, 108.

Corrall, takes scarres out of the eyes, p. 14. helps Rheumes, 20. spitting of bloud, 33. incarnates hollow ulcers, 115.

Corraline: helps the gout of the leggs, or feet, p. 88.

Costus, profits against the Spasme, p 8. paine in the sides, 38. expels urine, 66. increases Venery, 73. provokes menstrues, 76. helps the biting of Vipers, 119. take moles out of the face, 141. Sunne-spots, 141. and Freckles, 142.

Cotten-weed, good against Belly-ach, and wormes, p. 55.

Couch-grasse, kills wormes, p. 55. help pain-pisse, 70. breakes stones in the bladder, 72.

Coventrie-bells, provoke menstrues, p. 79.

Wild-Cowcumbers, profitable against the Head-ach, p. 2. paines in the eares, 22. Tooth-ach, 29. Squinancy, 31. shortnesse of breath, 35. swoundings of the heart, 40. Jaundise, 49. Sciatica, 90. Fellons, 97. Leprosie, 144. Tetters, and Ring-worms, 145. Morphew, 145. purge Choller, 150.

Garden-Cowcumbers, expell urine, p. 66. heale ulcers of the bladder, 71. oppose the malignity of Cantharides, and Henbane, 131, 133.

River-Crabs, or **Crey-fish**, good against the Tisick, p. 34. clefts and chaps of the fundament, 62. Kybes, 91. chaps of the feet, 91. against the bitings of Serpents, mad Doggs, &c. 120, 124, 125, 127, 128, 130.

Cramp-fish, good against the Head-ach, p. 1.

Cresses severall kinds, profit against Apostumes behinde the Eares, p. 22. Cough, 36. spitting putrified matter, 38, 40. inflammations of Womens Dugs, 41. vomiting, 43. Hickop, 46. Jaundise, 48. Wormes, 55. Strangury, 70. causes Venery, 73. cures the Sciatica, 88. Carbuncles, 97. Ulcers, 114. the biting and stinging of venemous Beasts, 121, 128. cures the malignity of Henbane, 133.

Crow-foot, or **Butter-flower**, causes sneesing, p 4. 26. helps the Tooth-ach, 28. causes viciate teeth to fall out, 29. heales Kybes, 91. causes rough nayles to fall off, 92. takes away skarres, 143. cures the scurfe, 147. warts, 148. and cornes, 148.

Cuckow-pinte, helps the Gout in the leggs or feet, p. 87.

Cummin, stanches bleeding at the nose, p. 24. profits against difficulty of breath, 39. Hickop, 46. wormes, 55. wind in the guts, 60. gravell in the reines, 65. Strangury, 71. pissing of bloud, 72. inflammations of the genitals, 74. restraines menstrues, 81.

Cuttle-fish, is profitable against sharpnesse of the eyes, p. 12. web in the eye, 16. makes teeth cleane, 27. loosen, 60. heale burnes, 113.

D

DAffodills, profitable against aches of the Sinewes, p. 11. cut sinewes, 12. causes vomiting, 45. expels urine, 67. help the Gout in the hands, 90. draw splinters out of Wounds, 108. cures Ulcers, 113. burnes, 114. Dislocations, 116. take moles out of the face, 141. freckles, 142. helpe the Leprosie, 144. Morphew, 145.

Darnell, bindes, p. 59. helps persons who cannot keep their water, 72. restraines excesse of menstrues, 80. cause conception, 84. stanch bleeding of a wound, 107. profit against ulcers, 109. and the scurfe, 147.

Dates, and the Tree, mittigate Headach, p. 3. prevent vomiting, 43. stay the Bloudy-flux, 56. heale Emeroids, 64. expell urine, 67. restraine menstrues, 80. take superfluous flesh out of wounds, 108. heale ulcers, 109. colour haire black, 139.

Devills-bit, causeth ugly Dreames, p. 4. heales Fellons, 97. drawes splinters out of wounds, 108. purge Choller, 150.

Dill, and the Seed, increases milke, 42. helps the Hickop, 46. wormes, 55. binde, 58. expell wind out of the guts, 60. profit against Apostumes of the fundament, 62. expell urine, 68. diminish Venery, 74. helps paines and gripings of the matrix, 87.

Dittander, helps the tooth-ach, p. 28. diminisheth the Spleen, 52.

Dittanie, causes abortion, p. 83. expels dead Children, 84. heales venemed wounds, 107. drawes splinters out of wounds, 108. drives away venemous beasts, 128.

Dodder, cures melancholly, p. 7. purges flegme, 151.

Dogs-dung, bindes, 58. the Liver is good against the biting of a mad Dog, 124.

Doves-foot, helps wind in the Matrix, p. 86.

Gum-Dragagant, or **Tragacantha,** profits against Rheumes of the head, p. 8. sharpnesse of the throat, 32. Cough, 36. paine in the reines, 64.

Dragons great and small, cure Rheumes of the head, p. 7. Spasm, 9. cut sinews, 12. spots in the eyes, 14. dimnesse of sight, 15. paines in the eares, 21. *Noli me tangere,* 25. Cankers, 25. Cough, 36. difficulty of breathing, 39. expell urine, 67. augment Venery, 73. cause abortion, 82. helpe maligne ulcers, 110, 111. Ruptures, 117. *Anthonies* fire, 143.

E

EAgle, the Gall mittigates sharpnesse of the Eye-lids, p. 13. to take blemishes out of the eyes, 14.

Ebonie, profitable against dimnesse of sight, p. 15. rheumes of the eyes, 20.

Eggs, good against paines in the eyes, p. 17. spitting of bloud, 32. Apostumes of the fundament, 62. corrects Coriander, 135. cleares Sun-burning, 140.

Eglantine, cures the Bloody-flux, p. 56.

Egrimonie, removes obstructions of the Liver, p. 48. profits against the Bloudy-flux, 57. cicatriseth ulcers, 115. cures the biting of Serpents, 122. is an Antidote against Mandragore, 135.

Elder, mollifies hardnesse, p. 86. helps the Gout of the leggs and feet, 88. Burnes, 114. bitings of Vipers, 120. and Dogs, 125.

Eleomelie, helps aches of the sinewes, p. 11.

Elicampane, good against the Spasme, p. 9. Cough, 35. expels urine, 66. provokes menstrues, 77. Ruptures, 117. biting and stinging of venemous beasts, 118.

Elme, good for broken bones, p,. 116. corrects Ceruse, 136. beautifies the face, 140. cures scabbinesse, 146.

Emerie, stayes watering of the gums, p. 30.

Endive, allayes inflammations of the eyes, p. 18.

Euphorbium, takes away the pinne or web out of the eye, p. 19. cures the Sciatica, 89. drawes out broken bones, 116. helps the biting of Serpents, or Aspes, p. 121.

F

FEarne, diminishes the Spleen, p. 53. kills wormes, 61.

Fennell, garden and wilde, is profitable against dimnesse of sight, p. 15. for nose bleeding, 24. increases milke, 42. helps inflammations of the stomach, 46. Jaundies, 49. bindes, 58. mittigates paine in the Reines, 65. expels urine, 68. voydes the stone of the bladder, 72. provokes menstrues, 78. is good for women in labour, 85. and persons bitten with venemous beasts, 120, 121.

Fenugreek, heales the scurfe on the head, p. 8. scarres in the eyes, 14. wind in the guts, 60. mollifies hardnesses and cures ulcers in the secret parts, 85, 86. cleanses the head from dandriffe, 138.

Ferula, or **Fennel-gyant**, mittigates head-ach, p. 3. stanches bleeding at the nose, 24. helpes spitting of bloud, 33. Rheumes of the stomach, 49. belly-ach, 54. biting of Vipers, 120. the malignity of meddow-saffron, 132.

Feverfew, good against shortnesse of breath, p. 35. gravell in the Reines, 65. inflammations of the matrix, 85. hardnesse of Womens naturall parts, 86. Holy fire, 99.

Figgs and the Tree, helpe Rheumes of the head, p. 8. Spasme, 9. aches of the sinewes, 11. itch of the eye-lids, 13. noyse of the eares, 24. Tooth-ach, 27. inflammation of the jawes, 31. the Tisick, 34. shortnesse of breath, 34. cough, 36. Rheumes of the stomach, 44. clotted milke, or bloud, 131. Dropsie, 51. diminish the spleen, 53. loosen, 60. prevent Gangrenaes, 98. help venome, 118. take away red pimples, 141.

Filbirds, good against Rheumes of the head, p. 7. Cough, 36.

Five-leaved grasse, vid. **Cinque-foile**.

Tode-flax, helpes inflammations of the Lungs, p. 38. Jaundise, 49. provokes menstrues, 79.

Fleawort, profits against Head-ach, p. 2. Falling-sicknesse, 6. spasme, 10. Apostumes behinde the eares, 22. ordure in the eares, 23. wormes in the eares, 24. Jaundise, 49. wormes in the belly, 55. strangury, 71. provokes menstrues, 79. causes abortion, 83. dissolves clottered milke, or bloud, 132.

Flints, stop the bloudy flux, p. 57. binde, 58. cure ulcers in the guts, 62. and in the naturall parts of women, 85.

Flos salis, takes blemishes out of the eyes, p. 14. helps dimnesse and weakness of sight, 16, 19. filth in the eares, 23. ulcers in the secret parts, 74. and else-where, 111.

Flower-de-luce of Illyria, profitable against paines in the head, p. 1. to provoke sleep, 3. help Rheumes of the head, 7. Spasme, 8. Cough, 35. excrements difficult to spit, 39. inflammations of the Spleen, 52. shedding seed, 74. provokes menstrues, 76. ulcers, 111. stinging and biting of venemous beasts, 118. takes away red pimples and freckles, 141, 142.

Fork-fish, helps the Tooth-ach, p. 27. causes viciate teeth to fall out, 29.

Foxes grease, eases paines of the eares, p. 21.

Frankincense and the tree, heales scurfe on the head, p. 8. sharpnesse of the eyes, 12. dimnesse of sight, 15. ulcers and inflammations in the eyes, 16, 17. Rheumes of the eyes, 19. filth of the eares, 22. bleeding at the nose, 24. tooth ache, 28. inflammations of duggs, 41. ulcers in the fundament, 62. restrains menstrues, 80. heales kybes, 91. Apostumes on the roots of the nayles, 92. bleeding of wounds, 106. burnes, 113. hollow ulcers, 115. is a remedy against the drinking of Cantharides, 131. cures tetters and ring-wormes, 144.

Froggs, mittigate Tooth-ach, p. 27. inflammation of the jawes, 31. stops bleeding of wounds, 106. biting of Serpents and Aspes, 120. helps persons who have drunke Salamanders, 131. stayes shedding of haire, 137.

Fullers earth, vid. **Cimolian earth**.

Fullers-thistle, good against quartaine feavers, p. 94. vid. Teasell.

G

GAlbanum, helps vertiginosities, p. 4. the spasme, 9. aches of the sinewes, 11. Tooth-ach, 28. shortnesse of breath, 35. cough, 36. paines of the sides, 38. paine-pisse, 70. provokes menstrues, 78. causes abortion, 83. expels dead children, 84. cures ruptures, 117. bitings of Vipers, 119. of Shrew-mice, 123. stinging of Scorpions, 128. drives away all venemous beasts, 128. is a remedy against poyson, 133. takes away freckles, 142.

Gallingall, heals Cancers in the mouth, p. 26. stayes watering of the gums, 29. provokes menstrues, 76.

Galls, stayes watering of the Gums, 29. helps rheumes of the stomach, 44. bloudy-flux, 56. excesse of menstrues, 80. falling of the matrix, 86. consumes superfluous flesh, 108. colour haire black, 139.

Garlick, cures the scurfe of the head, p. 8. Tooth-ach, 28. cough, 36. Dropsie, 50. wormes, 61. expell urine, 67. menstrues, 77. helps the biting of Vipers, 120. of Serpents, 122. of mad Dogs, 125. stayes shedding of haire, 137. cleanseth the head from Dandriff, 139.

Garum, stops the bloudy-flux, p. 57.

Gentian, good against the Spasme, p. 9. inflammations of the eyes, 18. paines of the sides, 38. vomitting, 43. diminishes the spleen, 52. causes abortion, 82. helps Fistulaes, 112. great bruises, 116. biting and stinging of venemous beasts, 118, 123.

Germander, good against the Spasme, p. 10. against dazeling of the eyes, 20. diminishes the spleen, 53. helps a cough, 36. excrements difficult to spit, 40. inflammations of the precordiall parts, 41. gripings of the stomach, 45. Dropsie, 50. hardnesse of the spleen, 51. diminishes the spleen, 52. cures the Bloudy-flux, 58. paine-pisse, 70. provokes menstrues, 78. causes abortion, 83. profits against old inveterate, ulcers, 111. ruptures, 117. and the biting and stinging of venemous beasts, p. 118, 121.

Ginger, takes blemishes out of the eyes, p. 14. helps digestion, 47.

Gith, profitable against head-ach, p. 2. dropping of the nose, 25. Tooth-ach, 28. shortnesse of breath, 35. increases milke, 42. helps the Jaundise, 49. kils wormes, 61. expels urine, 68. menstrues, 78. drives away venemous beasts, 128. takes away freckles. 142.

Stinking Gladdon, profits against the Spasme, p. 10. diminishes the spleen, 53. expels urine, 68. helps the Strangury, 71. Sciatica, 89. inflammations 96. drawes splinters out of wounds, 108. broken bones, 116. is usefull in ruptures, 117.

Glaux, increaseth milke, p. 42.

Goate, the gall helps purblinde persons, p. 18, 19. warts on the fundament, 64. the urine helps the Dropsie, 50. the suet, the Bloudy-flux, 57. as also the bloud, 57. and is a preservative against poyson, 129. the dung cures Apostumes behinde the eares, 22.

spitting of bloud, 33. paines in the sides, 38. provokes menstrues, 77. helps the Gout, 87. stenches bleeding of wounds, 106.

Goats-beard, restraines the menstrues, p. 80.

Goose, the grease, provokes menstrues, p. 77. eases paines and gripings of the matrix, 86. persons who have drunke Cantharides, 131.

Goose-grease, helps paines in the eares, p. 21.*{{note-small kind of bur}}

Gourds, profitable against inflammations of the braine, p. 7. of the eyes, 18. paine in the eares, 21. Gout in the leggs, 87.

Graines of Paradise, good against the Falling-sicknesse, p. 5. Spasme 8. cough, 35. wormes and belly-ach, 54. paines in the reines, 64. expell urine, 66. breake stones in the bladder, 72. profit against the Sciatica, 88. ruptures, 116. stinging and biting of venemous beasts, 118, 123, 126.

Grapes, purge the braine, p. 3. good against a Cough, 37. inflammations of duggs, 41. draw forth duggs, 41. profit against Rheumes of the stomach, 49. Bloudy-flux, 57. paines in the reines, 64. gravell in the reines, 65. ulcers in the bladder, 71. excesse of menstrues, 81.

Gromell, expels urine, p. 68. breakes the stone in the bladder, 72.

Grasse-hoppers, profit against the pain-pisse, p. 69.

Groundsell, helps aches in the sinewes, p. 11. and cut sinewes, 12. paines of the stomach, 45. inflammations of the fundament, 63. and of the Genitalls, 74.

Gudgeons, loosen, p. 60. help the bitings of mad doggs, 125.

Gum-Lac, profits against the Falling-sicknesse, p. 5. blemishes of the eyes, 13. skarres out of the eyes, 14. weaknesse of sight, 19. rotten putrified, gums, 30. shortnesse of breath, 35. expels menstrues, 77.

H

HAlcionium, makes teeth cleane, p. 27. diminishes the spleene, 53.

Hare, and the curd, profitable against the Falling-sicknesse, p. 5. Rheumes of the stomach, 44. bloudy-flux, 57. loosenesse, 59. excesse of menstrues, 80. helps conception, 84. bitings of Vipers, 120. poysons, 129. bloud of Hares takes blemishes and freckles out of the face, 141. the braines helpe trembling of the sinewes, 10.

Harts-horne, heales ulcers of the eyes, p. 16. Rheumes, 20. make Teeth cleane, 27. helps spitting of bloud, 32. the Jaundise, 48. Bloudy-flux, 57. paine-pisse, 69. excesse of menstrues, 80. biting of Vipers, 120. drives away venemous beasts, 128.

Harts-tongue, stayes the Bloudy-flux, p. 57. bindes, 58. is profitable against the biting of Serpents and Aspes, 121.

Haver-grasse, heales hollow ulcers of the eyes, p. 17.

Hawk-weed, helps gripings of the stomach, p. 45. inflammations of the same, 47. bitings and stingings of Serpents, Aspes, and Scorpions, 121, 127.

Hawthorne and the Hawes, stay the Bloudy-flux, p. 56. excesse of menstrues, 80. drawes splinters out of wounds, 108.

Heath, is profitable against the biting and stinging of venemous beasts, p. 118.

Hellebore white and black, causes sneesing, p. 4. 26. is good against the Falling-sicknesse, 6. melancholly, 7. dazeling of the eyes, 20. deafnesse of the eares, 23. provoke menstrues, 79. help the Gout, 90. poysons, 129. Leprosie, 144. Tetters, and Ring-worms, 144.

Hemlock, puts away milke, p. 42. hinder womens duggs from growing, 43. hinder Venery, 74. cure Holy fire, 99. and ulcers, 110.

Hemp, good against paines of the eares, p. 22. hinders Venery, 74. takes away knobs and nodosities of the joynts, 90.

Hen-bane, provokes sleep, p. 4 helps Rheumes of the head, 8. inflammations of the eyes, 18. paines of the eares, 22. Tooth-ach, 28. Cough, 37. winde in the guts, 60. inflammations of the genitalls, 75. excesse of menstrues, 77. paines and gripings of the matrix, 87. Gout, 88. Feavers, 94. bleeding of wounds, 107.

Herbe-mastick, helps ulcers, p. 109.

Herbe-patience, or sharp-pointed Dock, is good against Apostumes, p. 22. restraines menstrues, 80. causes rough nayles to fall off, 92. helps tetters and ring-worms, 144. scabbinesse, 147.

Hinde, the Gall, good against sharpnesse of the eyes, p. 13. the curd resolves milke, or bloud clotted in the stomach, 47.

Hippophestus, profits against the Falling-sicknesse, p. 6. aches of sinewes, 11. difficulty of breath, 39.

Hisope, helps Rheumes of the head, p. 8. Apostumes behind the eares, 22. Tooth-ach, 28. squinancie, 31. shortnesse of breath, 34. Cough, 36. 37. Dropsie, 50. expell urine, 68. causes a good colour, 140.

Hogge, the gall, good for ulcers in the eares, p. 23. the heele good for belly-ach, and wormes, 55. the grease or Lard good against Plurisies, 37. Apostumes of the fundament, 63. ulcers, 111. burnes, 113.

Hedge-hogs, help aches of the sinewes, p. 11. Dropsie, 50. loosen, 60. expell urine, 67. take away superfluous flesh, 108. stay shedding of haire, 137.

Sea-holly, is profitable against the Falling-sicknesse, p. 5. Spasme, 9. obstructions of the Liver, 48. Belly-ach, and wormes, 55. expell urine, 68. preserve against venemous wounds, 118. and poyson, 129.

Holly-rose, good against the bloudy-flux, p. 56. excesse of menstrues, 80. falling of the matrix, 86. ulcers, 109. 110. Burnes, 113.

Hony, profitable against the Falling-sicknesse, p. 6. Pin and Web in the eye, 19. paines in the eares, 21. noyse in the eares, 24. Squinancy, 30. inflammation of the jawes, 31. difficulty of breathing, 34. 39. Cough, 36. 37. inflammation of the lungs, 38. ulcers in the reins, 66. expels urine, 67. helps the Gout of the hands and joynts, 90. filthy maligne ulcers, 113. 115. the biting and stinging of venemous beasts, 118. 121. Night-shade, 132. Henbane, 132. *Apium risus*, Mandragore, and Tad-stoooles, 135.

Horse, the hoofe, profits against the Falling-sicknesse, p. 5. the curd, helps Rheumes in the stomach, 44. milk and bloud clotted in the stomach, 47. Bloudy-flux, 57.

Horse-foote, helps the Cough, p. 37. sharpnesse of the breast, 37. takes wrincles out of the face, 140.

Horse-taile, is profitable against the Cough, p. 37. difficulty of breath, 39. Bloudy-flux, 57. wounds in the guts, 61. wounds in the bladder, 71. expells urine, 69. restraines menstrues, 80. helpe falling of the Guts, 93.

Horse-tongue, mittigates the Head-ach, p. 2.

Hore-hound, good against dimnesse of sight, p. 16. paines in the eares, 21. Tisick, 34. shortnesse of breath, 35. Cough, 36. paines in the sides, 38. excrements difficult to spit, 40. Jaundise, 49. Apostumes of the fundament, 62. expells the after-birth, 82. dead children, 84. helps ulcers growing on the fingers ends, 92. and else-where, 110. 112. biting of Serpents, 121. Water-Adder, 123. and of mad dogs, 125.

Hounds-tongue, helps Burnes, p. 114. the biting of doggs, 125. the shedding of haire, 138.

Housleeke, helps the head-ach, p. 2. inflammations of the eyes, 18. Blear-eyednesse, 20. Bloudy-flux, 57. worms, 61. excesse of menstrues, 80. Gout of the leggs and feete, 88. ulcers, 110.

I

IAcynth, helps Rheumes of the stomach, p. 44. the Jaundise, 49. bindes, 59. expels urine, 69.

Idea, stayes the Bloudy-flux, p. 57. bindes, 59. restraines the menstrues, 80. heales wounds, 107.

Jet, vid. **Stone Gagates**.

Indian-leafe, expels urine, p. 66. allayes inflammations, 96.

St. *Johns*-**wort,** helps the Spasme, p. 10. expels urine, 68, provokes menstrues, 79. profits against the Sciatica, 89. tertian feavers, 94. and quartaines, 94. burnes, 114.

Iron-rust, is good against sharpnesse of the eyes, p. 13. watering of the gums, 30. impostumes of the fundament, 62. excesse of menstrues, 81. hinder conception, 84. is profitable against the Gout, 88. ulcers on the fingers ends, 92. the malignity of Aconitum, 133. shedding of haire, 138. scailes of Iron diminish the spleene, 54.

Ivie and the berries, profit against Head-ach, p. 1. paines of the eares, 21. noyse in the eares, 24. ulcers of the nose, 25. stench of the same, 25. Tooth-ach, 28. Spleen, 52. Bloudy-flux, 58. provoke menstrues, 78. cause abortion, 82. hinder conception, 84. helps ulcers, 110. 112. burnes, 113. poyson, 126. 129. causes shedding of the haire, 138.

Juniper and the berries, good against the Spasme, p. 9. Tisick, 34. Cough, 35. suffocation of the matrix, 76. Ruptures, 117. biting of Vipers, 119. drives away venemous beasts, 128. cures scabbinesse, 146.

Ivorie, helps ulcers on the fingers ends, p. 92.

K

KNeeholme, profitable against the Head-ach, p. 2. expels urine, 69. voyds the stone of the bladder, 72. provokes menstrues, 79.

Knot-grasse, helps paines in the eares, p. 22. filth in the eares, 23. spitting of bloud, 33. griping of the Stomach, 46. bindes, 58. profits against the Strangury, 71. ulcers in the secret parts, 74. excesse of menstrues, 81. feavers, 95. inflammations, 96. Holy fire, 99. corrosive ulcers, 110. biting of venemous beasts, 119.

L

LAbdanum, good against the Falling-sicknesse, p. 6. paines in the eares, 21. Cough, 35. Bloudy-flux, 56. expels urine, 67. mollifies, 86. stayes shedding of haire, 137.

Labruske, helps Cancers in the mouth, p. 26. putrified gums, 30. spitting of bloud, 33. inflammations of the Stomach, 46. bindes, 59. heales clefts in the fundament, 62. ulcers of the genitals, 75. excesse of menstrues, 81. ulcers on the fingers ends, 92. inflammations of wounds, 108.

Ladies Bed-straw, increase Venery, p. 73. stay bleeding of wounds, 107. heales burnes, 114.

Ladies-navell, good against filth of the eares, p. 23.

Larkes, help the Collick, p. 54.

Larkes-spur, helps the stinging of Scorpions, p. 127.

Laser, helps aches of the sinewes, p. 11 vid. **Asa-fetida**.

Laserwort, antidotary against poyson, p. 129. is good for persons which have swallowed Horse-leeches, 130.

French Lavender, good against shortnesse of breath, p. 34. Cough, 36.

Spurge-Laurell, causes sneezing, p. 4. helps inflammations of the Stomach, 46. belly-ach, and wormes, 55. expels urine, 69. purges menstrues, 79. and phlegme, 151.

Lead, helps Rheumes of the eyes, p. 20. clefts in the fundament, 62. ulcers in the same, 62. Apostumes in the same, 63. Emeroids, 64. consumes superfluous flesh, 109. stinging of venemous beasts, 124.

Leekes, profitable against paines in the eares, p. 21. noyse of the eares, 24. bleeding at the nose, 24. spitting bloud, 33. Tisick, 34. excrements hard to spit, 40. malladies of the breast, 40. expell urine, 67. increase Venery, 73. provoke menstrues, 77. help Carbuncles, 97. stinging and biting of venemous beasts, 118. 120. 123. take pock-holes and scarres out of the face, 141.

Lees of oyle, help the Tooth-ach, p. 27. cause viciate teeth to fall out, 29. good against the Dropsie, 50. clefts of the fundament, 62. Gout of the legs and feet, 87.

Lees of Wine, take skarres out of the eyes, p. 14. cure dimnesse of sight, 16. drives milk out of the breast, 43. binds, 59. restraine menstrues, 81. cause rough nayles to fall off, 92. colour haire black, 139.

Lemnian earth, helps the Bloudy-flux, p. 58. the biting and stinging of venemous beasts, 119. poyson, 130.

Lentils, cause horrible dreames, p. 4. resolve curdled milke, 42. helpe turnings of the Stomach, 43. binde, 58. good against the Gout, 87. Kybes, 91. Gangrena, 98. Holy fire, 98.

Lettice, provokes sleepe, p. 3. takes blemishes out of the eyes, 14. helps dimnesse of sight, 15. increases milke, 42. good against vomiting, 43. loosens, 60. causes chastity, 74. purges menstrues, 77. profits against burnes, 113. stinging and biting of venemous beasts, 123. 125. 127.

Wood-lice, good against paines in the eares, p. 21. squinancie, 30. Jaundise, 48. paine-pisse, 69.

Licium, vid. Juyce of Box-thorne.

Lillies, help the scurfe of the head, p. 8. aches of the sinewes, 11. cut sinewes, 12. inflammations of the genitals, 74. provoke menstrues, 79. mollifie, 86. good against Ulcers, 111. Burnes, 114. Dandriffe on the head, 139. Leprosie, 143.

Water-Lillies, good against head-ach, p. 2. Rheumes of the Stomach, 44. paines of the Stomach, 45. diminish the spleen, 53. stay the Bloudy-flux, 57. losing of the seed, 74. menstrues, 81. shedding of haire, 138. helps *Anthonies* fire, 143.

Lime, cicatriceth ulcers, p. 115.

Lin-seed, good against Apostumes behinde the eares, p. 22. Cough, 36. belly-ach and wormes, 56. increaseth Venery, 73. purges menstrues, 77. allayes gripings of the matrix, 86. causes rough nayles to fall off, 92. is good against ulcers, 109. takes away Sun-spots, 141.

Lions-leafe, helps the Sciatica, p. 89. biting of Serpents, and Aspes, 121.

Liquorice, takes the web out of the eye, p. 16. is profitable against Cancers in the mouth, 26. sharpnesse of the throat, 32. of the breast, 37. all malladies of the breast, 40. inflammation of the Stomach, 46. obstructions of the Liver, 48. paines of the reines, 65.

Liriconfancie, good against inflammations of womens duggs, p. 41. burnes, 113.

Lithargie, consumes superfluous flesh, p. 109. cicatriseth ulcers, 115.

Liverwort, cures the Jaundise, p. 49. inflammations, 96. bleeding of wounds, 107.

Lizard, mittigates Tooth-ach, p. 27. drawes splinters out of wounds, 108. helps the stinging of Scorpions, 127.

Lote-tree, colours haire yellow, p. 139. is good against Morphew, 145. and scurfe, 146.

Lovage, expels winde out of the Stomach, p. 46. help digestion, 47. profits against belly-ach, and wormes, 55. expels urine, 68. provokes menstrues, 78. is profitable against the biting and stinging of venemous beasts, 119.

Lupines, profitable against hardnesse of the spleen, p. 51. wormes, 61. expels urine, 67. purges menstrues, 77. is good against inflammations, 96. Carbuncles, 97. makes the face smooth, 140. helps Leprosie, 143.

M

Macer, helpes the Bloudy-flux, p. 56.

Madir, good against the Palsie, p. 10. Jaundise, 49. diminish the spleen, 53. expell urine, 68. purge menstrues, 79. expell the after-birth, 82. cause abortion, 83. help the Sciatica, 89. biting of Vipers, 120. Leprosie, 143.

Mad-wort, helps the Hickop, p. 46 biting of mad Doggs, 125. blemishes caused by the Sun, 141.

Mallowes, profit against the scurfe, p. 8. ulcers in the eyes, 17. incease milke, 42. loosen, 60. help pain-pisse, 69. mollifie, 86. good against Holy fire, 98. burnes, 113. stinging of Waspes, 128. Lime, or Arsenicke, 137. Dandriffe, 138.

Marsh-mallowes, profitable against trembling of the sinewes, p. 10. aches of the sinewes, 11. Apostumes behinde the eares, 22 Tooth-ach, 28. spitting of bloud, 33. inflammations of the Dugs, 41. Bloudy-flux, 57. binde, 59. good against inflammations of the fundament, 63. Stone and gravell in the reines, 65. paine-pisse, 69. helps women in Labour, 85. inflammations of the matrix, 85. Sciatica, 89. burnes, 114. ruptures, 117. stinging of Waspes, 128. Leprosie, 143.

Mandragore, and the Apples, provoke sleep, p. 4. good against inflammation of the eyes, 18. provoke menstrues, 79. cause abortion, 83. helps paines and gripings of the matrix, 87. Gout of the hands and joynts, 90. inflammations, 96. Holy fire, 99. biting of Serpents, and Aspes, 122. purges melancholly, 152.

Serpentine Marble, helps paines in the head, p. 3. biting of Serpents, and Aspes, 122.

Marjerome, good against the Spasme, p. 9. aches of the sinewes, 11. inflammations of the eye-lids, 13. Dropsie, 50. Paine-pisse, 69. provokes menstrues, 78. is profitable against dislocations, 115. stings of Scorpions, 127.

Marigolds, helps the Jaundise, p. 49.

Marrow, loosens, p. 60. incarnates hollow ulcers, 115. corrects the malignity of Poppie, 134.

Mastick, and the Tree, sweetens the breath, p. 26. fastens loose teeth, 29. helps the Cough, 35. Bloody-flux, 56. falling of the fundament, 63. expels urine, 66. restraines excesse of menstrues, 80. is good against ulcers, 109. makes the face smooth, 140. kils Tetters and Ring-wormes, 144.

Maudlein, expels urine, p. 68. mollifies hard places, 86.

Mayden-haire blacke and white, helps scurfe on the head, p. 8. spitting of bloud, 33. shortnesse of breath, 35. Rheumes of the Stomach, 44. Jaundise, 49. Dropsie, 50. opens the Spleen, 52. diminishes the Spleen, 53. bindes, 59. good against the Stone, and the gravell in the reines, 65. pain-pisse, 70. Stone in the bladder, 72. excites the menstrues, 79. expell the after-birth, 82. helps the biting of Serpents, and Aspes, 122.

Wheate-meale, is good against rheums falling upon the sinewes, p. 11. spitting of bloud, 33. Cough, 36. biting and stinging of beasts, 118.

Medlers, cure the Bloudy-flux, p. 56.

Melian-earth, takes away blemishes caused by the Sun, p. 142. help scabbinesse, 147.

Melilot, profitable against the head-ach, p. 2. scurfe on the head, 8. blemishes of the eyes, 14. dimnesse of sight, 15. inflammation of the eyes, 18. dazling of the eyes, 20. paines in the eares, 21. paines of the Stomach, 45. inflammations of the fundament, 63. and of the matrix, 85.

Mercurie, takes away warts on the genitall members, p. 75. purges Choller, 150. helps the Dropsie, 153.

Mice, good against the stinging of Scorpions, p. 127. their dung, voyds the Stone in the bladder, 71.

Millet-graine, good against the belly-ach, and wormes, p. 55.

Milke of Women and Kine, helps fresh wounds in the eyes, p. 16. inflammations of the jawes, 31. sharpnesse of the throat, 32. gripings of the Stomach, 45. loosens, 60. heale ulcers in the reines, 66. and in the bladder, 71. Gout of the leggs and feet, 87. Fistulaes, 112. is good against the malignity of Henbane, 132. of Apium risus, 135. of Ceruse, 136. of Quick-silver, 137. of Lime, and Arsenick, 137. blisters, wheales, and heat pushes, 145.

Milkwort, increases milke abundantly, p. 42.

Minte, garden, wild and water, mittigates the head-ach, p. 1. paines of the eares, 21. is profitable against the sharpnesse of the tongue, 27. spitting of bloud, 33. setling of milke in the breast, 43. Hickop, 46. increases Venery, 73. hinders Conception, 84. heales the biting of a mad Dogge, 125.

Mirtle-tree and fruit, prevent Drunkennesse, p. 7. help ulcers in the eyes, 17. inflammations of the eyes, 17. filth of the eares, 23. Bloudy-flux, 56. ulcere of the bladder, 71. excesse of menstrues, 80. falling of the matrix, 86. kybes, 91. Holy fire, 98. burnes, 113.

Misseltoe, good against Apostumes behinde the eares, p. 22. diminishes the spleen, 53. causes rough nayles to fall off, 92. heales old ulcers, 111.

Moone-fearne, diminishes the spleene, p. 53.

Morrell, or **garden Night-shade**, helps the head-ach, p. 2. ulcers in the eyes, 17. paines of the eares, 22. Apostumes growing behinde the eares, 22. inflammations of the Stomach, 46. excesse of menstrues, 81. Holy fire, 99. corrosive ulcers, 110.

Mosse, restraines excesse of Womens monthly purgations, 79.

Mothweed, helpes Rheumes of the head, p. 8. milke clotted in the Stomach, 47. Strangury, 71. those which pisse small clots of bloud, 72. purges menstrues, 79. is good against the Sciatica, 89. ruptures, 117. biting of Serpents and Aspes, 122.

Mouse-eare, helps ulcers in the eyes, p. 17. inflammations of the eyes, 18.

Mugwort, good against paines of the Stomach, p. 45. Stone, and gravell in the reines, 65. expels urine, 68. the after-birth, 82. causes abortion, 83. helps inflammations of the matrix, 85.

Mulberries and the Tree, mittigates the Tooth-ach, p. 27. helps rheumes of the Stomach, 44. loosen, 60. kill wormes, 61. profit against burnes, 113.

Mullein, profitable against the Spasme, p. 10. inflammations of the eyes, 18. tooth-ach, 29. sharpnesse of the throat, 32. Cough, 37. paines of the sides, 38. bindes, 59. is good against the Sciatica, 90. burnes, 114. broken bones, 116. ruptures, 117. stinging of Scorpions, 127.

Muskles, make the eye-lids thin, p. 13. helps dimnesse of sight, 15. make Teeth cleane, 27. profit against burnes, 113. cicatrise ulcers, 115. heale the biting of a mad Dogge, 125.

Mustard, profitable against the Lethargy, p. 3. provokes sneezing, 4, 26. is good against the Falling-sicknesse, 5. sharpnesse of the eyes, 13. weaknesse of sight, 19. paines in the eares, 21. noyse in the eares, 24. sharpnesse of the throat, 32. suffocation of the matrix, 76. Sciatica, 89. intermitting Feavers, 95. malignity of Henbane, 133. and of Tadstooles, 136.

Myrrhe, takes blemishes out of the eyes, p. 13. skarres out of the eyes, 14. helps ulcers in the eyes, 16. filth of the eares, 22. sweetens the breath, 26. good against sharpnesse of the throat, 32. paines of the sides, 38. Bloudy-flux, 56. provokes menstrues, 76. expels the afterbirth, 82. reincarnates bones, 107. stayes shedding of haire, 137. takes pockholes and scarres out of the face, 141.

N

SEa-navell-wort, helps the Dropsie, p. 50.

Nayle-wort, or **Whit-low-grasse,** good against ulcers growing on the fingers ends, 92.

Nettles, profit against Apostumes behinde the eares, p. 22. bleeding at the nose, 24, 25. inflammation of the jawes, 31. of the Lungs, 38. diminish the Spleen, 53. increase Venery, 73. purge menstrues, 79. helps falling of the matrix, 86. Gout of the hands and joynts, 90. Fellons, and small Apostumes, 97. prevent Gangrena's, 98. good against filthy ulcers, 113. members out of joynt, 116. biting of dogs, 125. the malignity of Henbane, 133.

Garden Night-shade, vid. **Morell.**

Binde-weed Night-shade, expels the after-birth, p. 82.

Sleepy Night-shade, causes sleepe, p. 4. helps weaknesse of sight, 19. Tooth-ach, 28. expels urine, 68.

Niter, good against ulcers on the head, p. 8. belly-ach and wormes, 55. swallowing of Horse-leeches, 131. Henbane, 133. black Poppy, 134.

O

HOlme-oake, good against the biting of Serpents, p. 123. colours haire black, 139.

Oake of Jerusalem, helps difficulty of breathing, p. 39.

Oates, sweeten the breath, p. 27. helps a Cough, 36.

Oker, helps obstructions of the Liver, p. 48. bindes, 59. is profitable against knobs and nodosities on the joynts, 90.

Oleander, good against the biting of Serpents and Aspes, p. 122.

Olives and the Tree, profits against head-ach, p. 1, 2. rhumes of the eye, 20. filth in the eares, 23. loose teeth, 29. watering of the Gums, 29. rheumes of the Stomach, 44. excesse of menstrues, 80. ulcers on the fingers ends, 91. Carbuncles, 97. Holy fire, 98. corrosive ulcers, 109. 112. scurfe, 112.

Onions, purge the braine, p. 3. good against the Lethargie, 3. Itch of the eye-lids, 13. blemishes in the eyes, 14. dimnesse of sight, 15. pin or web in the eye, 19. filth in the eares, 23. deafnesse, 23. noyse in the eares, 24. to purge the Humors of the Braine by the Nose, 26. squinancie, 30. Emeroids, 64. expell urine, 67. help the Strangury, 71.

provoke menstrues, 77. heale blisters and inflammations of the feet, 91. biting of mad Dogs, 125. shedding of haire, 137. pock-holes, and scarres in the face, 141. Leprosie, 143.

Opium, good against paines in the eares, p. 21. biting of Cockatrices, 124.

Opobalsamum, takes blemishes out of the eyes, p. 13.

Orage, cures the Jaundise, p. 48. loosens, 60, 153.

Finger-Orchis, helps Cancers in the mouth, p. 26.

Organie, profitable against the spasm, p. 9. paines of the eares, 21. purges the braine, 25. helps Cancers in the mouth, p. 26. inflammation of the jawes, 31. Cough, 36. inflammation of the Lungs, 38. causes vomiting, 45. helps digestion, 47. cures the Jaundise, 49. Dropsie, 50. diminishes the spleen, 53. expels urine, 68. allayes inflammations of the genitals, 74. purges menstrues, 78. helps ruptures, 117. stinging and biting of venemous beasts, 119, 123, 128. the malignity of meddow Saffron, 132. of Aconitum, 133. of Hemlock, 134. of Carline-th[i]stle, 134. of Tad-stooles, 136. of plaster, 136.

Orkanet, good against the Jaundise, p. 49. diminishes the spleen, 53. binds, 59. kils wormes, 61. profits against paines in the reines, 65. causes abortion, 83. allayes the Holy fire, 99. cures burnes, 114. dislocations, 116. biting of Vipers, 120. Leprosie, 143.

Orpine, vid. **Arsenick**.

Oxe-eye, helps the Jaundise, p. 49.

Oyle, profitable against the pin and web in the eye, p. 19. the malignity of Coriander, 135. of Plaster, 136.

P

PAlma Christi, helps inflammations of the eye-lids, p. 13. of the eyes, 18. drawes forth womens duggs, 41. makes the face smooth, 140. purges phlegme, 151.

Parsley, allayes inflammations of the eyes, p. 18. resolves curdled milk, 42. is good against inflammations of the Stomach, 46. Collick, 54. expels urine, 66. helps pain-pisse, 69. Stone in the bladder, 72. provokes menstrues, 78. expels the after-birth, 82. is an antidote against poyson, 129.

Parsenep, meddow and wilde, good against Head-ach, p. 2. Lethargy, 3. Frensie, 7. filth in the eares, 23. difficulty of breathing, 39. the Jaundise, 48. expels urine, 67. Stone in the bladder, 72. causes abortion, 82. helps corrosive ulcers, 110. biting of Serpents and Aspes, 121.

Partridges gall, good against the sharpnesse of the eyes, p. 12. for blemishes of the eyes, 14.

Passe-flower, helps filthy salt ulcers, p. 112.

Peaches, loosen, 60. correct the malignity of Ceruse, 136.

Peares, stay the bloudy-flux, p. 56.

Pellitory of Spaine, and the wall, purge the braine, p. 3. profit against paines in the eares, 22. Tooth-ach, 28. inflammations of the jawes, 31. Cough, 37. Apostumes of the fundament, 62. gout of the legs and feet, 88. shaking feavers, 95. inflammations, 96. Holy fire, 99. biting of Shrew-mice, 123.

Penniroyall, helps the Spasm, p. 9. watering of the Gums, 30. shortnesse of breath, 34. swoundings of the heart, 40. gripings of the Stomach, 45. helps digestion, 47. provokes menstrues, 78. expels the after-birth, 81. causes abortion, 82. helps inflammations of the matrix, 85. sciatica, 89. inflammations of any part, 96. corrosive ulcers, 110. biting and stinging of venemous beasts, 119. those who have drunk Cantharides, 131. take pock-holes and scars out of the face, 141.

Penni-wort, allayes inflammations of the Stomach, p. 45. profits against the Stone, and gravell of the reines, 65. expels urine, 69. heales kybes, 91. inflammations in any diseased part, 96.

Peonie, prevents vomiting, p. 43. profits against gripings of the Stomach, 45. Jaundise, 49. belly-ach, and wormes, 55. bindes, 59. helps paines in the reines, 65. pain-pisse, 70. suffocation of the matrix, 76. provokes menstrues, 79. is beneficiall for Women in labour, 85.

Pepper, good against the Falling-sicknesse, p. 5. squinancie, 31. Cough, 36. procures an appetite, 47. diminishes the spleen, 52. profits against the belly-ach, and wormes, 55. causes abortion, 82. hinders conception, 84, helps intermitting Feavers, 95. stinging and biting of venemous beasts, 118. the malignity of Hemlock, 134. Leprosie, 143.

Periwinckle, profitable against Head-ach, p. 2. Tooth-ach, 28. increases milk, 42. cures the bloudy-flux, 57. bindes, 59. helps the biting and stinging of venemous beasts, 119. 121.

S. *Peters*-wort, good against the Sciatica, p. 89. and burnes, 114.

Pidgeons bloud, helps wounds in the eyes, p. 16. helps the pur-blinde, 19. the dung cures Carbuncles, 97. burnes, 113. the eggs, correct the malignity of Ceruse, 136.

Pimpernell, allayes inflammations of the eyes, p. 13. helps weaknesse of sight, 19. paines in the eares, 22. Tooth-ach, 28. Dropsie, 50. paines in the reines, 65. drawes splinters out of wounds, 108. cures ulcers, 110. biting of Vipers, 120.

Pine-tree, and the fruit, allayes the Tooth-ach, p. 27. 28. helps the Tisick, 33. gripings of the Stomach, 45. heat the Liver, 48. expell urine, 66. allay inflammations of wounds, 108. profit against ulcers, 109. drinking of Cantharides, 131. of Henbane, 133. heale tetters and ring-wormes, 144.

Ground-pine, mollifies hardnesse of duggs, p. 41. removes obstructions of the Liver, 48. cures the Jaundise, 49. belly-ach and wormes, 55. pain-pisse, 69. expels the after-birth, 82. is profitable against the Sciatica, 89.

Pistachoes, helps the Tisick, 33.

Pitch and the Tree, good against sharpnesse of the eye-lids, p. 12. inflammations of the eyes, 17. rheumes of the eyes, 20. odor in the eares, 23. Tooth-ach, 27. obstructions of the Liver, 48. bloudy flux, 56. incarnates hollow ulcers, 115.

Plantaine, profitable against the Falling-sicknesse, p. 5. ulcers in the eyes, 17. bleareyednesse, 20. paines in the eares, 21. Apostumes behinde the eares, 22. Cancers in the mouth, 26. makes teeth cleane, 27. cures putrified gums, 30. spitting of bloud, 33. Tisick, 34. shortnesse of breath, 34. rheumes of the Stomach, 44. Dropsie, 50. bloudy-flux, 57. bindes, 58. heales ulcers in the reines, 66. suffocation of the matrix, 76. excesse of menstrues, 80. 81. Tertian Feaver, 94. Quartane Feaver, 94. inflammations, 96. Holy fire, 98. bleeding of wounds, 107. corrosive ulcers, 110. 111. hollow Fistulaes, 111. biting of dogs, 125.

Plum-tree leaves, stay watering of the gums, p. 30. fasten the pallat of the mouth, 31. the gum, helps dimnesse of sight, 15.

Poley, good against the Jaundise, p. 49. Dropsie, 50. diminishes the spleen, 52. purges menstrues, 78. helps the stinging and biting of venemous beasts, 119. drives away all venemous beasts, 128.

Polipodie, or **Oake-fearne**, good against the Dropsie, p. 50. dislocations, 116. causes shedding of haire, 138. purges choller, 150. and phlegme, 151.

Pomegranats, and the Tree, prevent Drunkennesse, p. 7. helps dimnesse of sight, 15. paines in the eares, 21. watering of the gums, 30. bloudy-flux, 56. binde, 59. cure ulcers of the fundament, 62. expell urine, 67. stay excesse of menstrues, 80. cure ulcers on the fingers ends, 91. falling down of the guts, 93.

Pompions, good against inflammations of the braine, p. 7. cause vomiting, 44. helpe ulcers, 114. make the face smooth, 140. keeps the body faire, 142.

Poplar-tree, profitable against weakenesse of sight, p. 19. paines in the eares, 21. expels urine, 67. cures the Sciatica, 88.

Poppy, wild, black, horned, & c. good against head-ach, p. 2. provokes sleep, 4. profits against the Falling-sicknesse, 6. Spasme, 9. inflammations of the eyes, 18. tooth-ach, 28. rheumes of the throat, 44. cough, 37. rheumes of the Stomach, 44. stopping of the liver, 48. diminish the spleen, 53. stay the bloudy-flux, 57. bindes, 59. helps the Stone and gravell in the reines, 65. pain-pisse, 70. excesse of menstrues, 80. sciatica, 89. inflammations, 96. Holy fire, 99. burns, 114. biting and stinging of venemous beasts, 118. poyson, 129. Leprosie, 143.

Privet, mittigates headach, p. 2. aches of the sinewes, 11. expels urine, 67. purges menstrues, 77. cures the Holy fire, 98. burnes, 113. colours haire yellow, 139.

Pullets gall, helps sharpnesse of the eyes, p. 13.

Punies, helps pain-pisse, p. 69. suffocation of the matrix, 76. Quartain Feavers, 94. biting of Serpents and Aspes, 121.

Purple-fish, makes the teeth clean, p. 27. consumes superfluous flesh, 109. cicatriseth ulcers, 115.

Purslaine, mittigates the head-ach, p. 2. is good against the Spasme, 9. inflammations of the eyes, 18. Blear-eyedness, 20. Teeth set on edge, 29. spitting of bloud, 33. increases milk, 42. allayes inflammations of the Stomach, 45. profits against belly-ach and worms, 54. bloudy-flux, 57. Emeroids, 64. pain-pisse, 69. paines and gripings of the matrix, 86. languishing feavers, 95. biting of Lizards, 124.

Q

Quinces and the tree, allay inflammations of the eyes, p. 18. of the duggs, 41. stay vomiting, 43. rheumes of the Stomach, 43. 47. mollifie hardnesse of the spleen, 51.

stay the bloudy-flux, 56. heale Apostumes of the fundament, 62. help falling of the matrix, 86. preserve against poyson, 133.

R

Radish, helps the Squinancy, p. 31. Cough, 36. excrements difficult to spit, 40. Dropsie, 50. hardnesse of the spleen, 51. expels urine, 67. the menstrues, 77. prevent Gangrenaes, 98. heal corrosive ulcers, 109. the biting of Vipers, 120. of Serpents, 122. the malignity of Tad-stooles, 135. shedding of haire, 137. take away freckles, 142. cause vomiting, 152.

Ramne-thorne, allayes the Holy fire, p. 98. heales corrosive ulcers, 109. Tetters and Ring-wormes, 144.

Rampions, diminish the spleen, p. 53. expels urine, 69. the after-birth, 82.

Raspis-bush, allay inflammation of the eyes, p. 18. Holy fire, 99.

Ethiopian Reed, provokes sleep, p. 3.

Rest-harrow, or **Cammock**, heales Emeroids, p. 64. expels urine, 68.

Rhapontick, cures the spasme p. 9. spitting of bloud, 33. shortnesse of breath, 34. hardnesse of the Midriffe, 40. rheumes of the Stomach, 44. paines of the Stomach, 45. hickop, 46. stopping of the Liver, 48. diminishes the spleen, 52. profits against the belly-ach & worms, 55. obstructions of the reines, 66. paine-pisse, 70. sciatica, 89. inflammations, 96. stinging and biting of venemous beasts, 118. Tetters and Ring-wormes, 144.

Rice, bindes, p. 58. and corrects the malignity of Lime or Arsenick 137.

Ring-doves bloud, cure wounds in the eyes, p. 16.

Rocket, increases milke, p. 42. helps digestion, 47. expels urine, 67. increases venery, 73. cures the biting of shrew-mice, 123.

Roses, good against Head-ach, p. 1, 2. paines in the eares, 21. watering of the gums, 29. bloudy-flux, 56. inflammations, 95. Holy fire, 98. members out of joynt, 115. poyson of Toads, 130.

Rosemary, profitable against the spasm, p. 10. dimnesse of sight, 16. malladies of the breast, 40. Jaundise, 49. belly-ach, and wormes, 54. Apostumes of the fundament, 62. bleeding of Emeroids, 64. purges menstrues, 78. is good against the Gout, 87. filthy ulcers, 112. ruptures, 117. biting of Serpents, and Aspes, 121. Leprosie, 143.

Rose-wood, helpes Cancers in the mouth, p. 26. bloudy-flux, 56. expels urine, 66. is good against ulcers in the naturall places of women, 85.

Rosewort, mittigates the Head-ach, p. 2.

Rue, profits against head-ach, p. 2. falling-sicknesse, 5. dimnesse of sight, 15. paines in the eyes, 18. weaknesse of sight, 19. paines in the eares, 21. bleeding at the nose, 24. shortnesse of breath, 34. 35. Dropsie, 50. Collick, 54. belly-ach and wormes, 54. bindes, 59. kils wormes, 61. expels urine, 68. helps persons which cannot keep their water, 72. hinders Venery, 74. allayes inflammations of the genitals, 74. helps suffocation of the matrix, 76. wind in the matrix, 86. sciatica, 89. gout of the hands and joynts, 90. Quartaine Feavers, 94. intermitting feavers, 95. Holy fire, 99. burns, 113. biting of Serpents and Aspes, 121. stinging of Scorpions, 128. Leprosie, 143.

Rushes, good against a Cough, p. 37. and the venome of Spiders, 126.

S

Saffron, good against the Frensie, p. 6. Drunkennesse, 7. dimnesse and weakness of sight, 15, 17. inflammations of the eares, 22. Collick, 54. belly-ach and wormes, 54. Apostumes of the fundament, 63. expels urine, 66. increaseth Venery, 73. cures the Holy fire, 98.

Meddow-saffron, mittigates tooth-ach, p. 28.

Gum sagapene, profitable against the Falling-sicknesse, p. 6. Spasme, 10. scars in the eyes, 14. pin or web in the eye, 19. Cough, 36. Plurisie, 37. diminishes the spleen, 52. voyds the stone in the bladder, 72. helps the suffocation of the matrix, 76. provokes menstrues, 78. cures ruptures, 117. biting of Serpents and Aspes, 121.

Sage, profits against spitting of bloud, p. 33. expels urine, 67. allayes itching of the genitals, 75. purges menstrues, 78. expels dead Children, 84. stayes the bleeding of wounds, 107.

Salamander, causes shedding of haire, p. 138. cures the Leprosie, 147.

Salt, takes blemishes out of the eyes, p. 14. mittigates paines of the eares, 22. helps Cancers in the mouth, 26. watering gums, 30. Squinancy, 31. inflammations of the jawes, 31. belly-ach and wormes, 55. gout of the leggs and feet, 88. ulcers on the fingers ends, 92. corrosive ulcers, 110. members out of joynt, 116. biting of Serpents, and Aspes, 122. 128. the malignity of Poppy, 134. of Tad-stooles, 136. wild scab, 146. scabbinesse, 147.

Samian-earth, good against inflammations of the duggs, p. 41. of the genitals, 75. excesse of womens termes, 81. biting of Serpents and Aspes, 122. drinking Cantharides, 131.

Samphire, cures the Hickop, p. 46. Jaundise, 48. pain-pisse, 69. expels menstrues, 77. purges choller, 150.

Sand, cures the Dropsie, p. 51.

Sarcocolla, helps rheumes of the eyes, p. 20.

Satirion, good against the spasme, p. 10. aches of the sinews, 11. bindes, 59. increases venery, 73.

Savine, profits against Carbuncles, p. 97. corrosive ulcers, 109. takes moles out of the face, 141.

Saverie, good against weaknesse of sight, p. 19. shortnesse of breath, 35. malladies of the breast, 40. worms, 61. expels urine, 68. takes away warts off the genitall members, 75. expels the afterbirth, 82. helps the sciatica, 89. resolves clotted bloud, 107.

Saxifrage, stayes the bloudy-flux, p. 57. expels urine, 68. breakes the stone in the bladder, 72. provokes menstrues, 79. drawes splinters out of wounds, 108.

Scabious, stanches bleeding of wounds, p. 106.

Scale-fearne, hinders Conception, p. 84.

Scalions, good against the scurfe of the head, p. 8. bruised eares, 123. excrements difficult to spit, 40. paines of the Stomach, 45. Dropsie, 50. gout of the leggs and feet, 87. Sciatica, 89. bruised nayles, 93. splinters, 108. scabs on the fundament, 114. members out of joynt, 115. ruptures, 117. biting of Doggs, 125. Dandriffe, 139. rases pock-holes, and scarres out of the face, 141. Sun-spots, 141. freckles, 142.

Scammonie, mittigates Head-ach, p. 2. helps the Sciatica, 90. fellons and small apostumes, 97. scabbinesse, 147. purges choller, 150. phlegme, 150.

Scarlet-graine, helps aches of the sinewes, p. 11. cut sinews, 12.

Scorpeno, the gall, helps sharpness of the eyes, p. 12. dimnesse of sight, 15. pin or web in the eye, 19.

Scorpions grasse, cures the stinging of Scorpions, p. 127.

Sea-grape, helps spitting of bloud, p. 33. rheumes of the Stomach, 44. bloudy-flux, 57. the malignity of Lime and Arsenick, 137.

Seale-fish, helps the suffocation of the matrix, p. 76.

Sea-water, good against the head-ach, p. 2. aches of the sinewes, 11. Dropsie, 51. belly-ach, and wormes, 55. biting of Serpents and Aspes, 122. 127. Tetters and Ring-wormes, 145. Wild Scab, 146.

Serapinum, vi d. **Gum Sagapene.**

Serpents skin, helps paine in the eares, p. 21. Tooth-ach, 27.

Services, stay the Bloudy-flux, p. 56.

Sesaminum, aches of the sinewes, p. 11 to subtilize the sinewes, 12. allayes inflammations of the eyes, 18. paines of the eyes, 18. paines of the eares, 21. inflammations of the eares, 22.

Seselios, helps the Cough, p. 36. difficulty of breath, 39. malladies of the breast, 40. digestion, 47. belly-ach and wormes, 55. paines in the reines, 65. pain-pisse, 70. strangury, 70. provokes menstrues, 78.

Shave-grasse, stanches bleeding at the nose, p. 25.

Sheeps-dung, takes away warts of the fundament, p. 64. of the genitall members, 75. helps burnes, 113. hardnesse of the skin, 148.

Siler, good against the Falling-sicknesse, p. 5. suffocation of the matrix, 76. causes abortion, 83.

Silver-weed, cures old ulcers, p. 111.

Silurus, stayes the Bloudy-flux, p. 57. loosens, 60. is good against the sciatica, 88. drawes out splinters, 108.

Sison, diminishes the spleen, p. 53.

Skink, increases venery, p. 73.

Skirrets, expell urine, p. 67.

Sloes, stay the bloudy-flux, p. 56

Smallage, expels urine, p. 68. helps the strangury, 71.

Snake-weed, cures Cancers in the mouth, p. 26. inflammations of the jawes, 31.

Snayles, helps cut sinewes, p. 12. Falling of haire off the eye-lids, 12. blemishes in the eyes, 13. scars in the eyes, 14. bleeding at the nose, 24. cleans teeth, 27. causes vomiting, 44. good against the Collick, 54. bloudy-flux, 56. provoke menstrues, 77. profit against the gout of the leggs and feet, 87. drawes splinters out of wounds, 108. take away Sun-spots, 141.

Sneesing-wort, causes sneesing, p. 4. 26.

Snow, helps persons who have swallowed Horse-leeches, p. 131.

Solomons-seale, makes the face smooth, and gives it a luster, p. 140.

Sope-wort, causes sneesing, p. 4. 26.

Sorrell, mittigates the Tooth-ach, p. 27. helps rheumes of the Stomach, 44. bloudy-flux, 57. bindes, 58.

Sory, mittigates the tooth-ach, p. 29. fastens loose teeth, 29. is good against the sciatica, 90. takes pock-holes and scars out of the face, 141.

Southern-wood, profits against the spasme, p. 9. inflammations of the eyes, 18. difficulty of breathing, 39. purges menstrues, 77. is good against the sciatica, 89. ruptures, 117. biting of Vipers, 119. Serpents and Aspes, 121. of Shrew-mice, 123. stinging of Scorpions, 127. drives away venemous beasts, 128. stayes shedding of haire, 138.

Sow-bread, purges the braine, p. 3, 25. is profitable against the scurfe of the head, 8. pin or web in the eye, 19. Apostumes of the Lungs, 34. diminishes the spleen, 52. helps falling of the fundament, 63. provokes menstrues, 77. causes abortion, 82. is good against the Gout of the legs and feet, 87. kybes, 91. members out of joynt, 115. shedding of haire, 137. Sun-burne, 140. Sun spots, 142.

Sow-fennell, mittigates the head-ach, p. 2. profits against the Lethargy, 3. vertiginosities, 4. Falling-sicknesse, 6. frensie, 7. spasme, 10. Palsie, 10. aches of the sinewes, 11. paines of the eares, 21. Tooth-ach, 28. shortnesse of breath, 35. Cough, 36. belly-ach and worms, 54. paines in the reines, 64. pain-pisse, 70. suffocation of the matrix, 76. purges menstrues, 78. is good for women in Labour, 85. helps filthy ulcers, 113. drawes out broken bones, 116. drives away venemous beasts, 128.

Sow-thistle, increases milk, p. 42. helps gripings of the Stomach, 45. inflammations of the fundament, 63. of the matrix, 85. stinging of Scorpions, 127.

Sparagus, cures the frensie, p. 6. tooth-ach, 27. Jaundise, 48. bloudy-flux, 57. loosens, 60. expels urine, 67. helpes the pain-pisse, 69. hinders conception, 84. is good against the Sciatica, 89. members out of joynt, 115.

Speed-well, stayes the bloudy flux, p. 57.

Spelt-corne, bindes, p. 58.

Spicknell, mittigates head-ach, p. 3. helps rheumes of the head, 7. winde in the Stomach, 46. belly-ach, and wormes, 54. expels urine, 66. is good against suffocation of the matrix, 76. purges menstrues, 76. profits against the Gout of the leggs and feet, 87. Sciatica, 88.

Spider, cures the Tertian feaver, p. 94.

Spider-wort, is good against the belly-ach and wormes, p. 55. stinging of Spiders, 126. and of Scorpions, 127.

Spikenard, stayes the falling of haire from the eye-lids, p. 12. vomiting, 43. helps gripings of the Stomach, 45. wind in the Stomach, 46. obstructions of the Liver, 48.

Jaundise, 48. inflammations of the spleen, 52. heats the Liver, 51. diminishes the spleen, 52. expels the stone and gravell of the reines, 65. urine, 66. restraines excesse of menstrues, 78. allayes inflammations of the matrix, 85. heales the biting and stinging of venemous beasts, 118.

Plow-mans Spikenard, mittigates head-ach, p. 1. provokes sleep, 3. is good against the spasm, 9. ulcers and inflamations in the eyes, 17, 18. shortnesse of breath, 35. Cough, 36. drawes forth womens duggs, 41. helps the pain-pisse, 69. stone in the bladder, 72. purges menstrues, 78. helps ruptures, 117. causes abortion, 83. is good for women in labour, 85.

Spleen-wort, diminishes the spleen, p. 53. expels urine, 68. helps the strangury, 71. breakes the stone in the bladder, 72. allayes inflammations, 96.

Sponges, profitable against blear-eyednesse, p. 20. bleeding of wounds, 107. ulcers, 111.

Spurge, takes blemises out of the eyes, p. 14. and scarres, 14. mittigates the Tooth-ach, 29. cures the Jaundise, 49. warts on the genitall members, 75. sciatica, 90. ulcers on the fingers ends, 92. and elsewhere, 112. stinging of Scorpions, 127. purges choller, 150. phlegme, 151. causes vomiting, 152. cures the Dropsie, 153.

Squill, helps the Falling-sicknesse, p. 5. shortnesse of breath, 34. cough, 36. excrements difficult to spit, 40. wambling of the Stomach, 43. digestion, 47. Jaundise, 48. Dropsie, 50. belly-ach and wormes, 55. kybes, 91. biting of Vipers, 120. hardnesse of the skin, 148. purges phlegme, 151.

Squinants, good against the spasme, p. 8. gripings of the Stomach, 45. expels urine, 66. provokes menstrues, 76. allayes inflammations of the matrix, 85.

Staphis-acre, purges the braine, p. 3. helps cancers in the mouth, 26. Tooth-ach, 29. watering of the gums, 30. scurfe, 112. kils Lice and Nits, 139. cures the wild scab, 145.

Star-wort, allayes inflammations of the eyes, p. 18. helps the falling of the fundament, 63. kernels and inflammations in the groine, 93.

Steele, stayes rheumes of the stomach, p. 44. diminishes the spleen, 53.

Stock-doves bloud, helps purblinde eyes, p. 19.

Stoebe, cures fresh wounds in the eyes, p. 16. filth of the eares, 23. bloudy-flux, 57.

Arabian-stone, or **white Marble**, makes the teeth cleane, p. 27. heales Emeroids, 64.

Asian-stone, helps the Tisick, p. 34. diminishes the spleen, 54. cures the gout of the leggs and feet, 88. fellons, 97. ulcers, 110, 111, 113.

Bloud-stone, good against sharpnesse of the eyes, p. 13. scarres of the eyes, 14. wounds of the eyes, 16. rheumes of the eyes, 20. blear-eyednesse, 20. spitting of bloud, 33. pain-pisse, 70. excesse of menstrues, 81.

Eagle-stone, profits against the Falling-sicknesse, p. 6. causes abortion, 83. preserves the Childe till the limitted time, 85.

Stone Gagates, or **Jet**, helps the suffocation of the matrix, p. 76. drives away venemous beasts, 128.

Galactitus, or **the Milk-stone**, cures ulcers in the eyes, p. 16. rheumes of the eyes, 20.

Stone Geodes, helps dimnesse of sight, p. 16. inflammation of womens duggs, 41. of the genitalls, 74.

Jasper-stone, causes abortion, p. 83.

Stone-Judaicus, helps the pain-pisse, p. 70. breakes stones in the bladder, 72.

Marchasite, or **Fire-stone**, helps dimnesse of sight, p. 16.

Stone Morochthus, helps rheumes of the eyes, p. 20. spitting of bloud, 33. rheums of the Stomach, 44. pain-pisse, 70. excesse of menstrues, 81.

Naxion-stone, or **Whet-stone**, good against the Falling-sicknesse, p. 6. keeps duggs from growing, 43. hinders shedding of Haire, 138.

Stone-Ostracites, allayes inflammations of the duggs, p. 41. stayes excesse of womens purgations, 81. hinders conception, 84. heales maligne ulcers, 111.

Phrigian-stone, cures burnes, p. 114.

Pumice-stone, helps dimnesse of sight, p. 16. rheumes of the eyes, 20. makes teeth cleane, 27. good against rotten gums, 30. incarnates hollow ulcers, 115.

Samius-stone, heales ulcers in the eyes, p. 16. rheumes of the eyes, 20. makes teeth cleane, 27. causes abortion, 83.

Saphire-stone, takes scarres out of the eyes, p. 14. helps dimnesse of sight, ulcers of the eyes and buds in the eyes, 16. 17. ulcers in the guts, 62. stinging of Scorpions, 128.

Stone-Schistos, helps ruptures, p. 117.

Specular-stone, good against the Falling-sicknesse, p. 6.

Sponge-stone, helps pain-pisse, p. 70. stone in the bladder, 72.

Stone-thyites, helps dimnesse of sight, p. 16.

Storax, mittigates the head-ach, p. 3. good against rheumes of the head, 7. cleares the voyce, 37. provokes menstrues, 77. mollifies, 86.

Storkes-dung, profitable against the Falling-sicknesse, p. 5.

Succorie, stayes falling of haire from the eye-lids, p. 12. panting and throbbing of the heart, 40. bindes, 58. provokes menstrues, 77. cures the gout of the leggs or feet, 87. Holy fire, 98 stinging of Scorpions, 127.

Sugar, allayes inflammations of the eyes, p. 18.

Sumacke, good against filth in the eares, p. 23. sharpnese of the tongue, 27. rheumes of the Stomach, 44. bloudy-flux, 56. Emeroids, 64. excesse of menstrues, 80. ulcers at the fingers ends, 92. inflammations, 96. prevent Gangrenaes, 97. colours haire black, 139.

Swallowes, profitable against the Falling-sicknesse, p. 5. dimnesse of sight, 15. squinancie, 30. 31.

Swallaw-wort, helps ulcerated duggs, p. 42. belly-ach and wormes, 55. ulcers in the secret parts, 85. biting and stinging of venemous beasts, 119.

Sweet-cane, good against the Spasme, p. 8. dimnesse of sight, 15. Cough, 35. paines of the sides, 38. Dropsie, 50. pains in the Liver, 51. inflammations of the Spleen, 52. diminishes the Spleen, 52. cures belly-ach and wormes, 54. expels urine, 66. helps the Strangury, 70. provokes menstrues, 76. cures ruptures, 116.

Sycamore, profits against rheumes of 'the eyes, p. 20. Tooth-ach, 27. gripings of the Stomach, 45. hardnese of the spleene, 51.

T

TAmariske, mittigates the Tooth-ach, p. 27. helps rheums of the Stomach, 44. Jaundise, 49. inflammations of the spleen, 52. kills Lice and Nits, 139. cures the Leprosie, 148.

Tarre, good against the squinancie, p. 30. Tisick, 34. clefts of the fundament. 62. tumours of the fundament, 63. kybes, 91. causes rough nayles to fall off, 92. profits against Carbuncles, 96. filthy salt ulcers, 112, 115. stinging and biting of venemous beasts, 118. 119. Tetters and Ring-wormes, 144.

Teasell, heales clefts of the fundament, p. 62. takes away cornes, 148.

Bastard-thistle, helps the stinging of Scorpions, p. 127.

Cotton-thistle, cures the spasme, p. 9.

Thistle-gentle, helps veines puffed and swelled with bloud, p. 93.

Lady-thistle, good against the spasme, p. 9. Tooth-ach, 28. paines of the sides, 38. vomiting, 43. sciatica, 89. ruptures, 117.

White-thistle, profits against the spasm, p. 9. tooth-ach, 28. spitting of bloud, 33. rheume of the Stomach, 44. expels urine, 68. heales the biting of Serpents and Aspes, 121.

Time, profitable against the Head-ach, p. 1. spasme, 9, 10. weaknesse of sight, 19. spitting of bloud, 33. shortnesse of breath, 34. difficulty of breath, 39. malladies of the breast, 40. belly-ach, and wormes, 55. 61. expels urine, 68. takes away warts, 75. provokes menstrues, 78. expels the after-birth, 81. causes abortion, 83. helps the sciatica, 89. clotted bloud, 107. ruptures, 117. biting of Serpents and Aspes, 121. 127. the malignity of meddow saffron, 132. of plaster, 136.

Tormentill, cures the biting of Shrew-mice, p. 123.

Tortoise, good against the Falling-sicknesse, p. 5. sharpnesse of the eyes, 14. Squinancy, 30. Corrosive ulcers, 109. stinging and biting of venemous beasts, 118.

Trefoile severall kindes, profits against the head-ach, p. 2. Falling-sicknesse, 6. shortnesse of breath, 35. paines of the sides, 38. bindes, 59. expels urine, 69. helps suffocation of the matrix, 76. expels the after-birth, 82. allayes inflammations of the groine, 93. cures the Tertian Feaver, 94. stinging and biting of venemous beasts, 119. 122. 128.

Tunnie-fish, helps the biting of Vipers, p. 120.

Turbith, purges Melancholly, p. 152.

Turmericke, causes shedding of haire, p. 138.

Turne-sole, allayes inflammations of the braine, p. 7. kils wormes, 61. takes away warts, 75. purges menstrues, 79. causes abortion, 83. helps Tertian Feavers, 94. members out of joynt, 116. stinging of Scorpions, 127. hardnesse of the skinne, 148. takes away Cornes, 148.

Turnips, increase venery, p. 73. is good against the Gout of the hands, and feet, p. 87. kybes, 91. all sorts of poyson, 129.

Turpentine and the Tree, heales ulcers in the eyes, p. 16. odor in the eares, 23. profitable against the Tisick, 33. paines of the sides, 38. expels urine, 66. cures itching of the genitals, 75. salt ulcers, 112. scabbines, 147.

Bloud of Turtle-doves, helps wounds in the eyes and the pur-blinde, p. 16, 19.

Tutie, cures fistulaes in the eyes, p. 20. rheumes of the eyes, 20. filthy salt ulcers, 113.

V

VAlerian, expels urine, p. 66. menstrues, 76. stinging and biting of venemous beasts, 118. preserves against poyson, 129.

Verdigrease, takes scars out of the eyes, p. 14. helps dazling of the eyes, 20. deafnesse of the eares, 24. *Noli me tangere*, 25. rotten putrified gums, 30. rheumes of the throat, 32. inflammations of wounds, 108. proud flesh, 109. corrosive ulcers, 110. 112. 113. cicatriseth ulcers, 115. helps scabbinesse, 147.

Verjuyce, good against sharpnesse of the eye-lids, p. 13. dimnesse of sight, 15. ulcers in the corners of the eyes, 17. filth in the eares, 23. watering or rotten of the gums, 30. fasten the Vvula, 31. rheumes of the throat, 32. spitting of bloud, 33. bloudy-flux, 58. excesse of womens menstrues, 81.

Vermillion, helps pain-pisse, p. 69.

Vernish, heales old ulcers, p. 111.

Verveine, helps Cancers in the mouth, p. 26. rheumes of the throat, 32. Jaundise, 49. paines and gripings of the matrix, 87. Tertian Feavers, 94. Quartane Feavers, 94. inflammations, 96. Holy fire, 99. corrosive ulcers, 110. 113.

Vetches severall sorts, mollifies hardness of the Duggs, p. 41. helps belly-ach and wormes, 55. expels urine, 67. 69. heales kybes, 91. Carbunckles, 97. prevents Gangrenaes, 98. stenches bleeding of wounds, 107. cures old ulcers, 109. biting of Vipers, 120.

Vine, good against the head-ach, p. 3. spitting of bloud, 33. vomiting, 43. inflammations of the Stomach, 45. 47. bloudy-flux, 57. Stone of the bladder, 72. loathing of meate, 85. bruised joynts, 90. windy ruptures, 93. members out of joynt, 116. biting of Vipers, 120. and Serpents, 122. of Doggs, 125. the malignity of meddow saffron, 132. of Tadstooles, 136. causeth shedding of haire, 138. takes away warts, 148. and cornes, 148.

Vinegar, profits against inflammations of the braine, p. 7. noise or wormes in the eares, 24. bleeding at the nose, 25. Tooth-ach, 29. rotten gums, 30. Squinancie, 30. procures and appetite, 47. takes away warts on the fundament, 64. helps falling of the matrix, 86. inflammations, 96. ulcers, 92. 110. poyson, 130. clotted milke, 131. the malignity of Hemlock, 134. of Tadstooles, 136. blisters, wheales, and heat pushes, 145.

Squill Vinegar, helps vertiginosities, p. 4. Falling-sicknesse, 6. aches of the sinewes, 11.

Violets, allayes inflammations of the eyes, p. 18. heales Cancers in the mouth, 26. squinancie, 31. inflammations of the Stomach, 47.

Viper, helps aches of the sinewes, p. 11. dimnesse of sight, 15. pin or web in the eye, 19.

Vitrioll, purges the braine, p. 3. *Noli me tangere,* 25. kils wormes, 61. helps the evill quality of Tadstooles, 136.

Unquis Odoratus, good against the Falling-sicknesse, p. 5. to clean teeth, 27. blemishes of the eyes, 13. ulcerated duggs, 42. suffocation of the matrix, 76. proud flesh, 109. filthy ulcers, 112. burnes, 113.

Urine, heales ulcers in the head, p. 8. blemishes of the eyes, 14. scars of the eyes, 14. dimnesse of sight, 15. filth of the eares, 23. wormes in the eares, 24. difficulty of breathing, 39. Dropsie, 50. suffocation of the matrix, 76. paines and gripings of the matrix, 86. Holy fire, 98. biting of Vipers, 120.

W

Wall-flowers, diminish the spleen, p. 53. heales clefts in the fundament, 62. provoke menstrues, 79. expell the after-birth, 82. allay inflammations of the matrix, 85.

Wall-nuts, mittigate Head-ach, p. 3. heale ulcers in the eyes, p. 17. inflammations of the duggs, 41. belly-ach, and wormes, 54. 60. Carbuncles, 97. prevent gangrenaes, 98. is an antidote against poyson, 129. the gum of Carline-thistle, 135.

Wall-wort, helps sharpnesse of the throat, p. 32. spitting of bloud, 33. malladies of the breast, 40. Dropsie, 50. paines in the reines, 65. falling down of the guts, 93.

Wax, profits against Colds, p. 36. milke curdled in the breasts, 42. belly-ach and wormes, 55. bloudy-flux, 57. tetters and ring-wormes, 144.

Weesill, good against the Falling-sicknesse, p. 5. gout of the leggs and feet, 87. biting of Serpents and Aspes, 120. poyson, 129.

Whey, profitable against the Falling-sicknesse, p. 5. loosens, 60. heales blisters, wheales, and heat-pushes, 145. Leprosie, 148.

Widdow-waile, purges choller, p. 150. and phlegme, 151.

Willow, helps paines in the eares, p. 20. hinders conception, 83. cure the gout, 87. dandriffe, 138. hardnesse of the skin, 148.

Willow-herbe, stayes bleeding at the nose, p. 24. spitting of bloud, 33. bloudy-flux, 57. drives away venemous beasts, 128.

Winde-flower, purges the braine, p. 3. allayes inflammations of the eyes, 18. increases milke, 42. provokes menstrues, 78.

Wine of Germander, cures the spasme, p. 10.

Wine of Hisope, helps shortnesse of breath, p. 34. cleares the voyce, 37. expels putrified matter, 39. helps difficulty of breath, 39.

Wine of French Lavender, cures aches of the sinewes, p. 11.

Wine of Mirtle, helps vomiting, p. 43. and rheumes of the Stomach, 44.

Wine of Mulberries, cures the Squinancy, p. 30.

Wine of Goates-Organy, helpes the Spasme, p. 10.

Wine of Quinces, stayes the bloudy-flux, p. 58. expels urine, 69.

Wine of Squill, good against vertiginosities, p. 4. Falling-sicknesse, 6. Spasme,10. Palsie, 10. vomiting, 43. Jaundise, 49. Dropsie, 51. diminishes the spleen, 53. provokes menstrues, 79.

Wine of Sumack, stayes the bloudy-flux, p. 58.

Wine of Time, cures aches of the sinewes, p. 11.

Wine of Worm-wood, kils round worms, p. 61.

Withiwind, purges choller, p. 150. vid. **Bindweed**.

Woad, diminishes the spleen, p. 52. cures the Holy fire, 98. bleeding of wounds, 107. corrosive ulcers, 110.

VVood of Aloes, fortifies the braine, p. 8. helps the belly-ach and wormes, 54.

Woodbinde, helps shortnesse of breath, p. 35. difficulty of breathing, 39. hickop, 46. paine of the Liver, 51. diminishes the spleen, 53. expels urine, 68. causes abortion, 83. hinders conception, 84. helps the shaking of Feavers, 95.

Wooll, mittigates the head-ach, p. 1. restraines falling of haire from the eye-lids, 12. ulcers in the eyes, 17. cures Apostumes behind the eares, 22. ulcers in the eares, 23. ulcers in the fundament, 62. ulcers in the secret parts, 74. provokes menstrues, 77.

Earth-wormes, helps cut sinewes, p. 12. Tooth-ach, 27. expels urine, 67. cures Tertian Feavers, 94.

Wormseed wort, kils round wormes, p. 61.

Wormwood, mittigates head-ach, p. 3. prevents Drunkennesse, 7. helps paines in the eyes, 18. weaknesse of sight, 19. paines of the eares, 21. filth in the eares, 23. Tooth-ach, 28. Squinancie, 31. panting and throbbing of the heart, 40. paines of the Stomach, 45. wind in the Stomach, 46. procures an appetite, 47. helps digestion, 47, the Jaundice, 48. Dropsie, 50. paines of the Liver, 51. stone and gravell in the reines, 65. obstructions in the reines, 66. expels urine, 68. provokes menstrues, 77. heales the biting of Shrew-mice, 123. cures the malignity of Hemlock, 134. of Carline-thistle, 134. of Tadstooles, 135. purges choller, 149.

Y

Yarrow, stayes bleeding at the nose, p. 25. spitting of bloud, 33. excesse of womens menstrues, 80. allayes inflammations of wounds, 96.

Appendix:
Table of Medicinal Ingredients

The ingredients listed in *The Ladies Dispensatory* are representative of the wide variety of simple and compound pharmaceuticals available in the mid-seventeenth century. This table contains an alphabetical list of ingredients in the classification format used by the College of Physicians in the 1653 edition of the *Pharmacopeia Londinensis: or the London Dispensatory*.[1] This system divided medicinal preparations broadly into simple and compound medicines (see Introduction). These categories were then subdivided further into categories such as roots, woods, barks, herbs, and seeds for the simples, and types of medications for the compounds. To facilitate a comparison of these ingredients with other seventeenth-century texts, superscript notations have been added to indicate ingredients used in the following sources:

The 1633 edition of Gerard's *The Herbal* ([G] John Gerard, *The Herbal or General History of Plants. The Complete 1633 Edition as Revised and Enlarged by Thomas Johnson*. [Facsimile of edition published by Adam Aslip, Joice Norton, and Richard Whitakers, London, 1633], New York: Dover Publications, 1975).

Culpeper's *Herbal* ([C] Nicholas Culpeper, Complete Herbal (London: W. Foulsham & Co., Ltd., 1923)).

Turner's *A New Herbal* ([H] William Turner, *A New Herbal* [Volume I (facsimile and transcript of 1551 edition), ed. G.T.L. Chapman and M. N. McTweedle, and indexed by by F. McCombie; Volume II (facsimile and transcript of Parts II

---

[1] Nicholas Culpeper, *Pharmacopœia Londinensis: or the London Dispensatory: further adorned by the studies and collections of the Fellows, now living of the said Colledg*. (London: Printed for Peter Cole, 1653).

[1562 edition] and III [1568 edition], ed. G.T.L. Chapman, F. McCombie, and A. Wesencraft), New York: Cambridge University Press, 1995]).

John Goodyer's 1652–1655 English translation from the Greek of Dioscorides's *Materia medica* (ᴰ *The Greek Herbal of Dioscorides, illustrated by a Byzantine A.D. 512, Englished by John Goodyer A.D. 1655, edited and first printed AD. 1933* (ed. R.T. Gunther; New York: Hafner Publishing Co., 1959).

The 1653 edition of the *Pharmacopoeia Londinensis* (Nicholas Culpeper, *Pharmacopoeia Londinensis: or the London Dispensatory: further adorned by the studies and collections of the Fellows, now living of the said Colledg.* London: Printed for Peter Cole, 1653). Two different symbols are used for this reference. The Old List, an English translation of the 1618 Latin edition of the *Pharmacopoeia*, is indicated by*, whereas the modified New List is indicated by⁺.

Italics indicate ingredients that did not also appear in *The Skilful Physician*. Selected ingredients are also described from the following sources:

Bate's Dispensatory: William Salmon, *Pharmacopœia Bateana or Bates Dispensatory. Translated from the last Edition of the Latin copy . . .* fifth ed. (London: William and John Innys, 1720).

Blancard: Stephen Blancard, *The Physical Dictionary. Wherein the Terms of Anatomy, the Names and Causes of Diseases, Chirurgical Instruments, and their Use are Accurately Described* (London: John and Benj. Sprint, 1726).

Ges: Conrad Gesner, *The Treasure of Evonymus, cotyninge the wonderfull hid secretes of nature, tochinge the most apte formes to prepare and destyl Medicines, for the conseruation of helth: as Quintessece, Aurum Potabile, Hippocras, Aromatical wynes, Balmes, Oyles, Perfumes, garnishyng waters, and other manifold excellent confections. Wherunto are ioyned the formes of sondry apt Fornaces, and vessels, required in this art. Translated (with great diligence, & laboure) out of Latin, by Peter Morvving felow of Magdaline Coleadge in Oxford.* (London: Iohn Daie, 1559). Fascimile edition of copy from Beinecke Rare Book and Manuscript Library, Yale University. New York: Da Capo Press/ Theatrum Orbis Terrarum Ltd., Number 97, The English Experience, 1969.

OED2: OED2: Oxford English Dictionary II [database online] Available from: BRS Software Products, McLean, VA; BRS/Search Full-Text Retrieval System, Revision 6.1, 1992.

Salmon: William Salmon, *The Compleat English Physician or, The Druggist's Shop Opened.* (London: Mathew Gilliflower 1693).

SIMPLES

Roots

Acanthium [Cotton thistle, White cotton thistle, Wild white thistle, Argentine, Silver thistle] roots^{GTD}

Aconitum [Wolf's bane]^{GD}

All-heale [Hercules wound-wort, Panax]^{GD}

Arabian thistle [Spina arabica; Acantha arabike], roots of^D

Aron roots [Aron=Wakerobbin or Cuckoo-Pint^G]^{G+*CD}

Asarabacca^{G+D}

Asphodil^{G+D}

Bastard Satyrion, roots of [Bird's nest, Goose nest, Satyrium abortirum, Nidus avis]^{G—"not used in Physicke", p. 229}

Bay, root of^{G*+D}

Bear's ear [Alisma=water plantain, Mountain cowslips]^{GD}

Beets, roots of^{GT*+D}

Betony roots^{GCD}

Bitter almond tree, roots of^D

Bramble roots

Brank ursine [Acanthus] roots^{G+D}

Briony^D

Buglosse^{G*+D}

Buglosse, Wild [Orkanet, Alkanet, Anchusa]^{G*+D}

Burnet [Pimpinella, Bunium] root^{*D}

Burre dock [Burdock, Clote burre, Arcion, Lappa]^{GT+D}

Burre-reed [Sparganium] (seeds listed in other sources)^D

Butchers broom roots [Knee-holme, Ruscus, Bruscus, Myrtus sylvestris]^{GT*CD}

Cammock roots [Camock, Rest Harrow, Petty Whinne, Ground furze, Anonis]^{GD}

Candy Alexander [Smyrnium or Thorow bored Parsley]^{GD}

Carline thistle root [Carlina, Chameleon albus of Dioscorides]^{GD}

Carrot, stinking deadly [Thapsia, Stinking carrot, deadly carrot]^{GD}

Carrot, yellow^{GD}

Celandine [Cellendine, Chelidone, Chelidonium] roots^{G*+CD}

Centaury, Great [Great Centory] roots^{GTD}

Chameleon thistle root [Crocodilium, Crocodilion, Carduus niger, "the Thistle that changeth it selfe into many shapes and colours"]^{GD}

Christ's Thorne roots [Paliurus, Rhamnus, Ramme of Lybia, "Christ's thistle" Paliuris of Dioscorides is jujube and root is medicinal^D*]*^G

Cinquefoile [Cinkfoil, Cinqfoil, Five finger grass, Pentaphyllum, Quinquefolium] roots^{GT*+CD}

Clote burre [Burre dock Burdock, Arcion, Lappa]^{GT+D}

Comfry [Consilida, Symphytum] roots^{GT*+CD}

Corn-flag [Xyphion], first and highest root of^{GD}

Corn-flag [Cladiolus, Gladiolus], second and lowest root of[GD]

Costus[G*+D]

Cotton thistle [Acanthium, White cotton thistle, Wild white thistle, Argentine, Silver thisle] roots[GTD]

Coventrie-bells, Blew Medium, the term in The Ladies Dispensatory *is in error according to Gerard*[G, p. 448]*, Viola mariana is Gerard's term; root of Medium is found in Dioscorides Book IV.18], root of*[GD]

Cowcumber roots, wild [wild cucumber[G]][GT*+D]

Crow-foot [Butter-flower, Ranunculus, King Kob, Gold cups, Gold knobs] roots[GTD]

Cuckow pint [Aron, Arum] root[G*+CD]

Daffodil [Narcissus] roots[GTD]

Devil's-bit [Morsus diabili, Pycnocomum] roots[G+CD]

Dittander [Pepper-wort, Lepidium] root[GD]

Dragon root[G*+CD]

Elder [Sambucus, Acte, Chamiacte] roots[D]

Elicampane root [*Enulacampana root, Enula campana roots*][GT*+CD]

Eringo roots [Sea-holly, Eryngium, *Erinringo roots*][GT*+CD]

Fennel root, red[GT*+CD]

Fern roots [male][GT*+CD]

*Finger fern roots [(?)Phyllitis multifida=*Finger harts-tongue[G]*]*

Finger-orchis [Serapias, Serapia's stones, Satyrions, Hares stones, Serapiades][G*+CD]

Flower-de-luce of *Illyria* [Ireos, "that is the roote of the white flowerdeluce" [iris][G]][GTD]

Galingal and Great Galingal [Galanga lesser and greater][G*+]

Galingal, Babilonish

Garlick[GT*+CD]

Gentian roots [Felwort][GT*+CD]

Ginger [*green Ginger, white Ginger*][G*+D]

Gum succory [Chondrilla, Rysshe Succorie, Cichorion, Seris (Dios. II.161] roots[GD]

Hawthorne [Oxyacantha, Pyrina (Dios. I.122)] root[D]

Hellebore, root of white [Neesewort, Neeping root, Helleborum album][TG+D]

Herb Patience, roots of [Sharp-pointed Dock, Lapathum acutum][GD]

*Holme-oak [Ilex, Scarlet oak, , Hulver oak, Holly oak, Cerris=*Great Holme-oak], *root/bark of root*[GD]

Horned poppy [Sea Poppy, Papaver cornutum] roots[GD]

Horse-tail roots [Shave-grass, Polygonon][GT]

Hounds-tongue [Hounds pisse, Dogs tongue, Cynoglossum] roots[G*+]

Idea roots ["it beareth leaves like Knee-holme, and is of a sharpe astringent taste"]

Jacynth roots [Iacynth, Hyacinth, Hyacinthus][G+D]

Knee-holme roots [Butcher's broom, Ruscus, Bruscus][GT*CD]

LIBER XX. .

Figura speciei cuiusdam Aconiti.

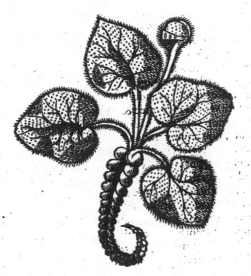

One species of Aconite

Ladies' Bed-straw [Gallium, Gallion, Cheese-renning, Maid's hair, pety Mugwort, wild Madder] root^{GTD}

Lady thistle [Our Lady(ies) Thistle, Leucæantha (mentioned in footnote of LD is Gerard's term for Carline thistle [p. 1150]), Carduus lacteus, Carduus Mariæ, Leucographus, Bedeguar, Spina alba, White Thistle, Milk Thistle] roots^{GT*+CD}

Laserwort [Laserpitium] root^{GD}

Liquorice *[Licoras, English Licoras, Glycyrrhiza]*$^{G*+CD}$

Lilly, root of *[Lilly roots]*$^{GT*+CD}$

Lilly, root of yellow *[Lilly roots, yellow]*$^{GT*+CD}$

Liriconfancie [May Lilly, Lilly in the Valley, Continual Lilly, Woodroof^{G}*]*

Lovage [Lygusticum, Levisticum]$^{G*+D}$

Madir [Madder] roots^{G+*CD}

Mandragory [Mandragore, Mandrake, Mandragon, Mandrage] root^{G*D}

Marsh mallow roots^{GT*+D}

Meadow Parsenep [Cow Parsnep, Madnep, Sphodylium] root^{D}

Milk vetch, root of [Astragalus]^{GTD}

Morsus diabili roots [Devil's-bit]$^{G+D}$

Mountain horse foot root [Cacalia]^{GD}

Mountain siler [Siler mountaine, Bastard Lovage] root^{GTD}

*Mullein [Verbascum, Woolen, Higta-
    per, Torches, Long-wort, Bul-
    lockes Long-wort, Hareweed,
    Tapsus barbatus, Mullin] root^{GD}*

*Oake fearne roots [Dryopteris, true oak
    fern, white oak fern, tree fern,
    Onopteris=*black oak fern]^{GD}

*Oleander [Rose bay, Nerium, Rose
    tree, Rose bay tree^G] roots*

Onions^{G*CD}

*Orkanet [Alkanet, Wild Bugloss,
    Anchusa]$^{G*+D}$*

Parsley roots [*Meadow Parsley root,
    Oreoselinon, Petroselinum
    sylvestre, Apium montanum*]^{GCD}

*Passe-flower [Pasque flower, Bastard
    Anemone, Pulsatilla, Flaw
    flower, Coventrie bells] root$^+$*

Peony[Pæonia, Aglaophotis] root^{G*+CD}

Pepper-plant roots^D

Plantaue [Plantago] roots^{G*+CD}

*Plow-mans Spikenard [Baccharis]
    roots^{GD}*

*Pompions [Melons, Millions, Popon,
    Pepo sp., Pumpkin], roots of^D*

*Reed cane [Arundo Cypria, Pole reed,
    Canes] roots^{G*D}*

Rest-harrow, rind of roots of [Camock,
    Cammock, Petty Whinne,
    Ground furze]^{GD}

Rhadish [Rabone, Raphanus, Sativa
    Radicula] roots^{GT*+CD}

*Rhapontick [Culinary or tart rhubarb,
    =Rhabarbarum = Rhubarb
    (Blancard), Rha Barbarum, Rha
    Ponticum =* Pontick Rubarh,
    Rha]$^{GT*+CD}$

*Rhodia radix [Roseroot, Rose-wort
    roots, Rose roots, Radix
    rhodia]$^{G+D}$*

*Rosemary [Rosmarinum, Libanotis]
    roots*

*Rose bushes [Rhodon, Rosa sp.], roots
    of*

*Rose-wort roots [Roseroot, Rose roots,
    Rhodia radiz, Radix rhodia]$^{G+D}$*

*Sope-wort [Bruise-wort, Saponaria,
    Struthium] roots^D*

*Satirion roots [Satyrion, Fox stones,
    Orchis sp., Testiculus sp., Sweet
    Cuilions, Serapia's stones. Seri-
    apias finger orchis, Serapias sp.,
    Fenny stones]^{GT*D}*

*Spleen-wort [Scale, Stone fern,
    Scolopendra, Spleen wort, Milt-
    waste, Asplenum, Lingua cervina,
    Lonchitis, Ceterach] roots^D*

Sea-holly root [Eryngium, Eringo,
    Iringo]$^{GT*+CD}$

*Sea-pimpernel [Sea ground pine,
    Anthyllis lentifolia] roots^{GD}*

Sea-Purslaine [Halimus] roots^{GTD}

*Seselios of Marseilles [Seseli Mas-
    siliense] roots^D*

*Silver-weed [Talychium, Wild Tansy,
    Argentina] root^C*

*Skirrets [Sisarm, Siser, Cher-
    villum]^{GT**CD}*

*Sleepy nightshade [Dwale, Deadly
    night shade, Raging nightshade,
    Solanum somniferum, Solanum
    lethule, Solanum manicum,
    Halicacabum], rind of roots
    of^{GD}*

Smallage [Marsh parsley, Water parsley, Eleoselinum, Paludiapium] roots^{G+CD}

Sorcerer's Garlick [Moly]^{GD}

Sow-bread [Cyclamen] roots^{G+CD}

Sow-fennel root [Peucedanum, Horestrange, Horestrong, Sulphurwort, Brimstone wort, Hogs Fennel]^{GD}

Sparage roots, Sparragus [Asparagus]$^{GT*+CD}$

Spatling-poppy [Frothy Poppy, Polemonia, Spumeum Papaver, Behen album, White Ben] roots^{G*D}

Spicknell [Spignell, Meon, Meum, Mew, Bearewort, Writhed Dill, Wild Dill] roots^{GT*+CD}

Spurge [Tithymalus sp., Esula sp., Peplus, Peplis, Apios, Chamæsyce] roots^{G}

Squills [Sea Onion, Scilla sp., Pancratium sp., Sea Daffodil]$^{GT*+CD}$

Squinanth [Camel's Hay, Squinanthum, Schœnanthum, Iuncus odoratus] roots^{D}

Stinking Gladdon [Xyris], roots of^{G+*D}

Succory roots [Endive, Seris, Cichorium sp., Intybus sp., *sallets of Succory roots*]$^{G*+CD}$

Swallow-wort [Asclepias], root of^{GT+CD}

Sycamore [Sycomorus] root

Teasell [Virga pastoris, Dipsacus sp., Labrum Veneris, Carduus Veneris, Card Teasell, Venus Bason, Fullers thistle] roots^{GT*CD}

Thistle-gentle [Circium, Cirsium] root^{D}

Tormentil [Chrisogonum, Setfoilc, Septifolium, Tormentilla] root^{G*+CD}

Trefoile [Common trefoile, Three-Leafed grass, Meadow trefoile, Suckles, Honey-suckles, Cocksheads, Shamrocks, Trifolium] roots^{D}

Turbith [Tripolium=Serapias Turbith=Sea-starwort; (Turbith of Antioch is a gummy plant stalk, Gerard, pp. 414–50)]$^{G*+D}$

Turmericke [Cyperus indicus, Curcuma, Crocus Indicus, Terra merita]$^{G+D(1,4)}$

Turnips [Rapum, Rape]$^{GT+CD}$

Viper's-Buglosse root [Echtum vulgare]$^{G+D}$

Wall flower [Viala lutea, Wull gilloflower, Yellow stock gilloflower, Winter-gilloflower, Cheiri] roots^{D}

Wall penni-wort [Ladies navell, Umbilicis veneris, Navel wort, Wall penniwort, Penniwort, Hipwort, Kidneywort, Scatum cæli, Scatellum, Wall penny grass, Cotyledon] root^{GD}

Wall-wort [Dane-wort, Dwarf elder, Ebulus, Sambucus humilis, Symphitum petreum] roots^{G*D}

Water lillies [Nymphea]$^{GT*+D}$

White Thistle [Bedegnar, Spina alba, Lady thistle, Our Lady(ies) Thistle, Carduas lacteus, Carduas Mariæ, Leucographus, Milk Thistle] roots^{GT*+CD}

Wild hemp roots [Nettle hemp, Bastard hemp, Cannabis sylvestris, Cannibis spuria sp.^G]^D

Wild meadow-saffron [Colchicum, Ephemerum] roots^D

Wild pomegranat tree roots

Wild Vine [Vitis sylvestris], roots of

Wind-flower [Anemone] roots^D

Barks

Bay tree^{GD}

Cinnamon [Cinnamome, Canell, Cinnamomum]^{G*+D}

Elme bark^{GD}

Frankinsence tree, bark of^{D(I.82)}

Juniper bark, burned^{GD(I.103)}

Macer [an Indian root] bark^{D(I.110)}

Mulberry [Morus] tree bark^{GD}

Pine tree bark^{GD}

Pitch tree [Picea sp.] bark^{GD}

Pomegranat, bark of^D

Poplar tree bark^{G+CD}

Rhadish [Rabone, Raphanus, Sativa Radicula], rind of^D

Sycamore [Sycomorus] bark

Willow bark, ashes of

Woods

Aloes wood [Lignum aloes, Agallochum, Xyloalloc]^{G(p.1622)*+D}

Ebonie [Ebony]^{+D}

Fennel giant, pith of [Corculum Ferulæ]^{GTD}

Ferula, pith of [Corculum Ferulæ]^{GTD}

Fig tree, ashes of^{D(I.186)}

Lignum aloes [Aloes Wood, Agallochum, Xyloalloe]^{G(p.1621)*+D}

Lote-tree [Nettle tree, Celtis, Lotus arbor]^{GTD}

Spurge flax [Thymelæa, Mountain Widow Waile], pith of^D

Tamarisk [Tamariscus, Tamaris, Myrica, Tamarix]^{GT*+CD}

Herbs

Acacia [Acatia]^{GD}

Agnus Castus [Chaste Tree leaves]^{GD}

Agrimony [Egrimony, Eupatorium] leaves^{G*+D}

Anthyllis [stinking ground pine]^{TG*+D}

Aristolochia [Aristologia=hartwort or birth-wort]^{GD}

Arsenicke [Orpinc, Liblong, Livelong, Crassula, Telephlum]^{G*+CD}

Asarabacca^{G+D}

Ash [Melia, Fraxinus] leaves^{GT+D}

Asp tree [Aspen, a poplar]^{G+}

Asphodil leaves^D

Barren-wort [Epimedium, "we have as yet no use hereof in Physicke."^{G, p. 481.}]^D

Basil [Ocimum]^{GT+D}

Basil, stone [Acynos]^{GD}

Basil, water

Basil, wild [Clinopodium in LD]^{GD}

Bastard parsley [Caucalis sp.]^{GD}

Bastard St. John's wort [Coris]^{G(p.544)}

Bastard stone parsley [Sison, Stone parsley of Macedonia]^{GTD}

Bastard Wild Poppy [Argemone, Wind-rose]^{GD}

Bastard Wood [Sesamoides Salamanticum]^D

Baulme [Balm; Melissa, Apiastrum]^{G*+D}

Bay-leaves [Bayes]^{G*+CD}

Bean trifoly [Bean trefoile, Anagyris, Laburnum] leaves^{GD}

Bear's ear [Alisma=water plantain, Mountain cowslips]^{GD}

Beets^{GT*+CD}

Ben or Behen [either Behen album (Spatling poppy^G) or the Catch-fly= Limewort^G]

Betony^{GT*+CD}

Binde-weed Nightshade [Binde-weed; Inchanter's Nightshade, Circæa; Gerard (p.351); "there is no use of this herbe either in physicke or Surgerel that I can reade of"]

Blites [Blitum]^{G+D}

Box-thorne [Lycium]^{GD}

Bramble [Bramble leaves, red Bramble leaves, red Brambles]^{GT+CD}

Briony, black^{GT+D}

Briony, branches or shoots of black^{G+D}

Briony, white^{GT+D}

Brooklime [Anagallis, Water pimpernel]^{G*+CD}

Broome [Genista sp., Orobanche(?)]^{G+D}

Broome, Spanish [Genista Hispanica, Spartium]^{GD}

Buck's horne [Cornu cervinum, Coronopus, Harts horne, Herb Ivy, Herb Eve]^{GD}

Buglosse^{G+CD}

Buglosse, wild [Alkanet, Orkanet, Anchusa]^{CD}

Burnet [Burnet leaves, Pimpinella, Bunium]^{GT+D}

Butchers broom [Knee-holme, Ruscus, Bruscus]^{GT*+D}

Butter burre [Petasitis in LD]^D

Cabbage [Brassica, Coleworts^G]^{G*+CD}

Calamint [Mountain mint, field calamint, callamint aromaticus]^{GT*+CD}

Caltraps, Land (Tribulus terrestris)^{GD}

Caltraps, Water (Tribulus aquaticus, Water Caltrops, Water Saligot, Water Nuts, Water Chesnuts)^{GD}

Cammel's Hay [Camel's Hay, Squinanth, Schænanthum, Iuncus odoratus]^{G+*D}

Camomile [Cammomile, Chamemelum, Anthemis]^{GT*+CD}

Caraway [Carum]^{GT}

Celandine, great [Cellendine, Chelidone, Chelidonium, great celadine=swallow-wort]^{G*+CD}

Celandine, lesser [Scrophularia minor, Chelidonium minus, Pile-wort, Figwort]^{G*+CD}

Centaury, Small [Lesser Centaury, Centory]^{GT*+CD}

Ceterach [Ceterach, Spleen-wort, Milt-wort, Lingua cervina, Scale fern, Stone fern, Asplenum]$^{GT*+CD}$

Chervil, Sweet [Myrrhis]$^{GT*+D}$

Christ's Thorne [Paliurus, Rhamnus, Ramme of Lybia, "Christ's thistle"]^{GD}

Cinquefoile [Cinkfoil, Cinqfoil, Five finger grass, Penta-phyllum]$^{GT*+CD}$

Clavers [*Clivers, Clivers artico, Tri-folium pratense*]$^{GT*+CD}$

Clote burre [Burre dock, Burdock, Arcion, Lappa]$^{GT*+D}$

Colewort leaves [Brassica, Garden colewort, Curled garden cole, Red colewort, White (or red or open) cabbage cole, cabbage, Coleflorey, Cauliflower, Savoy cole, Parsely colewort, English sea colewort, Wild cole-wort]$^{G*+CD}$

Colts foot [Horse foot, Tussilago, *coltsfoot*]^{G*CD}

Comfrey [*Great Comfrey*, Consilida, Symphytum, Great Confound^G]$^{GT*+CD}$

Common sweet cane ["The false adul-terated sweet Cane, a kinde of Corn-flag"]

Coriander [Coriandrum]^{GTD}

Corraline [Muscus marinus, Curraline, Corrallina*, = Coral moss; "Sea moss, that is Corralline"^{G}]^{G*D}

Cotton-weed [Gnaphaliion, Centuncu-lus, Cotton-weed, Cud-weed, Chaffe-weed, Petty cotton]^{GTD}

Cowcumber leaves^D

Crow-foot [Butter-flower, Ranunculus, King Kob, Gold cups, Gold knobs]^{GTD}

Crow garlick [Allium sylvestre]^D

Cyprus [Cypress, Cupressus] leaves^{GT+D}

Darnel [Lolium sp.]^{GTD}

Darnel, red [Phenix, Lolium rubrum, Great Darnell Grass]^{GTD}

Darnel, wild [(?) Darnel-grass-Gramen Sorghinum^G]

Devil's-bit [Morsus diabili, Pycnoco-mum]$^{GT*+CD}$

Dittander [Pepper wort, Lepidum, Dithander]$^{GT+CD}$

Dittony [Dittony leaves, Dictamnus]^{GT*CD}

Dodder [Epithymum]$^{GT*+CD}$

Dove's foot, Herb [Cranes-bill, Gera-nium columbinum^G, Geranium Herb Robert(?)]$^{G+D}$

Dragon^{GTCD}

Egrimony [Agrimony, Eupatorium]$^{G*+D}$

Elder [*Elder leaves, Sambucus*]$^{GT*+CD}$

Elme tree [Ptelea]^{GTCD}

Endive [Succory, Endive leaves]$^{GT+CD}$

Elecampane [Enula campane, Elicam-pagne]^{GT*CD}

Fennel [brown Fennel, red Fennel, Fennel spout, sweet red Fennel, Marathrum, Fœniculum]$^{GT*+CD}$

Fennel, wild [Marathrum sylvestre, Hippomarathrum, Fœniculum erraticum]$^{D(III.82)}$

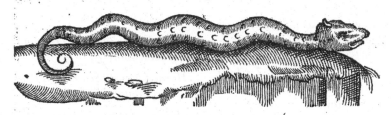

Hæmorrhoi serpentis effigies.

De Serpente seps dicto. **C A P. X V I I I.**

The Serpent called Emourrous

Fenugreek^GTD

Ferula [fennel giant]^GTD

Feverfew [Parthenium, Matricaria, Fedderfew, Featherfew or Fever-few]^GT*+CD

Fig-tree leaves^GD

Fleawort [Psyllium]^TGD

Garden cresses [Nasturtium hortense, N. hispanicum, N. latifolium, N. Petrœum]^GT+D(II.185)

Germander [Chamaedrys, Trissago major]^GT*+CD

Germander, Great [Teucrium, Tree Germander, Hungary Germander, Great Austrian Germander, Dwarf Rock Germander, Spanish Tree Germander, Rough headed Tree Germander]^GD

Glaux ["a kinde of Cytisus, or milke trefoile", Cytisus (8 kinds are noted in Gerard)]^GD

Great Water Parsenep [Sium maius latifolium]^GD

Ground pine [Herb-Ivy, Chamæpitys, Forget-me-not, Field Cypress]^G t+CD*

Gum succory [Chondrilla, Rysshe Succorie, Cichorion, Seris (Dios. II.161] leaves^GD

Hare foot trefoile [Lagopus, Harefoot]^GD

Harts-horn [Cornu ceruinum, Herbe Ivy, Herb Eve, Buckthorn^C]^G+CD

Harts-tongue [Phyllitis]^GT*+CD

Haver-grasse [Oats, Aigilops=Ægilops or Wild Oats]^GD

Hawk-weed [Hieracium majus=Great Hawk-weed, H. minus=Small Hares Hawk-weed= Yellow Devil's Bit, H. nigrum=Black Hawk-weed, H. Aphacoides= Succory Hawk-weed, H. intibaceum=Endives Hawk-weed, H. longius radicatum= Long-rooted Hawk-weed, H. asperum=Sharp Hawk-weed, H. falcatum Lobelij=Crooked Hawk-weed, H. falcatum alterum=The other crooked Hawk-weed, H. Latifolim montanum=Broad-leaved mountain Hawk-weed, H. montanum Latifolim minus=Lesser broad-

leaved mountain Hawk-weed]$^{TG+D}$

Hawk-weed, Clusius [Hieracium primum latifolium Clusij=First Hawk-weed of Clusius, H. 5. Clusij, H. 6. Clusij, H. 7. Clusij, H. parvum Creticum=Small Candy Hawk-weed, H. Dentis leonis folio hirstutum=Dandelion Hawk-weed]^{GD}

Heath [Hather [heather], Linge, Erica sp.]^{TGD}

Hellebore, black [True black hellebore, Wilde black hellebore, Great Ox-heel, Setter-wort, Bearfoot, Predalian, Lyon's claw, Black Master-wort=Black Hellebore of Dioscorides]^{GTD}

Hellebore, wild white [Epipactis recentiorum, Epipactis, Helleborine, Narrow-leafed wild neesewort]^{GD}

Hemlock [*white Hemlock, Herb Bennet, Homlock, Kexe*]$^{GT*+CD}$

Henbane [Hyoscyamus]^{G*CD}

Herb eve [Harts horn, Herb Ivie that is Buckes horne Plantaine^{G}]$^{G+CD}$

Herb-grace [Herb-grace that is Rue^{G}]$^{GT+*CD}$

Herb-Mastick [Marum]$^{G*+CD}$

Herb Patience [Sharp-pointed Dock, Lapathum acutum]$^{G*+D}$

Hisope [Hysop, Hyssop]$^{G*+CD}$

Holly-rose [Cistus]^{D}

Horehound [White Horehound, Marrubium]$^{GT*+D}$

Horehound, Stinking [Black Horehound, Marrubium niger, Ballota]$^{GT*+D}$

Horse foot [Colts-foot, Tussilago, coltsfoot]^{G*CD}

Horned poppy [Sea Poppy, Papaver cornutum]^{GD}

Horse-tail [Shave-grass, Polygonon]^{GTD}

Horse-tongue [Hippoglossum, Double-tongue, Tongue-blade, Laurel of Alexandria, Daphne Alexandrina, Laurus Alexandrina]$^{GT+D}$

Hounds-tongue [Hounds pisse, Cynoglossum]$^{G*+D}$

House-leek [*houseleek*, Sedum magnum, Sempervivum magnum, houseleek or sengreen^{+}]$^{GT*+CD}$

Indian-leaf [Malabathrum, Tamalapatra, Tembul]$^{G*+D}$

Ivy [Hedera] leaves^{G+D}

Juniper leaves^{D}

Knee-holme [Ruscus, Bruscus, Butcher's broom]^{GTD}

Knot grasse [Polygonum, Swine's grass, Bird's tongue]$^{GT*+C}$

Ladies navell [Umbilicis veneris, Navel wort, Wall penniwort, Penniwort, Hipwort, Kidneywort, Scatum cœli, Scatellum, Wall penny grass]$^{GT*+D}$

Larkspur, wild [Delphinium, Consolida regalis, Wild Larks heel, Wild Larks toes, Wild Larks claw]$^{GT+D}$

Laserwort [Laserpitium]^{GD}

Leeks [Headed or Set Leeks, Cut or Unset Leeks, Porrum, Porrus]^{GT+D}

Leeks, Wild [Ampeloprason, Porrum vitium, Vine Leek, French Leek]^{GTD}

Lettice [Latuca]^{GT*+CD}

Lilly leaf,^{GT*+CD}

Lions-leaf [Lions turnip, Leontopetalum, Leontopetalon (root^G)]^D

Liverwort [Hepatica, liver-wort, Bruon, Bryon, Lichen, Muscus]^{GT*+CD}

Long wort [Longwort is Pellitory of Spain^G]^{GCD}

Madwort [Galen's Madwort, Dioscorides' Madwort, Dioscorides' Moonwort, Alyssum, Healdog]^{GD}

Maidenhair, Black [Adiantum, Maydenhair, Polytricon, Capillis veneris, Venus hair, Black Maidenhair, Common Maidenhair, English Maidenhair=Trichomanes mas]^{GT*+CD}

Maidenhair [White maidenhair, Wallrue, Ruta muraria]^{GCD}

Maidenhair [see also Ladies' Bedstraw=Gallium, Gallion, Cheeserenning, Maid's hair, Maidenhair, pety Mugwort, wild Madder] flowers^{GTC}]

Mallowes [Malva, Hortensis, Mallow leaves, Mallow stalk]^{GT*+CD}

Mandragore [Mandrake, Mandragon, Mandrage]^{GT*+D}

Marjerom, great [Great Sweet Marjerom, Amaracus, Samsuchum]^{GCD}

Marjerom, Sweet [Great Sweet Marjerom]^{GCD}

Marsh mallows [Moorish Mallow, Marish Mallow, Althea, Alcea]^{GT*+D}

Mastick-tree, leaves of [Lentiske, Lentiscus]^{G*D}

Maydenhair, (Black or Common) [Maidenhair, Polytricon, Capillis veneris, Venus hair, Black Maidenhair, Common Maidenhair, English Maidenhair = Trichomanes mas]^{GT*+CD}

Meadow Parsenep [Cow Parsnep, Madnep, Sphodylium, Spondilium]^{GTD}

Meadow saffron [Colchicum ephemerum] leaves^D

Mellilot [Plaister Claver, Hart's Claver, Assyrian Claver, Italian Claver, Kings Claver, German Claver, Sertula campana, *melilot, mellilot herbs, mellilote*]^{GT*+CD}

Mercury, Dogs [Cynocrambe, wild Mercury]^{GD}

Milk trefoile [Cytisus, Shrub trefoile, Tretrifoly]^{GTD}

Milk-wort [Polygala, Cross flower, Gang week, Gang-flower, Procession-flower, Rogation week, Rogation-flower, vulgarly called "Hedge hyssop"]^{GD}

Mint [Mentha, Hedyosmus]^{GT*+CD}

Mint, water [Eduosmon agrion, Mentastrum, Mentha aquatica][GT+CD]

Mirtle [Myrtus] leaves[GT*+D]

Misseltoe [Viscum, Missel][GD]

Mock-privet [Phyllyrea][GD]

Moon-fearne [Moone-Ferne, Mule's Fern, Hemionitis][GD]

Morel [Solanum hortense, solanum nigrum, Strumum, Morrel, garden nightshade][GT*+CD]

Morsus diabili herb [Devil's-bit[G]][G*+CD]

Mosse of trees [e.g. moss of a Crab tree, Muscus][G*+D]

Mothweed, Golden [Helichryson, Elyohryson, Gold-flower, Golden mothwort][GD]

Mother time [Mother of time, Wild time, Serpillum][GT+CD]*

Mousear [Auricula murie, Pillosella][GT*+CD]

Mugwort [Artemesia][GT*+CD]

Mulberry [Morus] leaves[GD]

Mullein [Mullein, Woolen, Higtaper, Torches, Long-wort, Bullockes Long-wort, Hareweed, Tapsus barbatus, Mullin][G+D]

Mullein bearing yellow flowers [Male mullein, Woolen, Higtaper, Torches, Long-wort, Bullockes Long-wort, Hareweed, Tapsus barbatus, Mullin][G+D]

Mullein, Æthiopian [Æthiopus, Woolly Mullein][GD]

Nayle-wort [Whitlow grass, White low-grass, Paronychia sp.][GD]

Nettles [Urtica sp.][G*+CD]

Nightshade [Solanum hortense, Strumum, Solanum nigrum. Garden nightshade, morel, morrell][GT**CD]

Oak fernes [Petty fern, Mosse-Fern, Bryopteris, Dryoperis, Querna filix][G+D]

Oak of Jerusalem [Oak of Cappadocia, Oak of Paradise, Botrys][GT+D]

Orage [Orach, All seed, Atriplex, Aureum Olus][GSTCD]

Organie [Organy, Wild Marjerome, Bastard Marjerome, Grove Marjerome, Origanum][GT+CD]*

Organie, Goats [Goats Marjerome, Tragoriganum][GD]

Orkanet [Alkanet, Wild Bugloss, Anchusa][GD]

Orpine [Liblong, Live long, Crassula, Arsenicke, Telephium][G*+CD]

Oxe-eye [Buphthalmum][TD]

Palma Christi [Satyrion Royall=Finger Orchis (for roots[G, p.221]),Ricinis=Kik (for seeds[G, p.496])][D](Ricinis)

Parsley [*Parsly, Parslye, garden Parsley, mead Parsley, Petrosilinum*][GT+CD]

Pellamountain [Poley, Polium sp., Leucas][GT*+D]

Pellitory of Spain [*Pelitory of Spain*, Bertram, Pyrethrum][GCD]

Pellitory of the wall [Parietariam, Helxine parietaria, pellitory of the wal, pellitory on the wall, Wall pellitory, Sideritis][GT*+CD]

Penniroyal [Pudding grass, Pulliał
Royal, Pulegium,
Peniroyal]^{GT*+CD}

Peony [Pæonia, Aglaophotis] leaves^{CD}

Periwinkle [Clematitis]^{GT*+CD}

Petty morral [Morrell or petie Morrel,
that is Nightshade^G]^{GT*+CD}

Pimpernel^{GT*+CD}

Pine tree [Pinus] leaves^D

Pitch tree [Picea] leaves^{GD}

Plantain [Plantane, Plantago]^{GT*+CD}

Plow-mans Spikenard [Baccharis]^{GCD}

Poley [Pellamountain, Polium sp.,
Leucas]^{GT*+D}

Polypodie [*Ladies Dispensatory* uses
this term as a synonym for Oak
fern. A similar confusion of
names cited in Gerard (1633) p.
1134, Ceterach is described as
polypodium in Dioscorides]^{G+D}

*Poppy leaves [Garden Poppy (black
and white); Papaver
album/nigrum]^{GT*+CD}*

*Privet leaves [Prim Print, Print,
Ligustrum, Phillyrea]^{GTCD}*

*Purslaine [Purslane, Porcelane, Por-
tulaca]^{GT*+CD}*

*Ramne thorn [Harts Thorn,
Ramnum]^{G*+CD}*

Rocket [Eruca sp.]^{GT+CD}

Rose-leaves [*red Rose leaves*]^{G*CD}

Rosemary [Rosmarinus,
Libanotis]^{GT*+CD}

Rubarb^{GC}

Rue [*green Rew*, Rewe, Herb Grace,
Ruta sp., Harmala]^{GT*+CD}

Sage [Elaphoboscon, Salvia offici-
nalis, brown Sage, red Sage,
vertue Sage, wild sage]^{GT*+CD}

Saint Johns Wort [Hypericum, Saint
John's Grass]^{GT*+D}

Saint Peters Wort [Ascirum, Ascyron,
Square or Great St. Johns grass,
Hardhay, Androsæmum]^{GD}

*Samphire [Empetrum (LD note),
Crithmon, Herniaria, Herba
Turca, Rupture wort,
Burstwort]^{G+CD}*

*Savine [Savin, Garden Savin, Cypress
of Candy, Barren Savin, Sabina
sterilis, Savine bearing berries,
Sabina baccifera, Brathus]^{GT*+CD}*

*Savory, summer [Thumbra, Satureia
hortensis astiva]^{GT*+CD}*

Saxifrage [Saxiphragum]^{GT*+CD}

*Saxifrage, small [Tragium, Small Bur-
net Saxifrage, Small Burnet, Bipinella, Saxifraga minor]^{G*+CD}*

Scabious [Stœbe]^{GT*+CD}

Scale fearn [Scale fern, Stone fern,
Scolopendra, Spleen wort, Milt-
waste, Asplenum, Lingua cervina,
Ceterach]^{GT*+CD}

Scallions [Ascalonitides]^{GTD}

Scolopendria [Scale fern, Stone fern,
Scolopendra, Spleen wort, Milt-
waste, Asplenum, Lingua cervina,
Ceterach]^{GT*+CD}

Sciatica cresses [Iberia]^{G+D}

Scammony [Scammonia, Diagridy,
Rhasis, Coriziola]^{G*+CD}

*Scorpion's grass [Scorpioides, Myoso-
tis scorpioides, Caterpillers]^{GCD}*

Sea navell-wort [Androsace, Sea navell]GD

Sea-pimpernel [Sea ground pine, Anthyllis lentifolia]GD

Sea-pimpernel, second kind of [Many flowered ground pine, Stinking ground pine, Anthyllis marina, Anthyllis altera Italiorum]GD

Sea-Purslaine [Halimus] leavesGTD

Sea rushes, tender leaves growing at bottom of

Seselios of Candy [Harte-wort of Candy, Seseli Creticum sp., Tordylion]GD

Seselios of Marseilles [Seseli Massiliense]GD

Sison [Bastard stone parsley, Stone parsley of Macedonia]GTD

Smallage [Marsh parsley, Water parsley, Elcosclinum, Paludiapium]GT*+CD

Solomons seale [Polygonatum, Sigillum Salomonis]G*+CD

Southern-wood [Sowthernwood, Abrotanum]GT*+CD

Sow-bread [Cyclamen]GT

Sow-fennel [Peucedanum, Horestrange, Horestrong, Sulphurwort, Brimstone wort, Hogs Fennel]GD

Sow-thistle [Sonchus, Hares thistle, Hares colewort, Cicerbita]GT*+CD

Sneesing-wort [Ptarmica, Pyrethrum sylvestre, Pyrus sylvestre, Wild Pellitory, Bastard Pellitory, Field Pellitory]G*+CD

Sparagus [Sperage, Asparagus] (shoots)GTCD

Speedwel [=vervain in SP, Veronica]G*+CD

Spider-wort [Phalangium]GD

Spikenard [Nardus sp., Mountain set-wall]GTCD

Spikenard, Celtic [Nardus Celtica]GTD

Spikenard, French [Nardus narbonensis]G

Spikenard, Mountain [Nardus montana]GD

Spleen-wort [Scale fern, Stone fern, Scolopendra, Spleen wort, Miltwaste, Asplenum, Lingua cervina, Ceterach]GT*+CD

Spleen-wort [Lonchitis aspera (Gerard), Rough Spleen-wort], leaves of the second kind ofG

Spurge, petty [Exula rotunda, Peplus]GT+CD

Spurge-laurel [Daphnoides, Laureola, little Laurel, Daphnel leavesGT*+CD

Squinanth [Camel's Hay, Schœnanthum, Iuncus odoratus]G+*D

Staphis-acre [Staves acre, Staphis agria, Louse-wort, Lousepowder]GTCD

Star-wort [Aster atticus, Sharewort, Eubonium, Inguinalis, Asterion]G*+CD

Stinking trefoile [Treacle claver, Trifolium asphalteum, Trifolium bitumenosum Asphalteum, Bitumen] leavesG

Vermis in inteſtinis geniti & excluſi effigies.

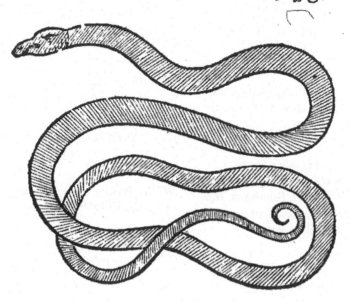

Long worms

Stinking bean trefoile [Anagyris fœtida, Laburnum]^GD

Succory [Endive, Cichorium sp., Intybus sp.]^GT*+CD

Sumack [Rhus Coriaria, Rhus myrtifolia, Coggyria Theophrasti, Venice Sumach, Cotinus Coriarius, Red Sumach] leaves^GD

Swallow-wort [Asclepias], leaves of^GD

Sweet cane [Acorum, Acoris, Sweet-smelling Reed, Aromatical Reed, Calamus aromaticus]^D

Tarre [Tare. Vetch, Fetch, Vicia sp., Lathyrus sylvestris, Black Milk Tare=Glaux of Dioscorides]^GTC

Time [garden Time, running Time^G, standing Time, unset Time]^GT+CD*

Trefoile [Common trefoile, Three-leafed grass, Meadow trefoile, Suckles, Honey-suckles, Cocks-heads, Shamrocks, Trifolium]^GT+CD

Turn-soile [Heliotropium, Tornsole] leaves^GD

Tutsan Saint John's wort [Androsæmon, Tutsan, Park-leaves], leaves of^GD

Valerian [Valeriana sp, Capons tail, Setwal]^GT+CD*

Verveine [Vervain, Verbena communalis (first kind), Verbena sacra (second kind)], Juno's tears, Mercuries moist blood, Holyherbe, Pigeon-grass, Columbine (by some)]^GT*+CD

Vine *[Vitis vinifera, Vitis sylvestris, Grape vine, Raisin vine] leaves and branches*[GT+CD]

Violet [Sweet Violet, Ion, Viola odorata], leaves[GT*+CD]

Viper's-Buglosse Echium vulgare][G+D]

Wall pellitory [Pellitory of the wall, Parietariam, Helxine parietaria, pellitory of the wal, pellitory on the wall][GT*+CD]

Wall penni-wort [Ladies navell, Umbilicis veneris, Navel wort, Wall penniwort, Penniwort, Hipwort, Kidneywort, Scatum cœli, Scatellum, Wall penny grass][GT+D]*

Wall-wort [Dane-wort, Dwarf elder, Ebulus, Sambucus humilis, Symphitum petreum][GT+D]*

Water betony[GD]

Water mints [Sisymbrium, also called 'water cresses']][GT+C]

Water-cresses [*watercresses, Nasturtium aquaticum*][G*+D]

Water germander [Scordium, Garlick germander][G+D]*

Widdow-waile [Chamelea, Spurge Olive, Mezereon][G+D]*

Wild bastard thistle [Colus agrestis, Atractylis, Colus Rustica, Fusus agrestis, Cnicus sylvestris, Ardactyla, Sylvestris Carthamus, Wild Bastard Saffron, Spindle Thistle][GD]

Wild Lettice [Thridax agria, Latuca sylvestris][GT+D]

Wild olive tree [Agrielaia, Olea Oleaster] leaves[GD]

*Wild pear tree [Pyrus sylvestis/stranulatorium, pedicularia/Corvina, Choke pear tree, wild hedge pear tree, Wild crab pear tree, Lowsie wild pear tree, Crow pear tree] leaves**

Wild rue [Ruta sylvestris, Harmala][GCD]

Wild time [Serpillum, Pullial Mountain, Pella mountaine, Running time, Creeping time, Mother of time][GT+CD]*

Willow [Withy, Salix, Sallow] leaves[GT*+CD]

Willow-herb, yellow [Lysimachia lutea, Loose strife, herb Willow][GT+CD]

Wind-flower [Anemone][GCD]

Winter cresses [Pseudobunium, Barbarea, herb Saint Barbara][GD]

Withy [Willow, Sallow, Salix] leaves[GT*+CD]

Woad [Isatus sativa, Garden: Glastum savitum, Wild: Glastum sylvestre][G+CD]

Worm-seed-wort [Sementina, Holy Wormewood][G]

Wormwood [wormewood, French Wormwood, Roman Wormwood, Romane Wormwood, Absinthium][GT*+CD]

Yarrow or Nose-bleed Yarrow [Nose-bleed, Millefolium, Common Yarrow (purple or white flowers), Red Yarrow, Milfoile, Thousand leaf][G*+CD]

Yarrow, Achilles [Achillea, Millefolium nobile][GCD]

Flowers

All-heale, Esculapius [Panaces Aesculapij][GD]

Asphodil flowers[D]

Broome [Spartium] flowers, Spanish[G*+CD]

Colewort flowers [Brassica, Garden colewort, Curled garden cole, Red colewort, White (or red or open) cabbage cole, cabbage, Cole-florey, Cauliflower, Savoy cole, Parsely colewort, English sea colewort, Wild colewort][G*+CD]

Feverfew flowers[D]

Heath flowers [Hather [heather], Linge, Erica sp.][TGD]

Holly-rose [Cistus][GTD]

Ivie [Ivy, Hedera] flowers[D]

Labruske [Labrusca, Vitis sylvestris, Vitis vinifera sylvestris, Brionia nigra, Wild Vine, Wild grape Vine, Black briony[GT]*; also, Viornia =Traveller's Joy =Vitis sylvestris of Dioscorides*[G]*] flowers*[D]

Ladies' Bed-straw [Gallium, Gallion, Cheese-renning, Maid's hair, Maidenhair, pety Mugwort, wild Madder] flowers[GTCD]

Marigold [*marygold*] flowers [Chrysanthemum= includes German Marigold, Corn Marigold][GT*+D]

Mullein [Mullein, Woolen, Higtaper, Torches, Long-wort, Bullockes Long-wort, Hareweed, Tapsus barbatus, Mullin] flowers[GD]

Oxe-eye flowers [Buphthalmum][GD]

Pimpernel, flowers of female [azure flower of Anagallis[D]*]*[D]

Pomegranat flowers[GD]

Pompion [Melons, Millions, Popon, Pepo sp., Pumpkin] flowers

Privet [Phillyrea, Ligustrum, Prim print, Print] flowers

Raspis-bush [Rubus Idæysm Framboise, Hindeberry], flowers of[G]

Rose flowers, red[GT*+CD]

Saffron[GT*+C]

Sneesing-wort [Ptarmica, Pyrethrum sylvestre, Wild Pellitory, Bastard Pellitory] flowers[D]

Spider-wort [Phalangium] flowers[GD]

Stinking trefoile [Treacle claver, Asphalteum, Bitumen] berries

Violets, Sweet [Violets, Violae, Ion, Viola odorata][GT*+CD]

Wall-flowers [Viola lutea, Wall gilloflower, Yellow stock gilloflower, Winter-gilloflower, Cheiri][GT*+CD]

Wild Pomegranat-tree flowers [Balastium][GD]

Woodbind [Honeysuckle, Periclymenum, Caprifoly] flowers[G+]

Fruits and Buds

Almonds, bitter[G*+TD]

Almonds, Jordan [or sweet; "long sweet almond, vulgarly termed Iordan almond"[GT]][D]

Apple, sweet[G+D]

Apple of Colliquintida [Coloquintida, or coloquint and his kinds^G; colo-cynthis]^{G*+D}

Arbute-berries [Arbutus or Strawberry tree]^{GD}

Bay berries^{G*+CD}

Briony berries^{GD}

Butcher's broom [Knee-holme, Ruscus, Bruscus] berries^{GTD}

Capers^{GT+D}

Cedar [Prickly cedar, Cedar Juniper] berries^{GD}

Cherries [Cerasum]^{G*+D}

Citrons [Pome citrons, Citrium malum, Malum Citrium, Malus medica]^{GT*+D}

Currans [*Berries of wild vines*]^{G*+CD}

Cyprus apples [fruit of Cypress tree, Pilulæ Cupressi, Nuces Cupressi, Galbuli, Nuces Cypressi, Cypress nuts or clogs, Cypresse pills]^{GT*+D}

Dates^{GT*+D}

Dates, Phenecian [fruit of Phoinix]^D

Dates, Thebane [fruit of Phoinix the-baikai]^D

Eglantine [Sweet briar, Rubis canis, Rosa syvestris odora, Kunosba-ton]^{GTD}

Figge^{GT*+CD}

Figs, burned^D

Figs, early ["The first figs which being too forward do not thrive"]^D

Galls [from Gall tree or Galla = oak galls^D]^{G*+D}

Goose-grease ["a small kinde of Burre"]

Hawthorn berries [Hawes, berry of Hawthorne^C, Oxyacanthus] ^{TG+C}

Hawes, berry of^{TG+C}

Ivy berries^{G+CD}

Juniper berries^{GT+CD}

Knee-holme [Ruscus, Bruscus, Butcher's broom] berries^{GTD}

Mandragore apples [Mandrake, Man-dragon, Mandrage]^{G*+D}

Medlars [fruit of Three grain Medlar, Neapolitan Medlar, Medlar of Naples, Mespilus sativa]^{GT**CD}

Mirtle [Myrtus] berries^{GD}

Mulberries [Morus, Mora[um] celsi], green^{G*+D}

Mulberries [Morus, Mora[um] celsi], ripe^{G*+D}

Mothweed, Golden [Helichryson, Ely-ohryson, Gold-flower, Golden mothwort], tops of^{GD}

Mountain horse-foot [Cacalia] berries^D

Olives, yellow^{G*+D}

Pears [Pirus sp., Pirum]^{GT+D}

Peony berries^{GCD}

Pepper, brown [prob. black pepper, Piper nigrum^{GT*+CD}]

Pepper, Long [Piper longus^{GT*+C}]

Pepper, white [Piper album]^{GT*+CD}

Pine apples [Pine cones, Strobili]^{G*+D}

Pistacho [Pistachia, Nux vesicaria, St. Anthonies nuts]^{G*D}

Pomegranat shell [pomegranat pill (peel)]^{G+CD}

Pompions [Melons, Millions, Popon, Pepo sp., Pumpkin]^{GT*CD}

Poplar tree, little balls when they begin to bud—pillulae [Poplar buds]^{GCD}

Poppy heads [Garden Poppy (black and white); Papaver album/nigrum]$^{GT*+CD}$

Quince^{GT*+CD}

Sharp-pricking Ivy [Hedera spinosa, Smilax aspera (or lenis)=Rough Bindeweed^G] berries^D

Sloes [Wild plums, fruit of Prunus sylvestris]$^{GT+D}$

Small Sea-grape [Tragus, Vua marina minor, Sea-Cluster, Sea Raison]^{GD}

Spurge flax [Thymelæa, Mountain Widow Waile, Granum Gnidum] berries, inward part of^{GD}

Sycamore [Sycomorus] berries^{GCD}

Turpentine tree [Terebintha] berries [Granum viride]^{GD}

Wall-nuts [Walnuts, Nux Regia, Kingly Nut, Nux Iuglans, Jupiters Acorn, Iuvans glans, Helping Acorn, Persica Nux, Persian nuts, Walsh nut]$^{GT*+CD}$

Wall-nut shells, ashes of^D

Wild pears [Achras, Choke pear, Wild crab pear, Wild hedge pear, Lowsie wild pear, Crow pear]^{GD}

Wild poppy heads [Red Poppy, Cornerose, Papaver sylvestre]$^{GT+CD}$

Wild rose [Eglantine, Sweet briar, Briar rose, Hep tree, Pimpinell rose, Dogs rose, Dogs Thorn] buds^D

Wild Vine [Vitis sylvestris] berries [Currants]$^{G*+CD}$

Winter cherries [Solanum Halicacabum, Halicacabum Peregrinum, Cor Indum/Indicum, Indian heart, Heart pease]^{GD}

Seeds

Acacalis ("The seed of an herb growing in AEgypt, much like the seed of Tamarisk."^{G})^D

Acorns [Balanoi]^{GD}

Acorns, innermost skin of^{GD}

Agnus castus [Chaste Tree] seeds^{*D}

All-heale [Hercules wound-wort, Panax heraculanum]^{GD}

All-heale, Esculapius^{GD}

Ameos [*Ammeos*], seed of [Ammi, Bishop's Weed^C]$^{G*+CD}$

Amomum [stone parsley of Macedonie] seeds^{G+CD}

Anniseeds [*Annis*]$^{G*+T}$

Asp tree seeds [Aspen, a poplar^G]

Asphodil seeds^D

Bank-cresses [Erysimum], seed of^{GTD}

Barley [French Barley]$^{*+D}$

Basil seeds^{+D}

Basil [Clinopodium in LD] seeds, wild

Bastard Saint John's wort [Coris], seed of$^{G (p. 544)D}$

Baulme seeds [Balm; Melissa, Apiastrum]

Beans [Greek bean, Kuamos hellenikos, peason]^{GTCD}

Beans, Ægyptian^G, meal of [Phaseolus Ægyptiacus]^D

Beans, French [Kidney bean, Phaseolus sp., Smilax hortensis sp.]^{GD}

The figure of a certaine kind of Aconite.

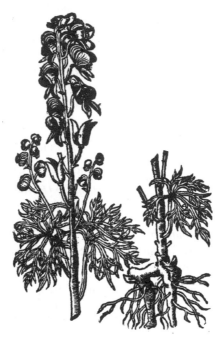

A second species of Aconite

Bean flower [flour ground from beans^C]

Bean meal^D

Binde-weed, seed of Great [Binde-weed Nightshade; Inchanter's Nightshade, Circæa; Gerard (p.351); "there is no vse of this herbe either in physicke or Surgerei that I can reade of"]^D

Box-thorne seeds^D

Briony seeds

Broome [Spartium] seeds, Spanish^{G+CD}

Buglosse seeds^D

Bull-rush seeds [Iuncus aquaticus maximus]^{GD}

Candy Alexander [Smyrnium or Thorow bored Parsley] seeds^{GD}

Caraway seeds [*Carum, carraway seeds, caraway*]^{GT*+CD}

Carob beans [Keratia, Siliquae]^{GD}

Coriander seeds [*Coriander*]^{G*+D}

Carrot, yellow, seeds of^{G*+D}

Chameleon thistle seeds [Crocodilium, Crocodilion, Carduus niger, "the Thistle that changeth it selfe into many shapes and colours"^G]^D

Chesnuts, inner skin/rind of [Chestnut, Castanea[GD]]

Christ's Thorne [Paliurus, Rhamnus, Ramme of Lybia, 'Christ's thistle'; seed of Paliurus (jujube) listed in Dioscorides[D,]][G]

Ciches [Cicer, Common Ciche, Ram Ciche, Black or Red Ciche, Sheepes Ciche Pease/Peason, Chich-pease][G*+D]

Clote burre [Burre dock Burdock, Arcion, Lappa], seed of small[GT*+]

Colewort seeds [Brassica, Garden colewort, Curled garden cole, Red colewort, White (or red or open) cabbage cole, cabbage, Cole-florey, Cauliflower, Savoy cole, Parsely colewort, English sea colewort, Wild colewort][G+D]

Columbine [Isopyrum (of Dioscorides [G. pp. 1095, 1194])] seeds[GTD]

Coventrie-bells, Blew [Medium, the term in The Ladies Dispensatory is in error according to Gerard[G, p. 448], Viola mariana is Gerard's term; root of Medium is found in Dioscorides Book IV.18], seed of[D]

Cowcumber, Garden [Cucumber], seed of[GT+]

Cumin seeds [Commin, Cuminum sativum, Cyminum][G*+D]

Cummin, Ethiopian [Cuminum sativum from Ethiopia][D]

Cummin, wild [Cuminum sylvestre][GD]

Darnel [Lolium] meal[GT+D]

Devil's-bit [Morsus diabili, Pycnocomum] seed[D]

Dill seeds[G*+CD]

Egrimony [Agrimony, Eupatorium] seeds[GD]

Ethiopian Reed [Æthiopian Reed, Aethiopical Iuncus, form of Dioscorides' Iuncus (IV.52)] seeds[D]

Fennel seed [Fennelseeds][GT*+CD]

Fennel giant seeds [ferula][GTD]

Fenugreek seed [Fenicreek][GT*+CD]

Fenugreek, meal of[GD]

Garden cresses, seed of[G*D]

Gith [Nigella romana, Melanthium][G*+D]

Hemp [Cannabis]seeds[GD]

Hen-bane seeds [Hyoscyamus][GT*+D]

Horned poppy [Sea Poppy, Papaver cornutum] seed[GD]

Jacynth seeds [Iacynth, Hyacinth, Hyacinthus][GD]

Leek seed[GTD]

Lentils [Lens major, Lens minor][GT*+D]

Lettice seed[G+D]

Linseed [flax seed, Linum seed][G*+CD]

Lovage [Lygusticum, Levisticum][G*+D]

Lupine [flat bean called lupine, Garden Lupine, Tame Lupine, Figbean, Lupinus, Thermos], meal of[GT*+D]

Mallows, seed of[D]

Mandragore [Mandrake, Mandragon, Mandrage], seed of[D]

Marsh mallows, seed of[GD]

Meadow Parsenep [Cow Parsnep, Madnep, Sphodylium, Spondilium] seed[GTD]

Millet [Milium][GTD]

Mirtle seeds

Mountain siler [Siler mountaine, Bastard Lovage] seed[GTD]

Mustard seed [Sinapi sp.][GT*+C]

Nettles [Urtica], seeds [tops] of[G*+CD]

Oats [Oaten bran, Oatmeal, Oatmeal grets, Avens, Avena][G+CD]

Palma Christi seed [Satyrion Royall=Finger Orchis (for roots[G, p.221]), Ricinis=Kik (for seeds[6, p.496])][GD]

Pine apple kernel [Pituides, pityides, pine cone kernels][GCD]

Peony seed [Piony seed][G*+CD]

Plantain [Plantane, Plantago] seeds[G*+CD]

Pomegranat kernels[GD]

Pompions [Melons, Millions, Popon, Pepo sp., Pumpkin], seeds of[G*CD]

Poppy seeds[G*+CD]

Purslaine [Purslane, Porcelane, Portulaca] seeds[GT*+C]

Radish [Rabone, Raphanus, Sativa Radicula] seeds[G*+D]

Rampions [Wild Bell Flowers, Rapunculus, Rapuntium, Erinus], seeds of[D]

Rice [Oryza sativa][GT+CD]

Rocket [Eruca sp.] seeds[G*+D]

Rose-campion seeds [Lychnis rubra, Lychnis coronaria][GD]

Rose-campion, wild, seeds [Lychnis sylvestris, Lychnis marina, Lychnis hirta, Lychnis caliculis][GD]

Rosemary [Rosmarinus] seed

Rue seeds[G*D]

Saint John's wort [Hypericum, Saint John's Grass], seed of[G*+D]

Saint Peters wort [Ascirum, Ascyron, Square or Great St. Johns grass, Hardhay, Androsæmum], seed of[GD]

Saxifrage, small [Tragium, Small Burnet Saxifrage, Small Burnet, Bipinella, Saxifraga minor] seed[G*D]

Scarlet grain [Scarlet berry, Coccus infectoria, Chesmes, Chermes, Kermes, Granum tinctorum sive Kermes, Coccus Baphicus][G*]

Sea Bull-rush seeds [Iuncus odoratus, Camel's hay, Squinanth, Squinants][GD]

Sesamum [Sesaminum, Sesami, Oily Pulse, Oily Grain, Turky Millet][GT*+]

Seselios of Marseilles [Seseli Massiliense] seeds[G*+D]

Seselios of Candy [Harte-wort of Candy, Seseli Creticum sp., Tordylion] seed[G*+D]

Sleepy nightshade [Dwale, Deadly night shade, Raging nightshade, Solanum somniferum, Solanum lethale, Solanum manicum], seed of[*[Semina Solanum sativum]]

Smallage [Mars parsley, Water parsley, Elcosclinum, Paludiapium] seed[D]

Southern-wood [Abrotanum] seeds-^{GTCD}

Sow-bread [Cyclamen hederifolium], seed of second kind of^{D(fruit)}

Spatling-poppy [Frothy Poppy, Polemonia, Spumeum Papaver, Behen album, White Ben] seeds

Spelt-corne [Zea, Spelta, Ador, Adoreum, Semen adoreum, Semen, Spelt Wheat, Rice-wheat, Greek Wheat]^{GT+D}

Spider-wort [Phalangium] seeds^{GD}

Spurge grains [Spurge seeds]^{G+CD}

Staphis-acre [Staves acre, Staphis agria, Louse-wort, Louse-powder] seeds^{G+*CD}

Stinking bean trefoile [Anagyris fœtida, Laburnum] seed^{GD}

Stinking Gladdon [Xyris], seed of^{GD}

Stinking trefoile [Treacle claver, Asphalteum, Bitumen] seeds^G

Sumack [Rhus Coriaria, Rhus myrtifolia, Coggyria Theophrasti, Venice Sumach, Cotinus Coriarius, Red Sumach] seeds^{G*+CD}

Treacle mustard [Thlapsi, Dish mustard, Bowyers Mustard, Churles mustard, Wild cresses] seed^{GTD}

Trefoile [Common trefoile, Three-leafed grass, Meadow trefoile, Suckles, Honey-suckles, Cocks-heads, Shamrocks, Trifolium], seed of^{CD}

Turnip [Rapum, Rape] seed^{G*+D}

Turn-soile [Heliotropium, Tornsole] seeds^{GD}

Tutsan Saint John's wort [Androœmon, Tutsan, Park-leaves], seed of^{GD}

Viper's-Buglosse^{GD}

Wall-flowers [Viola lutea, Wall gilloflower, Yellow stock gilloflower, Winter-gilloflower, Cheiri], seed of^D

Water-cresses [Nasturium aquaticum], seed of^{D*}

Water plantain [Limonium] seeds^D

Wild Turnip [Rapum sylvestre, Rapistrum sp.] seed^{GD}

Winter cresses [Pseudobunium, Barbarea, herb Saint Barbara] seeds^G

Wheat [*Wheat bran, wheaten bran, wheat flower/flour, Wheat flowers, wheat meal*]^{G+D}

White Thistle [Bedeguar, Spina alba, Lady thistle, Our Lady(ies) Thistle, Carduus lacteus, Carduus Mariæ, Leucographus, Milk Thistle] seeds^{GT+D}

Wild Lentils [(?) Dioscorides' Phasiolus (Book II, 130)]

Wild parsenep [Elaphoboscum, Pastinaca latifolia sylvestris, Mypes], seed of^{G+*D}

Wild poppy [Red Poppy, Corn-rose] seeds^D

Wild rue seeds^{*D}

Withiwind [Binde-weed, Hedge-bells, Convolulus, Smilax laevis]^{GT} *seed*^D

Woodbind [Periclymenum, Honey-suckle, Caprifoly] seed^{GCD}

Gums, Rosins

Æthiopian olive tree [wild olive tree, Cotinon], gum of [Dakruon elaias aithiopikes][D]

Aloes, Alloes sicatrina [a type of aloes yielding juice][GD] and Aloes hepatica[G*+TD]

Amilum [Amylum, Starch, white or Stirch, white[OED2]; Salmon p.949 (listed with Gums, Rosins and Balsams): "Amylum, *White Starch* . . . is made either out of *Wheat Bran* or *Wheat Meal*, by soaking it in water."][D(II.123)]

Amoniacum [*Armoniacum*, Gum from Herbe Ferula or Fennell Gyant[G]][GT+D]

Asa-foetida [Laser, sapor liquor from the roots of Laserpitium (Laserwort)[G]][G*+]

Bitter almond tree, gum of[D]

Bdelium*[+D]

Benzoin [Benjamin[OED2, Blancard]]*+

Birdlime [classified as a rosin[+, p.48]; dung of several birds listed in Dioscorides II.98]

Castorium [Euforbium castorium-gum from Euphorbia plant[G](?); Blancard: "'tis difficult to know what this is from foreigners; for our Merchants buy it of others, who have it from other countries. It comes from the Indies." See also Castoreum under Parts of Living Creatures][G+]

Cedar rosin ["Pitch of the Cedars of Greece"[+,p.48]][GD]

Cherry tree [Ceraus], gum of[GD]

Diagridy [=scammony[C]][G*+CD]

Dragon's blood [Sanguis draconis, a gum/rosin from the Dragon tree[G]][G*+D]

Eleomelie ["A sweet fat liquor issuing from the trunks of certaine trees in Syria."] (?)Elemni[*+]*[D]

Elme, liquor growing in certain purses upon[GD]

Euforbium castorium [gum from Euphorbia plant[G]][G+D]

Fig tree, milk of wild and garden[GD]

Frankinsence [*Frankisence, white*][G*D]

Galbanum ["Gum from Herbe Ferula, or Fennell Giant"[G]][G*+D]

Green pitch of Herb ferula [see amoniacum][D]

Gum of the Acacia tree[G] [gum arebeck][G*D]

Gum dragon [*Gum traganthum, Gumdragagant*; gum from Goats Thorne or Tragacantha[G]][G*D]

Gum lac [Gum lacca][G*+]

Gum sagapene ["It distills from a certain herb in Media", Serapinum, Sagapenum]*[+D]

Gum succory [Chondrilla, Rysshe Succorie, Seris, Condrilla (Dios. II. 161)], gum and milk of[GTD]

Hercules All-heale, gum of [Opoponax; a yellow gummy juice from the Hercules All-heale or Wound-wort[G, p.1003]][G*+D]

Labdanum [*Gums of labdanum*; Ladanum*; "There be divers sorts of Cistus [Ledon], whereof that gummy matter is gathered called in shops *Ladanum*, and *Lab-danum*, but vnproperly"[G, p. 1283], Gum cistus, Gum creticus][GT*+D]

Laser [Asa-foetida, sapor liquor from the roots of Laserpitium (Laser-wort)[G]][G+]*

Lees of vinegar [Foex of vinegar, Dios. V.132][D]

Lees of wine [Argall, Tartar, Tartarum][G+D]

Lees of oyle[+]

Lupines, sap of

Mastick [Gum of Mastick-tree][G+CD]*

Mulberry roots, gum of[D]

Myrrhe [Mirrh, Gum of mirrh, mir-rhe]*[+D]

Olive tree, gum of [Dakruon elaias][D]

Opium ["condensed iuice of Poppie heads"[G, p. 370 [misnumbered 400]]][G*+CD]

Opobalsamum [liquor flowing from Balsam tree=Balsami sp., Balsa-mum][G+D]

Pine tree rosin[D]

Pitch [Rosin of the Pitch tree, "Pitch of the Cedars of Greece"[+, p. 48]; Blancard: "*Colophonia*, Rosin-Pitch", p. 98; colophonia is the residue from distilling oil of tur-pentine[+]][G+D]

Pitch, soot of[D]

Plum tree gum[GCD]

Rosen ["Liquid and dry, rozin of firr tree, Larch tree, Pine tree"[+, p. 48]; Gesner: "Put .iiii pounde of Tur-pentin Rosin or larix in a larg crooked still" p. 29.][G+D]

Sanguis draconis [Dragon's blood, a gum/rosin from the Dragon tree[G]][G*+D]

Sarcocolla [Sarcacolla, "a bitter per-sian Gum" (LD)][+D]*

Serapinum ["It distills from a certain herb in Media", Gum sagapene, Sagapenum]*[+D]

Storax [*Storax cremitie*; Gum of the Storax tree[G, p. 1526]; Blancard: "see *Styrax*", p.323; Styrax calamita (resin)][G*+D]

Sugar [The iuyce of this Reed [sugar cane] is made the most pleasant and profitable sweet, called Sugar"[G, p. 38]][G+D]

Sycamore [Sycomorus] gum[GCD]

Tarre [(?)Stockholm tar=Pix liquida or Conum from fattest part of Pine or Pitch tree[D]]

Turpentine [*Best Turpentine, good Turpentine, Gore Turpentine, Ordinary Turpentine, Venice Tur-pentine*; Blancard: "*Terebinthina*, Turpentine; 'tis twofold, *Vulgar* and *Venetian*; the *Venetian* is also call'd *Chious* or *Cyprian*; the best is clear, pellucid, white and of a Glass-colour; it comes from *Chious, Cyprus, Libya* and many other places" pg. 335][G*+D]

Juices

Acacia, juice of[D]

All-heale [Hercules wound-wort], juice of[D]

Asphodil, juice of roots[GD]

Basil, juice of[D]

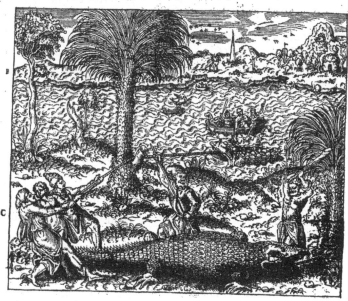

Jmago quæ Crocodilorum capturam oculis subiicit.

Crocodile

Basil, water, juice of

Bastard saffron [Cartamus, Carthamum, Mock saffron, Saffron d'orte], juice of seed of[G]

Bay-berries, juice of[D]

Baulme [Balm; Melissa], juice of[G]

Beets, juice of[D]

Box-thorne, juice of [Lycium, Licium][GD]

Bramble, juice of[GD]

Bramble-berries, juice of[GD]

Briony, juice of[GD]

Buck's horn [Coronopus], juice of

Calamint, juice of[G]

Caltraps (land or water), juice of[D]

Canary-grasse [Canary seed, Pety Panick, Phalaris], juice of[G]

Carrot, stinking deadly [Thapsia], juice of[D]

Carrot, stinking deadly [Thapsia], milk of

Celandine [Cellendine, Chelidonia], juice of[GD]

Clote burre [Burre dock Burdock], juice of[G]

Centaury, juice of Small[GD]

Chelidony [probably Great Celendine, Chelidonia, Gerard (p. 1070) states that juice sharpens vision], juice of[GD]

Cinquefoile [Cinkfoil, Cinqfoil, Five finger grass, Pentaphyllum], juice of[GD]

Cinquefoile [Cinkfoil, Cinqfoil, Five finger grass, Pentaphyllum] roots, juice of[GD]

Cinquefoile [*Cinkfoil, Cinqfoil, Five finger grass, Pentaphyllum*] *seed, juice of*

Coleworts, juice of[CD]

Cowcumbers, juice of [leaves of/ roots and rinds of] wild[GTD]

Dittany, juice of[GD]

Dragons, juice of the root of great[D]

Elme leaves, juice of

Fennel, juice of[D]

Fleawort [Psyllium], juice of[D]

Gentian roots, juice of

Goats-beard [Mead sweet, Trago-pogon[G]*], juice of*

Hawk-weed, juice of both kinds of [Hawk-weed, Clusius Hawk-weed, Hieracium sp.][D]

Hemlock, juice of[D]

Hemp [Cannabis], juice of[GD]

Hen-bane juice [Hyoscyamus][GD]

Hippophestus ["thought to be a kinde of Fullers Teasell", Hippophae-ston is Dioscorides IV.163], juice of[D]

Holly-rose, male [Cistus mas angusti-folius, Cistus mas cum Hypocis-tide], juice of [Hypocistus, grows about roots of Cistus][G*D]

Hore-hound, juice of[G]

Horse-tail [Shave-grass], juice of[G]

Ivie [Ivy, Hedera] berries, juice of[D]

Ivie [Ivy, Hedera] leaves, juice of[GD]

Juniper leaves, juice of[D]

Knot-grass [Polygonum, Swine's grass, Birds tongue], juice of[G]

Laserwort [Laserpitium], juice of

Leeks, juice of[GD]

Leek seed, juice of[D]

Licium [Lycium, Box-thorne], juice of[GD]

Lilly leaves, juice of[D]

Liquorice, juice of[GD]

Lupine, juice of

Madir [Madder] roots, juice of

Marsh mallows, juice of[G]

Mandragore [Mandrake, Mandragon, Mandrage], juice of[GD]

Mastick-tree, juice of[D]

Meadow Parsenep [Cow Parsnep, Madnep, Sphodylium], juice of flowers of[D]

Mellilot [Plaister Claver, Hart's Claver, Assyrian Claver, Italian Claver, Kings Claver, German Claver, Sertula campana, *melilot, mellilot herbs, mellilote*], juice of[GCD]

Mercury, juice of[GD]

Mints, juice of[D]

Mirtle-berries, juice of[G]

Mulberry [Morus] leaves, juice of[D]

Onions, juice of[GCD]

Organie, juice of[D]

Parsley, juice of[C]

Pellitory of the wall [Parietariam, Helxine parietaria, pellitory of the wal, pellitory on the wall], juice of[GCD]

Pimpernel [Anagallis], juice of[GCD]

Plantain [Plantane, Plantago], juice of[GCD]

Pomegranats, juice of[GTD]

Pomegranats, juice of sowre (sour)[GD]

Pompions [Melons, Millions, Popon, Pepo sp., Pumpkin], juice of the inner parts of[D]

Poppy juice [see Opium][G*+CD]

Purslaine [Purslane, Porcelane, Portulaca], juice of[GTD]

Rosemary [Rosmarinum], juice of roots and leaves of

Rue, juice of[CD]

Sage, juice of[C]

Saxifrage, small [Tragium, Small Burnet Saxifrage, Small Burnet, Bipinella, Saxifraga minor] juice of[GCD]

Scammony [Diagridy, Rhasis, Coriziola], juice of[D]

Shave-grass [Horse-tail], juice of[G]

Sleepy nightshade [Dwale, Deadly night shate, Raging nightshade, Solanum somniferum, Solanum lethale, Solanum manicum], juice of[GD]

Snake-weed [Bistorta sp., Britannica, Oisterloit, Passions], juice of[G]

Sope-wort [Bruise-wort, Saponaria, Struthium], juice of

Sow-bread [Cyclamen], juice of[GCD]

Sow-fennel, juice of[D]

Sow-thistle [Sonchus, Hares thistle, Hares colewort], juice of[GD]

Spurge, juice of[G]

Spurge, milk of [Caracias][G]

Spurge, milk of male

Spurge-laurel [Daphnoides, Laureola, little Laurel[GT*+]], juice of the leaves of

Spurge-time [Chamæsyce], juice of[G]

Sweet cane [Acorum, Acoris, Sweet-smelling Reed, Aromatical Reed, Calamus aromaticus], juice of[GD]

Sycamore [Sycomorus, juice[GCD]

Teasell [Virga pastoris, Dipsacus sp., Labrum Veneris, Carduus Veneris, Card Teasell, Venus Bason, Fuller's thistle] juice

Verjuice [Verjuyce; a condiment made with sour, acidic juice of unripe grapes, crab apples and other fruit[OED2]]

Vine [Vitis vinifera, Vitis sylvestris, Grape vine, Raisin vine] leaves, juice of[D]

Vinegar[+D]

Vinegar, honied[D]

Wall penni-wort [Ladies navell, Umbilicis veneris, Navel wort, Penniwort, Hipwort, Kidneywort, Scatum cœli, Scatellum, Wall penny grass], juice of[GD]

Water betony [Clymenon(?), Galiopsis ((?)], juice of[GD]

Water germander [Scordium], juice of[D]

Widdow-waile [Chamelea, Spurge Olive, Mezereon][G*+], juice of

Wild lettice, Milk [juice] of[GTD]

Wild olive leaves, juice of[GD]

Wild rue, juice of

Wild time [Serpillum, Pullial Moun-
tain, Pella mountaine, Running
time, Creeping time, Mother of
time], juice of^{GD}

Willow [Salix, Sallow, Withy]^G*, juice*
of leaves and bark of^D

Willow-herb, yellow [Lysimachia
lutea, Loose strife, herb Willow],
juice of^{GD}

Wind-flower [Anemone], juice of^{GCD}

Wormwood [Absinthium], juice of^{CD}

Plants [Plantarum Excrementa]

Agarick (fungus growing on Larch
tree)^{GT*+}

Living Creatures

Barbell, Great Sea [fish; Mullus bar-
batus (bearded mullet or goat-
fish?); Trigla]^D

Cantharides [described as a toxin,
appears as a drug^{+D}]

Cramp-fish

Crey-fish [River crabs, crayfish]^{+D}

Crey-fish [River crabs, crayfish],
ashes of^D

Cuttle fish, ashes of burned

Earth-wormes^{*+D}

Fork-fish

Frogs^{*+D}

Gudgeons [Kobios, Gobius niger]^D

Hedge-hogs⁺

Hens cleft alive^D

Larks^{+D}

Lizard^D

Mice^D

Muskles [Mussels]^D

Muskles [Mussels], ashes of^D

Punies ["a stinking worm so called"]

Purple-fish

Purple shell fish [Porphura;
Purpura]^D

Salamander^D

Scorpions^{*+D}

Seal-fish

Silurus [fresh water fish like
sturgeon]^D

Skink^D

Snayles^D

Spider^D

Swallowes, young [fledged]^{+D}

Tortoise⁺

Tunny-fish [Omotarichus]^D

Weesil^D

Weesil, powdered^D

Wood-lice [millipedes]^{*+D}

Worms found in Fullers thistle

Parts of Living Creatures

Asses dung^D

Asses grease

Asses hoof^D

Asses liver^D

Asses milk^D

Beaver stones^D

Bee wax^{*+D}

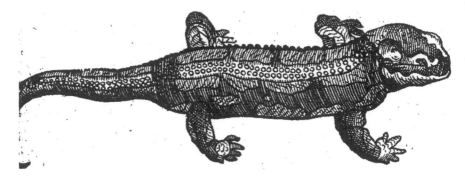

Salamander

Blood, bull's[+D]

Blood, dog[D]

Blood, hares[+D]

Blood, hart's[D]

Blood, he-goat's[+*D]

Blood of a Land Tortoise [Testudo][+D]

Blood, pigeon[+D]

Blood, ring-dove's

Blood of a Sea Tortoise[D]

Blood, she-goat's[+D]

Blood, stock-dove's

Blood, turtle-dove's

Blood, weesils[D]

Bonie excrescence growing on the Cronet of a Horses hoofe [Leichenes hippon; Spavins of horses][D]

Brains of hares[*D]

Buck skin

Butter[+D]

Butter, soot of [fuligo gathered out of butter][D]

Cackerell fish [Smaris[OED]*], head of*[D]

Calamarie fish shell

Castoreum[D]

Cockles[+]

Cobwebs[+]

Curd [rennet], hare's[+D]

Curd, hart's[D]

Curd, Sea-calfe's[D]

Dung, asses[D]

Dung, chickens [poultry dung[D]*]*

Dung, dog's[+D]

Dung, goat's[+D]

Dung, hens [poultry dung[D]*]*[+]

Dung, horses[D]

Dung of land crocodiles[D]

Dung, mans[+D]

Dung, mice[+D]

Dung, ox

Dung, pidgeons[+]

Dung of poultry[D]

Dung, rats, ashes of

Dung of a she-goat[D]

Dung, sheeps[D]

Dung of stock doves[D]

Dung, storks^D

Dung of wild she-goats^D

Eagle stone [stone found in nest of eagles]^D

Egg [egge]$^{+D}$

Eggs, hen's^{+D}

Eggs of land and sea tortoises

Eggs, pigeon's

Egg, reer [rear egg; rare egg; an undercooked egg(OED)]

Fat of a Fox^{*+D}

Gall of a bear^{+D}

Gall of a bull^{+D}

Gall of an eagle^D

Gall of a hind

Gall of a hogge$^+$

Gall, ox [*Oxe Gall*]

Gall, partridge's^D

Gall, pullet's

Gall of a Sea Hedge-Hog

Gall of a Sea Tortoise^D

Gall of a Sea Urchin

Gall, Scorpeno's ["A little dark green Fish found in the Marsellian Sea"; Scorpaena scrofa(?)]^D

Gall of a Tortoise^D

Gall of a white hen^D

Gall of a wild she-goat^{+D}

Gizern [gizzard], inner skin of chicken's$^+$

Gizern, cocks-Grease, bear^{+D}

Grease, foxes^{+D}

Grease, goose^D

Honey [hony, English Honey, Stone Honey]$^{+D}$

Hares head, ashes of a burned^D

Harts horn [*harts horne*]$^{+D}$

Horse's hoof

Ivory*

Lights [lungs] of a bear^D

Lizards head^D

Lizards liver^D

Marrow bones^{+D}

Marrow, deer's^D

Milk, cowes [*milk of a browne cow, milk of kine*]$^{+D}$

Milk, womans^{+D}

Oiliness of sheeps wool before it be washed [Oisupon; Oesypum; Wool fat; Lanolin]^D

Serpent's skin^{+D}

Suet, bull^{+D}

Turd, goose$^+$

Turd, dogs white$^+$

Unguis odoratus ("Blatta byzanzia, sive Unguis Odoratus, the shell of a Fish of a very sweet Scent, brown Colour, and oblong Figure" (Blancard, p.55); Sweet-hoof: "It is a Shell-fish breeding in Lakes full with Spiknard, on which they breed and live, and from thence the shell receives its smell; it is also said to be found on the Shoars of Tyrus the Metropolis of Phœnicia, where they first died Purple" (Salmon, p.641); Onux, Onyx]$^{*+D}$

Unguis odoratus [Onux], ashes of^D

Urine[D]

Urine of a boar[+D]

Urine of a bull[D]

Urine of a dog[D]

Urine, man's[+D]

Urine, man's, stale[D]

Urine, patients [Urine of the party
    grieved][+D]

Urine of a she-goat[+D]

Urine, stale[D]

Urine of a wild boar[+]

Urine, young child's[D]

Viper [flesh][+D]

Wax (Beeswax)*[+D]

Wax, virgin [Beeswax. Propolis: found
    at the entrance to the hive
    (Salmon, p. 654)]*[+D]

Wax, white (Beeswax)*[+D]

Weesil, ashes of[D]

Weesils cod, outward skin of

Weesils cod skin

Weesils, salted powder of[D]

Weesil, ventricle of[D]

Whey[+D]

Wool [*Shank Wool carded in flakes;
    Wool newly taken from the sheep;
    Black wool newly plucked from
    sheeps neck; Wool from flanks
    and codds; flank wool; black
    Wooll*][D]

Belonging to the Sea

Amber*[+D]

Corral [*Curral, Coral*][G*+D]

Flos salis [*"a brackish foam or scum
    floating on certain Lakes*][D]

*Halcyonium [Halcionium], fifth kind
    of* [*"a kind of seafoam indurate
    called also Spuma maris"*][+D]

*Halcyonium [Halcionium], third kind
    of*

Sea sand[+D]

Sea water[D]

Sponges[+D]

Metals and Stones

Allome*[+D]

Alabaster dust[+D]

Antimony*[+D]

*Arabian-stone [white marble, Lapis
    arabicus]*[+D]

Arsenicke [white and red][+D]

Asian-stone [Lapis asius][+D]

Bitumen ["Blancard: Bitumen is gen-
    erally taken for all sorts of fat
    Earth that are separated with dif-
    ficulty and easily burn; this is
    said to be the Fuel of all the Fires
    that are vomited out in burning
    Mountains. It comprehends sev-
    ersal kinds, but particularly a fat
    Juice that is found about the Red
    Sea, swimming upon it like a
    Froth, afterwards dried upon the
    Shore, it becomes harder than
    pitch."][D]

Bitumen Judaicum [Blancard:
    ="Asphaltos, Asphaltium, a sort
    of Pitch gather'd from the Lake
    Asphaltites, in Palestine."]*[D]

Bole armoniack[+] [Bolearmonick]

Bloodstone, prepared ["Blood-stone is a kind of Jasper of diverse colors, with red spots in it like blood, stops the Terms and bleeding in any part of the Body."[+, p. 54]]+D

*Borax**

Brass, burned [Chalkos kekumenos][D]

Brass, scales of [filed plates of brass, Lepis, Helitis]+D

Brass, dross of [Dyphriges; Diphriges]+D

Brimstone*+D

Bricks

Cadmia*+D

Calamine [*callaminaris stones, Lapis calaminaris*]+D

Ceruse [cerus, =white lead[OED2]. white lead*+][D]

*Chalcitis**[D]

Chalk, green mineral+D

Chio, Earth of [Chian earth, Terra chia, Chia terra][D]

Cimolian earth [Fuller's earth]+D

Cinnaber [Cinnabar, Cinnabaris, Cinabris]+D

Emerie [emery; "A black hard miner-all substance, where-with Iron-worke is polished, and precious stones and glasse cut."][D]

Fire-stone [Marchasite-stone]+

Flints+

Fuller's earth [Cimolian earth]+D

Galactitus [Milk-stone]+D

Iron-rust+D

Jaspar stone+D

DE VENENIS, &c.
Leporis marini effigies.

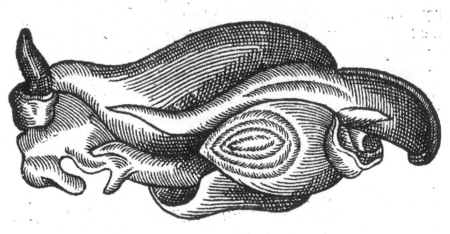

Sea hare

Jet [Stone gagates][+D]

Tutie, Alexandrian [Lapis tutiae, rock tutty][+D]

Lead, red[+]

Lead, washed[+D]

Lead, white [*lead, white-*]*[+D]

Lemnian earth[+D]

Lime[+D]

Lithargy [Littargy, Litharge]*[+D]

Marble, serpentine[+]

Marble, white [Arabian-stone][+D]

Marchasite-stone [fire-stone][+]

Melian earth[D]

Milk-stone [galactitus][+D]

Naxion-stone [whetstone][+D]

Niter[+D]

Oker [ochre, red or yellow][+D]

Phrigian-stone [Lapis phrygius][+D]

Pumice-stone[+D]

Red stone from a swallow ["Young swallows of the first brood, if you cut them up, between the time they were hatched, and the next full Moon, you shall find two stones in their ventricle [ventriculus = stomach[Blancard]], one reddish, the other blackish."[+, p.34]; "the Stone found in the Maw of a Swallow"[+, p.54]]*[+D]

Salt[D]

Samian earth (Earth of Samos][+D]

Samius-stone [Lapis samius][D+]

Saphire-stone[+D]

Sory ["A mettall like to Melanteria, but thinner and more spungie"][D]

Specular-stone

Sponge-stone [Lapis sponge, "found in sponges [LD"]*]*[+D]

Steel[+]

Stone gagates [Jet][+D]

Stone geodes[+D]

Stone-Judaicus [Lapis judaicus]][+D]

Stone Morocthus[+D]

Stone Ostracites[+D]

Stone Schistos [Lapis schistos][+D]

Stone Thyites [Lapis thyites][+D]

Tar (?)

Tuttie [*tucia, tutia,* tutty, Blancard: "is nothing but the Soot of Brass sticking to the Furnace in the fusion of that Metal." p.348][+D]

Verdigrease[+D]

Vermillion, Artificial ["Sandix, it is made of burnt Ceruse"(LD)][D]

Vitriol, white[+]

Whetstone [Naxion-stone][+D]

Simple Distilled Waters

Cowcumbers, smell of wild

COMPOSITA OR COMPOUND MEDICINES

Physical Wines

Wine of Gentian roots

Wine of Germander[G]

Wine of Hisope[D]

Wine of French lavender]Stichas, Stœchas, Stickado(ue), Cassidonie, Cast-me-down][D]

Wine of Goates-Organy [Tragoriganum][D]

Wine of Labrusk flowers [Oinos oinanthinos; Vinum Oenanthinum][D]

Wine of Mirtle[D]

Wine of Mulberries

Wine of Quinces[D]

Wine of Sour Pomegranats[D]

Wine of Squill[+D]

Wine of Sumack

Wine of Time[D]

Wine of Worm-wood[+D]

Physical Vinegars

Rose vineger[+]

Squill vinegar[+D]

Decoctions

Acacia, decoction of[D]

Acorns [Balanoi], decoction of[D]

Agnus castus, decoction of leaves and seeds of[D]

Asphodil, decoction of roots[G]

Bastard saffron [Carthamum, Cnicus], decoction of

Baulme [Balm; Melissa], decoction of[GD]

Bay leaves, decoction of[GD]

Bear's ear [Alisma=water plantain, Mountain cowslips], decoction of

Beets, decoction of[D]

Betony, decoction of[D]

Bramble, decoction of[D]

Bramble branches, decoction of[D]

Brimstone, decoction of

Burnet [Pimpinella], decoction of[G]

Calamint, decoction of[GD]

Cammock roots [Camock, Rest Harrow, Anonis], decoction of[D]

Cammomill [Anthemis], decoction of[GD]

Capers, decoction of

Capers, decoction of seed of

Carline thistle [Leucacantha, Carlina, Chameleon alba], decoction of[D]

Centaury, Small, decoction of[D]

Ceterach [Spleenwort, Asplenon, Scolopendrium], decoction of[D]

*Chameleon thistle roots [Crocodilium, Crocodilion, Carduus niger, "the Thistle that changeth it selfe into many shapes and colours" *[G]*], decoction of*

Christ's Thorne [Paliurus, Ramme of Lybia, 'Christ's thistle'][G], *decoction of leaves and roots of*[D (for Paliurus(jujube))]

Cinquefoile [Cinkfoil, Cinqfoil, Five finger grass, Pentaphyllum], decoction of roots of^{GD}

Cockles [Chamai, a broth from bivalves], decoction of^D

Colewort [Brassica, Garden colewort, Curled garden cole, Red colewort, White (or red or open) cabbage cole, cabbage, Coleflorey, Cauliflower, Savoy cole, Parsely colewort, English sea colewort, Wild colewort], decoction of^D

Colts-foot, decoction of^G

Coloquintida, decoction of^G

Common sweet cane ["The false adulterated sweet Cane, a kinde of Corn-flag"], decoction of

Cowcumbers, decoction of wild^D

Crow-foot [Butter-flower, Ranunculus, King Kob, Gold cups, Gold knobs], decoction of^D

Cyprus [Cypress] apples [Cypress pills], decoction of green^D

Dates, decoction of the rind or skin of

Dill, decoction of seeds and tops of^D

Dog's mercury [Cynocramhe], decoction of^D

Dragons, decoction of great^D

Elder [Sambucus, Akte, Chamaiakte, Arbor ursi], decoction of^D

Elecampane roots, decoction of^{GD}

Elme, bark of roots, decoction of^{GD}

Elme leaves, decoction of^{GD}

Fennel, decoction of^G

Feverfew, decoction of^{GD}

Figs, decoction of^D

Figs, decoction of dry^D

Figs and hisope [hyssop], decoction of dry^{GD}

Figs and rue, decoction of^D

Flower-de-luce of Illyria [Ireos, Iris], decoction of^{GD}

French lavender [Stichas, Stœchas, Stickado(ue), Cassidonie, Cast-me-down], decoction of^{GTD}

Golden tode-flax [Chrysocome], decoction of^{GT+D}

Galingall roots, decoction of

Galls, decoction of$^{D(I.146)}$

Garlick leaves, decoction of^D

Gentian, decoction of^{GD}

Germander, decoction of^{GD}

Gith [Nigella romana, Melanthium], decoction of^D

Goats organy [Tragoriganum], decoction of^{GD}

Ground pine, decoction of^{GD}

Heart of Pine, of Garlick, and of frankincense, decoction of [Garlic sod with Taeda (heart of pine) and frankincense, Dioscorides II.182)]^D

Hisope boiled with figgs, decoction of^{GD}

Hisope, figgs, hony and rue, decoction of^D

Hen-bane roots [Hyoscyamus roots$^+$], decoction of^D

Hen-bane seeds [Hyoscyamus seeds^{GT*+}], decoction of

Hisope [Hyssop], decoction of^{GD}

Horehound [Marrubium], decoction of^D

Horehound, Wild [Stachys], decoction of^{GD}

Horned poppy [Sea Poppy, Papaver cornutum] root, decoction of^D

Hounds-tongue [Hounds pissê, Cynoglossum, Dogstongue], decoction of^D

Lady thistle [Our Lady(ies) Thistle, Leucæantha (mentioned in footnote of LD is Gerard's term for Carline thistle [p. 1150]), Carduus lacteus, Carduus Mariæ, Leucographus, Bedeguar, Spina alba, White Thistle, Milk Thistle] roots, decoction of^D

Lentils, decoction of^{GD}

Linseed, decoction of^{GD}

Lupine [flat bean called lupine, Garden Lupine, Tame Lupine, Figbean, Lupinus, Thermos], decoction of^{GD}

Maidenhair, Black or Common [Maydenhair, Capillis veneris, Venus hair, Black Maidenhair, Common Maidenhair, English Maidenhair=Trichomanes mas], decoction of^{GCD}

Maidenhair [White maidenhair, Wallrue, Ruta muraria], decoction of^{GCD}

Mallows, decoction of^{GD}

Marsh mallows, decoction of^{GD}

Mandragore root, decoction of^D

Marjerom, decoction of^D

Marjerom, decoction of Great^D

Marigolds [Chrysanthemum= includes German Marigold, Corn Marigold], decoction of

Mastick-tree, decoction of^{GD}

Mastick-tree leaves, decoction of^D

Mellilot [Plaister Claver, Hart's Claver, Assyrian Claver, Italian Claver, Kings Claver, German Claver, Sertula campana, melilot, mellilot herbs, mellilote], decoction of^D

Mercury [French Mercury], decoction of^{GD}

Milk trefoile [Cytisus, Shrub trefoile], decoction of^{SGD}

Mirtle [Myrtus], decoction of^{GD}

Mugwort [Artemesia], decoction of^D

Mulberry [Morus], decoction of bark of^D

Mulberry [Morus], decoction of bark of roots of^{GD}

Mullein [Woolen, Higtaper, Torches, Long-wort, Bullockes Long-wort, Hareweed, Tapsus barbatus], decoction of^D

Mullein, Æthiopian [Æthiopus (Dios. IV.105), Woolly Mullein], decoction of^D

Oak leaves, decoction of

Organie, decoction of^{GD}

Organy boiled with figgs, decoction of

Orkanet [Alkanet, Wild Bugloss, Anchusa], decoction of roots of^{GD}

Parsley, decoction of

Pellitory of Spain [Pelitory of Spain, Bertram, Pyrethrum], decoction of^D

Penniroyal [Pudding grass, Pulial Royal, Pulegium, Peniroyal], decoction of^{GCD}

Pine hear [Toeda], decoction of^D

Pine tree leaves, decoction of^D

Plantain [Plantane, Plantago] root, decoction of^D

Plow-mans Spikenard [Baccharis], decoction of^{GC}

Plow-mans Spikenard [Baccharis] roots, decoction of^{GD}

Plum tree leaves, decoction of^{GD}

Poley [Pellamountain, Polium sp., Leucas], decoction of both kinds of^D

Polypodie [Ladies Dispensatory uses this term as a synomym for Oak fern. A similar confusion of names cited in Gerard (1633) p. 1134, Ceterach is described as polypodium in Dioscorides], decoction of^D

Pomegranat tree, decoction of the root of$^{D(1.153)}$

Poppy-heads, decoction of [Dia-codium]$^{G*+CD}$

Privet leaves [Prim Print, Print, Lagustrum], decoction of^{GD}

Purslaine [Purslane, Porcelane, Portulaca], decoction of^D

Quinces, decoction of^D

Rest-Harrow [Cammock, Cammock, Petty Whinne, Ground furze, Anonis], decoction of^D

Rosemary, decoction of^D

Roses [Rosa], decoction of dry^{GCD}

Rose-wood [Aspalathus, Lignum Rhodium], decoction of^D

Rue [Ruta sp., Herb-grace], decoction of^{GCD}

Rushes [Iuncus], decoction of

Sage [Elaphoboscon, Salvia officinalis], decoction of^D

Savine, decoction of

Savory, summer [Satureia hortensis astiva], decoction of^D

Scallions [Ascalonitides], decoction of^D

Sea-holly [Eryngium, Eringo, Iringo], decoction of

Sleepy nightshade [Dwale, Deadly night shate, Raging nightshade, Solanum somniferum, Solanum lethale, Solanum manicum], decoction of^D

Sory ["A mettall like to Melanteria, but thinner and more spungie"], decoction of

Southern-wood [Abrotanum], decoction of^{CD}

Sow-bread [Cyclamen], decoction of^{GCD}

Sparagus roots, decoction of^D

Sparagus roots, boiled with figgs and Cich pease, decoction of^D

Spicknell [Spignell, Meon, Meum, Mew, Bearewort, Writhed Dill, Wild Dill], decoction of^{GC}

Spikenard, decoction of^{GD}

Spleen-wort [Scale fern, Stone fern, Scolopendra, Spleen wort, Miltwaste, *Asplenum, Lingua cervina, Lonchitis, Ceterach], decoction of^G*

Squinanth [Camel's Hay, Schœnanthum, Iuncus odoratus], decoction of^D

Staphis-acre [Staves acre, Staphis agria, Louse-wort, Lousepowder], decoction of^{GD}

Sumack, decoction of^{GD}

Sweet cane [Acorum, Acoris, Sweet-smelling Reed, Aromatical Reed], decoction of^{GD}

Tamarisk [Tamariscus] decoction of^{GCD}

Time, decoction of^{GD}

Tode-flax [Osyris], decoction of^{GT+D}

Turnsole [Heliotropium], decoction of^D

Turnips [Rapum, Rape], decoction of^{GD}

Valerian [Valeriana sp, Capons tail, Setwal], decoction of^D

Wall-flowers [Viola lutea, Wall gilloflower, Yellow stock gilloflower, Winter-gilloflower, Cheiri], decoction of^{GD}

Wall-wort- [Dane-wort, Dwarf elder, Ebulus, Sambucus humilis, Symphitum petreum], decoction of^{GD}

Water Germander [Scordium], decoction of [. . . in wine]^{GD}

White Thistle [Bedeguar, Spina Alba, Lady thistle, Our Lady(ies) Thistle, Carduus lacteus, Carduus Mariæ, Leucographus, Milk Thistle] roots, decoction of^D

Wild Mercury [Cynocrambe = Dogs Mercury, Phyllon sp. = Childrens Mercury], decoction of^{GD}

Willow [Salix, Sallow, Withy]^G, decoction of leaves and bark of^D

Wormwood [wormewood, French Wormwood, Roman Wormwood, Romane Wormwood, Absinthium], decoction of^D

Conserves and Sugars

Organie confected in the Sun, in a copper vessell, with onions, and seed of Sumack drunk. It must have stood in the Sun all the Dog-dayes, and as many other as amounteth to forty.$^{D(III.32)}$

Electuaries (mixture of powdered herbs and clarified honey)

Bitter almonds, electuary of

Briony roots, electuary of [lohoc with honey^D]

Bank cresses [Erysimum], electuary of^D

Goats organy [Tragoriganum^G] and honey, electuary of [lohoc with honey^D]

Hisope [Hyssop] and honey, electuary of [lohoc with honey^D]

Linseed, electuary of^D

Pepper, Electuary of^D

Seselios of Candy [Seseli Creticum sp., Tordylion], electuary of root of

Squill [Sea Onion, Scilla sp., Pancratium sp., Sea Daffodil], electuary of^D

Storax, electuary of

Time, electuary of^D

Pills

Pills of Agarick^{+,p. 139}

Oils

Oyle^D

Simple Oils by Expression
Oyl of almonds^{+D}

Oyl of bayes [*Oyle of bayes*]⁺

Oyl olive [*Oyle olive*]^{G+D}

Oyle of wild olives^{GD}

Simple Oils by Infusion and Decoction
Oyle of cedar^D

Oyle of fenegreek^D

Oyle of galbanum

Oyl of lillies^{+D}

Oyle of [great] marjerome [Great sweet marjerom, Mariorana maior, Oleum Majoranæ]^{G+D}

Oyle of mastick^D

Oyl of mirtle [*myrtill*]^D

Oyle of Palma Christi [Cicinum]^D

Oyle of privet

Oyle of quinces^{GD} [*"There is boiled with Quinces oile which therefore is called in Greek Melinon, or oile of Quinces", Gerard, p. 1453]*^D

Oyle of roses [*Oyl of roses*]^{+,Ges 347–50}

Oyle of saffron [Crocomagna]^D

Oyle Sycionium [formula in text; "Made of wild Cowcumber roots and juyce, and oyle"]^D

Oyle of storax [(?)Unguentum styracinum^D*]*

Compound Oils by Infusion and Decoction
Oyle of Flower-de-luce [Oleum Irinum, Oyl of Orris]^{G+}

Ointments

Marjerom, ointment of [Great]^D

Privet [Prim print, Ligustrum, Print], ointment of

Other Processed Herbals

Garlick, ashes of, applied with honey^D

Mint suppository

Soot of frankicense [burned in a close pot, Fuligo of frankincense]^D

Vine [Vitis vinifera, Vitis sylvestris, Grape vine, Raisin vine] leaves and branches, ashes of^{GCD}

Liniments

Carro [Thapsia], stinking deadly, liniment of^D

Figgs, of Hisope, and of Niter, liniment of^D

Hisope [Hyssop], liniment of

Indian-leaf [Malabathrum, Tamalapatra, Tembul], liniment of^D

Lesser celandine [Scrophularia minor, Chelidonium minus, Pile-wort, Figwort], liniment of

Misseltoe, boyled with Cole-worts, and the stone Gagates, liniment made of[D]

Mustard and vinegar, liniment made of[D]

Myrrhe, Labdanum, and Myrtill wine, liniment of[D]

Organie, salt, hony, and hisope, liniment made of

Pellitory of the wall [Parietariam, Helxine parietaria, pellitory of the wal, pellitory on the wall], liniment made of cerus and juice of[CD]

Periwinkle, liniment of

Storax, liniment of[D]

Perfumes

Agnus castus, perfume of[D]

Brimstone, perfume of[D]

Calamint, perfume of[D]

Colt's foot, perfume of[D]

Darnell meale, myrthe, Frankincense, Bitumen, and Saffron, perfume of[D]

Garden cresses, perfume of

Gith [Nigella romana, Melanthium], perfume of[D]

Harts-horne [cornua cervina (animal product], perfume of[D(II.63)]

Hisope [Hyssop], perfume of[D]

Horse foot [Colts-foot, Tussilago, coltsfoot], perfume of[D]

Juniper plant, perfume of[D]

Maudlein [Ageratum, Balsamita fœmina, Herba Giula[G]*], perfume of*

Meadow Parsenep [Cow Parsnep, Madnep, Sphodylium, Spondilium], perfume of[D]

Poley [Pellamountain, Polium sp., Leucas], perfume of[D]

Sweet cane [Acorum, Acoris, Sweet-smelling Reed, Aromatical Reed, Calamus aromaticus], perfume of[D]

Unguis odoratus ("Blatta byzanzia, sive Unguis Odoratus, the shell of a Fish of a very sweet Scent, brown Colour, and oblong Figure" (Blancard, p.55)], perfume of[D]

Willow-herb, perfume of[D]

Wormwood [wormewood, French Wormwood, Roman Wormwood, Romane Wormwood, Absinthium], perfume of boiling[= =steam or vapor][D]

Foods/Drinks

Barley flower [flour]

Barley meal[GD]

Barley water[D]

Bean flower [flour ground from beans[C]]

Bean meal[D]

Bran, Wheaten[G+D]

Brine

Broth of wormwood, figs, niter, and darnell meale[D]

Cheese[D]

Ciches [Cicer, Ciche pease, Chich pease], meal of

Garum ['the pickle or brine of fish or flesh"][D]

Polenta ["Barly steeped in water, dried by a fire and after fryed for phisicall uses."[G]*]*

Miscellaneous Nonmedicinal Items

Snow

Glossary

Medical terminology of the mid-seventeenth century is a combination of popular lay health beliefs and scientific concepts based on humoral and iatrochemical medicine. Hence, the meanings of these terms are often alien to the modern reader. The modern reader faces two challenges. Firstly, many terms for diseases and symptoms have not been in common usage since the mid-nineteenth century. Secondly, some current disease terms (e.g., anthrax) had significantly different meanings to the practioners and patients of that era. This glossary presents contemporaneous definitions of key medical terms found in *The Ladies Dispensatory*. The original spellings and language have been preserved to convey both the denotation and connotation of the terms. When definitions vary between contemporary sources, the range of these definitions is presented. Since these terms are based on etiologic mechanisms and nosologies that differ significantly from a modern view, no attempt is made to bias the reader by relating these definitions directly to modern terminology.

A brief note is in order regarding the spelling and typography from sixteenth- and early seventeenth-century texts. The reader will note the equivalence of letters *i/y* and *u/v*, producing words such as *yf* [if], *receyue* [receive], *vnmouable* [unmovable], *vnquyete* [unquiet], and *vrine* [urine]. In addition, vowels followed by a nasal (m or n) are printed as ã, ẽ, õ, and ũ, producing words such as *secõde* [second], *chãceth* [chanceth], *Elephãcia* [Elephancia], and *sodẽ* [sudden]. Finally, spelling is phonetic, producing variants such as *cole* [coal], *hote* [hot], *hyer* [higher], and *fyer* [fire].

GLOSSARY REFERENCES

Banister

Richard Banister, *A treatise of one hundred and thirteene diseases of the eyes* (Amsterdam: Theatrum Orbis Terrarum; New York: Da Capo Press, 1971).

Billings

John S. Billings, *The National Medical Dictionary: Including English, French, German, Italian, and Latin Technical Terms Used in Medicine and the Collateral Sciences, and a Series of Tables of Useful Data* (Philadelphia: Lea Brothers & Co., 1890).

Blancard

Steven Blancard, *The Physical Dictionary. Wherein the Terms of Anatomy, the Names and Causes of Diseases, Chirurgical Instruments, and Their Use, Are Accurately Described* (London: John and Benjamin Sprint, 1726).

Borde

Andrew Borde, *The Breviary of Helthe* (London, 1547). Facsimile edition of British Museum Shelfmark: C.122.d.1.; Amsterdam: Da Capo Press, 1971.

Cullen

William Cullen, *First Line of the Practice of Physic* (New York: Samuel Campbell, 1793).

Dunglison (1839)

Robley Dunglison. *Medical Lexicon: A Dictionary of Medical Science* (Philadelphia: Lea and Blanchard, 1839).

Dunglison (1845)

Robley Dunglison, *Medical Lexicon: A Dictionary of Medical Science* (Philadelphia: Lea and Blanchard, 1845).

Dunglison (1895)

Robley Dunglison, *A Dictionary of Medical Science* (Philadelphia: Lea Brothers & Co., 1895).

Elyot

Sir Thomas Elyot, *The Castel of Helth Corrected and in some places augmented* (London, 1641). Facsimile edition; New York: Scholars' Facsimiles & Reprints, 1937.

Goeurot

John Goeurot, *The Regiment of Life, Whereunto is added a treatyse of the Pestilence, with the Booke of Children Newly Corrected and Enlarged* (London, 1546). Facsimile edition of Bodleian Library (Oxford) Shelfmark 8°.P.24 Med.; Amsterdam/Norwood, N.J.: Walter J. Johnson, Inc./Theatrum Orbis Terrarum, Ltd., 1976.

Guillemeau

Jacques Guillemeau, *A worthy treatise of the eyes: contayning the knowledge and cure of one-hundreth and thirteen diseases,* trans. A. H. (Special facsimile of 1622 edition; Birmingham, Ala.: Classics of Ophthalmology Library, 1989).

Harris

John Harris, *Lexicon technicum: or, An universal English dictionary of arts and sciences.* (London: D. Brown, 1704) (New York: Johnson Reprint Corp., 1966 [1704 edition]).

Hooper

Robert Hooper, *Lexicon-Medicum; or Medical Dictionary; Containing an Explanation of Terms in Anatomy, Physiology, Practice of Physic, Materia Medica, Chemistry, Pharmacy, Surgery, Midwifery, and the Various Branches of Natural Philosophy Connected with Medicine* (New York: Harper & Bros., 1847).

Lowe

Peter Lowe, *A Discourse on the Whole Art of Chyrurgerie* (London: R. Hodgkin-sonne, 1654).

Morton

Richard Morton, *Phthisiologia, or, A Treatise of Consumptions: Wherein the Diffenence, Nature, Causes, Signs, and Cure of all Sorts of Comsumptions Are Explained. . . .* (London: printed for Sam. Smith and Benj. Walford, 1694).

OED2

OED2: Oxford English Dictionary II [database online]. Available from BRS Software Products, McLean, Virg.: BRS/Search Full-Text Retrieval System, Revision 6.1, 1992.

Paré

Ambroise Paré, *The Workes of that Famous Chirurgion Ambrose Parey: Translated out of Latine and Compared with the French*, trans. Thomas Johnson (London: Thomas Coates and R. Young, 1634).

Quincy

John Quincy, *Lexicon Physico-Medicum; or, a New Medicinal Dictionary. Explaining the Difficult Terms Used in the Several Branches of the Profession, and in such Parts of Natural Philosophy, As are Introductory thereto* (London: T. Longman, 1787).

Skilful Physician

Balaban, Carey D., Jonathon Erlen and Richard Siderits (eds) *The Skilful Physician* (Amsterdam: Harwood Academic, 1997).

ABORTION

Borde: "*Abhorsus* or *Abhortus* be the latyn wordes. In englysh it is named Abhorsion. And ye is whã a woman is delyuered of her chylde before her tyme. Or els Abhorsion is also, whan a chylde is cut out of the mothers bely.

The cause of Abhorsion.

Abhorsion dothe come many wayes. Fyrste it may come by vetosyte and lubrycyte of humours in the matryx Or it may come by a great feare or by extreme thoughte, or by extreme sicknesse, or death, it doth come also by a strype or a stroke or a fall,. Also it may come by receptes of medecines as by the extreme purgacions, pocions, and other laxatyues drynkes, of the whiche I dare nat to speke of at this tyme lest any lyght womã shulde haue knowledge, by the whiche wylful Abhorsion should happen. Also Abhorsion maye come of the multitudenes of the flowers of a woman."

AGUE, BURNING OR BURNING FEVER

Harris: "CAUSUS, or a *burning Fever*, is that which is attended with a greater heat than other continued Fevers, an intolerable Thirst, and other Symptoms, which argue an extraordinary accension of the Blood."

AGUES

Blancard: "*Intermittens Febris*, is call'd a Fever or Ague that ceaseth and returns at certain times; 'Tis either Quotidian, Tertian, Quartan, and some add the Quintan.

Intermittens Morbus, a Disease which comes at certain times and then remits a little. Intermittent *Fevers* or *Agues* proceed not from any fictitious *Focus*, but only from a wrong assimilation of the Chyle."

Harris: "*Intermittent Feavers*, commonly called, *Agues*; have certain Times of intermission, beginning for the most part with Cold or Shivering, ending in Sweat and running exactly at set Periods."

APOSTUMES (SEE ALSO **BOTCH, IMPOSTHUME, ULCER,** AND **WHITLOW**)

Borde: "Agria is the greke word. In latyn it it named vlcera. In englyshe it is named byles or botches or such lyke apostumations. A dyfference is betwyxe Acria & Agria [see **WILD SCAB**] for the one is with swelling and the other is with skabbes without swellinge."

"Apostema is the latyn worde. In greke it is named Apostima. In englyshe it is a postume. A postume is no other thynge but a collection or a connynge togyther of euyll humours. And some be interyall, and some be exteryall. The interyall apostumes be other in the heed, in the stomake, in the lunges, in the splene, or in the bowels. The exteryall apostumes be in the flesshe under the skynne.

The cause of this infyrmyte.

All apostumations do come by corrupt blode or els by congeyled fleume or fleume vnnaturall Or els by coler, or els by melancoly. If the impostume do come of corrupt & infectiouse blode, then the impostume is named *Flegmon*. An if it come by congyled or vnnaturall fleume the imposthume is named *zimie* and some do name it *zumma*.

And yf the impostume do come by coler the impostume is named *Herisipula*. And if ye impostume do come of melãcoly, or coler adusted, than the impostume is named *Cancri* or *scliros*. Yet there be many other impostumes the whiche do come of myxt humours, as the boch and byte, and such like. These impostumes that be interyall and can nat be sene be more periculus then they the whiche a mã may se and feie. For this matter and for a remedy loke in ye proper names of the impostumes & specially in the capytle named suffocation or *suffocatio*."

"Bvbo is the latin word. In englyshe it is named a grosse impostume. And there be certeyn kyndes some be pestiferous & some be nat pestiferous."

"The 131. Capytle doth shewe in generall of all appostumacions.

Exitura is the latyn worde. Upon what worde it is grounded I can nat tel, but they the whiche hath writen vpon this worde doth say it is named euery appostumacion, in the which is matter and fylth, and there be many kyndes of these appostumacions. The fyrst is named Cammarate Caurine, the seconde is named Albir or Toplaria, and the thyrde is named Talpa, the fyrste is named as I haue sayd Camarate and that is ingendred of an euyl and corrupt flesshe, the seconde is named Albir or Toplaria the which is most comonly in chyldryns heedes, the thyrde is named Talpa the which is ingendred in the heed vpon the skyn penytratynge the flesshe." (fol. xvii v.)

"Fvgilla is the latyn worde. In englyshe it is named an harde impostume vnder a man or womans arme hole, or there about. . . . This infyrmyte doth come of a melancoly humour, and other while it maye come of a fleumatyke matter couerted to hardnes." (fol. lxix)

"Natta or Narra be the latyn wordes. In englysh it is a great flesshy impostume lyke a wenne & is soft & it doth grow on the back or ye shulders. . . . This impediment doth come of reume, and of the grosnes of blode." (fol. lxxxxviii v)

". . . an harde or dence appostumacion. Sephiros is the greke worde. In englyshe it is named an harde appostumacion in the flesshe under the skyn. . . . This impediment doth come of either a grosse or viscus fleume, or els of a melacholy humour, and if it be whitishe it doth come of fleume, yf it be swart it doth come of melancholy."

"Vndimia is the latyn worde. And some doth say it is a barbarous worde. In englyshe it is named a cold appostumacion white and soft." (fol. Cxxxviii)

APOSTUME, FLAT CALLED IN GREEK *PANOS*

Blancard: "*Panus*, a sort of Botch or Sore under the Arm-pits or Jaws, Ears and Groins, that is in the Glandulous Parts. 'Tis also taken for *Phygethlus*."

APPETITE

Borde: "Apetitius is the latyn worde. In engyshe it is a mans apetyde to meat. There be dyuers apetydes, some be natural, and some be vnnaturall. And one apetyde is w'out order, and that is whan a man wold eat and can nat. And some hathe lost theyr apetyde that they haue lytle stomake or none to eat any meat. A natural apetyde is to eat in dewe order and dewe tyme after a digestiõ. An vnnaturall apetyde is to eat and drynke at all tymes without dewe order, or to desyre to eate raw and vnleful thynges as women with chylde doth and such lyke."

APPOPLEXIE

Borde: "Apoplexis is the greke worde. Apoplexia is the barbarous word. In latyn it is named Percussio. In englysh it is named a sodeyn stryking downe takynge away a mannes wyt, reson and mouynge.

The cause of this infyrmyte.

This infyrmyte doth came of a colde humour the whiche doth opylate or stop ye ventrycles of the brayne and doth fyl the celles of the heed. And some say it is a colde and grosse appostomacion that lyeth in the hinder part of the heed."

BELCHING

Borde: "Eructuacio is the latyn worde. In englishe it is named an eructuacio or belchynge.

The cause of this infyrmyte.

This impedimẽt doth come of ventosyte or a sower humour in the stomacke." (fol. lv v.)

BELLY-ACH

Borde: "Colirica passio as Alexander saythe is deriued out of a worde of greke named *Colides* yᵉ whyche is named the inwardes of a man. Some Greciõs doth name this sicknes *Colidica* or *Ciliaca* or *Cocliaca passio.* And some grekes wᵗ the latenystes doth name it *Cholera.* In latyn it is named *Ventralis passio.* In englyshe it is named the bely ache or a passion in the bely.

The cause of this impedyment.

This impedimẽt doth come for lacke of perfite digestion for a man shal exonerat or discharge by egestion and vomet both his body and stomake in one houre vpwarde and downewarde." (fol. XXXIX)

BITING (BY AN ANIMAL)

Borde: "Morsus is the latyn worde. In greke it is named Digma. In englishe it is named a bytinge the which may come in many wayes, as by bytyng of an adder or styngynge of a scorpion, snake, or waspe, pissinge of a tode, or spyder and such lyke, the venym of all the whiche maye hurt man." (fol. lxxxxv v)

BLEAR-EYEDNESSE

Banister: *"Of the Tettar, Ringworme, or Scabbes on the Eye-liddes, or sharpe fleumy blearednesse, called in Greeke,* Psoropthalmia. *In Latin,* Lippitudo pruriginosa.

Psoropthalmia is, when the Eye-liddes are red, and salt-biting teares issue from them, the corners of the eyes hauing vlcerations and red-nesse, with much itching." [Diseases of the Eye-liddes, Chap. 2]

"Of the itching or dry Rringworme, or blearednesse of the Eyes, called in Greeke, Xeropthalmia, *in Latin,* Arida lippitudo.

Xeropthalmia is a dry blearednesse, wherein the eyes are neither puffed vp, nor send foorth teares, but are onely redde and heauy with paine, and in the night the eye-liddes sticke fast, & are as it were glewed together with thick fleume: whidh disease is of the longer con-tinuance, sith the matter is tough and heauy." [Diseases of the Eye-liddes, Chap. 3]

Borde: "Liptitudo is the latyn word. In englyshe it is named blere eyes whiche is whan the underlyd of the eye is subuerted. Rasis doth say ye Liptudo is whan ye white of ye eye is turned to rednes." (fol. lxxxiii)

Blancard: *"Lippitudo,* a certain roughness within the Eyes, as if Sand had got in 'em. Blearedness, Blearey'd."

BLISTER

Borde: "Noma is used for a latyn worde. In englyshe it is for a certayne kynde of a blyster or blysters the which doth ryse in the nyght vnkyndly." (fol. lxxxxvii)

BOTCH (SEE ALSO **APOSTUME**)

Borde: "The 58. Capytle dothe shewe of a Carbocle or a botche.

Carbunculus is the latyn worde. Altoin is the araby worde. In englyshe it is named a Carbocle or a botche. Carbunculus is deryued oute of a worde of latyn named Carbo the which is a cole in englyshe, for this infyrmyte hath the propertie of a cole that is hote burnynge, for a carbocle dothe burne & prycke."

Blancard: "*Phlegmone*, or *Inflammatio*; a Tumour of the Blood in the Flesh or Muscles, causing Heat, Redness, Beating and Pain."

BRAINE, DISEASES OF

Elyot: "Brayne hot and moyste distempered hath:
The head akynge and heuye [heavy].
Fulle of superfluities in the nose.
The southern wind greuous.
The Northern wind holsome.
Slepe deepe, but vnquyete, with often wakynges, and straunge dreames.
The senses and wytte vnperfecte.

Brayne hot and drye dystempered hath:
None aboundaunce of superfluities, whyche may be expelled.
Senses perfecte.
Moche watche.
Sooner balde than other.
Moche heare in chyldehoode and blacke or browne, and coutlyd.
The head hot and ruddye.

Brayne colde and moist distempered hath:
The senses and wytte dulle.
Moche sleape.
The head sone replenysshed with superfluouse moysture.
Distillations and poses or murres.
Not shortly balde.
Soone hurte with colde.

> Brayne cold and dry distempered hath:
> The head colde in felynge and with out colour.
> The vaynes not appearynge.
> Soon hurte with colde.
> Often discrased.
> Wytte perfecte in childhode, but in age dulle.
> Aged shortly and bald." (pp. 4–5)

BRAINE, TO PURGE THE

Borde: "Emunctoria is the latin word. In englishe it is named the emunctory or cleansing places of mans body. Here is to be marked that man hath .iii. principall mēbers the hert, the brayne, and the liuer, and euery one of these principall members hathe emunctory places to clense them selfe as the hertes emunctory places be under the arme holes there where ye heres dothe growe. The brayne hath many emunctory places to purge him selfe, as the eyes, the eares, the nose, the mouth, the heres, and the poores of the heed." (Extrauagantes section)

BREATH, DIFFICULTY AND SHORTNESSE OF (SEE ALSO LUNGS, STOPPING OF THE)

Goeurot: "Shortness of the wind procedeth oftentymes of fleume, that is tough and clāmishe, hangynge vpon ye longes [lungs] or stoppinge ye conduits of ye same, being in the holowenes of the brest, or of catarrous humours yt [that] droppeth downe into the longes, and thereby cōmeth straitnesse in drawing of the breth, whych is called of phisitions dispnoea or asthma, & when a pacient can not bend his necke down for drede of suffocation it is called orthopnoca." (fol. xxviii)

Borde: "Hoccomia or Occomia be the latyn wordes. In englyshe it is named rotlyng in the throte or shortnes of wynde . . . . This infyrmyte doth come whan that Asthma and Disma be joyned together." (fol. lxxv)

"Orthopnoisis is the greke worde. In latyn it is named Recta spiracio. In englysh it is named an euyl drawynge of a mannes brethe, for yf he do lye in his bedde he is redy to sound, or the brethe wylbe stopped. . . . This impediment dothe come either of the malice of the lunges or of opilacions of the pypes or els it may come thorowe viscus fleume." (fol. ciiii–ciiii v.)

Blancard: "*Dyspnoea*, a difficulty of breathing, which proceeeds from vitiated, obstructed, or irritated Organs."

BREST, STOPPING IN THE

See LUNGS, STOPPING OF THE

BURSTINGS (SEE RUPTURE)

CANKER

Borde: "Cancer is the latyn word. In englyshe it is named a canker the which is a sore the which both corode & eat the flesshe corruptynge te Arters the vaynes & the sinewes corodyng or eatyng the bone and doth putryfy & corrupt it. And then it is seldome made whole."

"Carcinodes is the greke word. In latyn it is named Cancer in naso. In englyshe it is named a Canker in the nose."

Lowe: "Of Pustules and Ulcers in the mouth.

Those Pustule and Ulcers with oftentimes possesse the upper part of the mouth and gums, are namee by the Greeks *Apthe* and by Avicen *Altolla*, in vulgar the Water Canker, and are of a white fiery quality, for the most part incident to young children, sometime to those of elder age.

The Signes are evident to the sight, and are known by the colour. Those which are doe proceed of blood, the colour is red, hot, the part tumified; if it proceed of Flegm, the colour is white, with little dolour; if of choller, it is jawnish [yellowish] colour, with som tumour, punction, and heat; if of Melancholy, the colour appeareth blackish, which is worst of all: thos which be black and scurfy like the crust of bread, it sheweth great corruption and adustion of humours, very dangerous, and for the most part deadly: those which be red or white, are not malignant: such as are superficial, are easily cured, those which penetrat more profunditie, are difficile." p. 200

PET.	What are those six kindes of Ulcers?
JOS.	The first is sanious, 2. virulent, 3 filthie, 4 cancrous, 5. putrid or stinking, 6 corrosive or rotten away . . .
PET.	How take they their names of the accidents?
JOS.	. . . of the cankers or hardnesse turned over it called cancrous." p. 326

Quincy: Eroding gingival ulcers, formed without a previous tumor.

CANKER IN THE NOSE

Borde: "Carcinodes is the greke word. In latyn it is named Cancer in naso. In englyshe it is named a Canker in the nose

CANNOT KEEPE THEIR WATER (SEE ALSO **PISSING**)

Borde: "The .98. Capytle doth shewe of them that can nat kepe theyr water but doth pysse as much as they do drynke.

Diabete is the greke worde. And some grekes doth name it *Dipsacos* or *Sipho*. The latyns do name it Afflictio renum. The barbarus men do name it *Diabetica passio*. In englyshe it is named an immoderate pyssinge." (Marginal printed notation: "Inordinate pyssinge", fol. xlv)

"Mictus or Mictura be ye latyn wordes. In greke it is named Vria. In englyshe it is named pissinge, and there be many impediments of pissing for some can nat holde theyr water & some can nat pysse or make water, some doth pysse blode, & some in theyr pyssinge doth auoyde gravel & some stones, and som whan they haue pyssed it doth burne in the issewe as well in woman as in man."

CARBUNCLE

Borde: "Altoin is the araby worde. In greke it is named Althaca. In latyn it is named Carbunculus. In englyshe it is named a Carbocle or a botch Carbunculus doth take his name of Carbo whiche is to say in englyshe a cole. For a cole beynge a fyre is hote, as so is a Carbocle . . . . This vlceration & infyrmyte most comonly doth brede in the emunctory places, there where ye .iii. pryncypal members hath theyr purgynge places the whiche be under ye eare or throte, or els about the arme holes or brest, or els about the secret partes of a man or woman, or in the share, or thyghe or flanke. And of Carbocles there be .iiii. kyndes. The fyrst is blacke. The secde is reed. The third is of a glase or grenyshe colour. And the fourth is of a swarte or dym colour."

Lowe: "There is small difference betweene Anthrax and Carbuncle, saving that Anthrax is the greeke word, and Carbuncle the Latine, and is so called because it burneth the place where it is, like unto coales. Carbuncle is defined to be a pustule, inflamed, black, burning the place, it is sore with many blisters about it, as if it were burnt with fire or water. The cause is divers, according to the sundry kinds thereof; the cause of the simple Carbuncle is an ebulition of grosse blood, thick and hot, where it falleth in any place it burneth and maketh ulcers, with a scale accompanied with great inflammation and dolour.

The signes of the simple Carbuncle are these, there appeareth many little black pustules not eminent, sometime pale, which groweth sodainly red, with great inflammation about the place where it is, and is harder than it ought to be, the sick loseth appetite and coveteth sleep, accompanied with cold sweat and fevers.

The signes of the maligne, are vomiting continually, weak appetite, trembling, sweunding, beating of the heart, the face wareth white and livid."

Harris: "CARBUNCULUS, the same with *Anthrax*."

"ANTHRAX, *Carbo*, *Pruna*, or *Carbunculus*, is defined to be a Tumour that arises in several places, surrounded with hot, fiery and most sharp pimples, accompanied with acute Pains, but without ever being separated, and when it spreads it self farther, it burns the flesh, throws off lobes of it when it is rotten, and leaves an ulcer behind it, as if it had been burnt in with an Iron."

CATARRHE

Blancard: "But there are no such things as Catarrhs, for there is nothing falls from the Head to those parts [below]. But the glandules of the Nostrils, and those that are about the parts of the Mouth, are often obstructed, and hence, come those Disorders. It is thus distinguish'd, if it fall on the Breast, the *Cattarh* is call'd *Rheum*; if on the Jaws, *Branchus*; if on the Nostrils, *Coryza*."

Cullen: "The cattarh is an increased excretion of mucus from the mucus membrane of the nose, fauces and bronchiae, attended by pyrexia." Frequently treated under title of tussis (cough) paragraph 1045, p.48.

Harris: "CATARRHUS, is a Defluxion of Humours from the Head towards the Parts under it, as the Nostrils, Mouth, Lungs, &c. Some distinguish it by the Name of *Loryza*, when it falls on the Nostrils, by that of *Bronchus* when on the Jaws; and by the word *Rhume*, when it falls on the Breast."

Quincy: "Catarrhus, . . . a defluxion of sharp serum from the glands about the head and throat, . . . commonly called a *Cold*."

C. Bellinsulanus=mumps; C. Suffocatus (Barbadensis)=croup; C. Vessicae="glus"="a kind of dysuria, called *dysuria mucosa*, purulent urine. It consists of a copious discharge of mucus with the urine."

CATHERICK (CATARACT [*SIC*]; SEE ALSO WEB)

Borde: "Catharacta is the barbarous worde. In greke it is named Ypechima. In englysh is is named a catharact the which doth let a man to see yfuely. . . . This impediment doth come of a grosse and a wateryshe humour the whiche doth lye before the syght lettynge a man to se clerely, for he can nat deserne a far of, a crowe from a man, nor a beest from a bushe, and of one thynge he shall se .ii. thynges although it be but one thynge."

CHOLER

Lowe: "Pe. What is Choller?
Jo. It is an Humour, hot and drie, of thinn and subtill substance, black coloured, bitter tasted, proper to nourish the parts hot, and drye, it is compared to the fire."

Harris: "Bile . . . .BILE, or the *Gall*, is a Liquor partly Sulphureous and partly Saline, which is separated from the Blood of Animals in the Liver"

CLEANSE OR PURGE (BACK, BRAINS, CHOLER, EVIL SAVOR OF THE NOSE, GUMS, GUTS, HEAD, MELANCHOLY, MELT, PHLEGME, STOMACH, TEETH, VEINS, OR WIND)

Borde: "Emunctoria is the latin word. In englishe it is named the emunctory or cleansing places of mans body. Here is to be marked that man hath .iii. principal mbers the hert, the brayne, and the liuer, and euery one of these principall members hathe emunctory places to clense them selfe as the hertes emunctory places be under the arme holes there where ye heres dothe growe. The brayne hath many emunctory places to purge him selfe, as the eyes, the eares, the nose, the mouth, the heres, and the poores of the heed. The liuer hathe emunctory places, as the bladder, the foundment and the flanks or the share." (Extrauagantes section)

CLEFTS OR CHAPS IN THE LIPS OR FEET

Borde: "Fissura is the latyn worde. In Englyshe it is named a chappe or chappes beynge in the lyppes tonge, handes and fete in a

man . . . .This infyrmyte dothe come of a drye humour of a march
wynde, or els of some other hote cause or hote wines, or hote wyndes." (Fol. lxvii v.)

CLEFTS OR CHAPS OF THE FUNDAMENT

Borde: "Ragades is the greke word. Ragadie is the barbarous worde. In
latin it is named Fissure or Rime. In englyshe it is named chappes in a
mannes foundment and in the secret place of a woman. . . . This
impediment doth come of acidite or of a drye coleryke humour."

COLICK/COLLICK (SEE **STONE** FOR DIFFERENTIAL DIAGNOSIS)

Goeurot: "Against disease of the raynes of the backe, and the loynes. Payne
of the reynes is called nephretica passio, & cmeth of some one or
grauel, & it is most lyke vnto the colicke in cure, but in causes they be
cleane contrarie: for the colicke beginneth at the lower partes on the
righte side, and goeth vp to the hyer partes on the left side, of the
belly, and it lyeth rather more forwarde then backewarde, but nephretica passio begynneth contrarywise aboue, descendyng downewarde,
and euer lieth more towarde the backe.

Also nephretica is paynfuller afore meat, and the colicke is euer
more greuous after. And often the colicke chaceth sodenlie, but
nephretica contrarie, for commonlie it commeth by litle and litle, for
euermore before, one shal fele payne of ye backe wt difficultie of
vrine.

Item there is more difference, for the colicke sheweth vrynes
[urines] as it were coloured, but nephretica in the begynuinge is
cleare, and white like water, & after waxeth thycke, and then
appeareth at the bottom of the vessel leke red sande or grauel." (Fol.
lxiii)

Borde: "Colica passio be the latyn wordes. In englyshe it is named the
Colycke and is named a passion, forasmuche ast he payne is very
extreme. The Cdolycke doth take his name of a gout which is in man
named Colon." (Fol. XXXVIII)

Harris: "COLICK, is a vehement pain in the Abdomen or lower Belly, and
takes its Name from the part chiefly affected, *viz.* the Gut *Colon*,
which is stretch'd, prick'd, and corroded by Winds or Excrementious
Humours, either remaining within its Cavity or fixt to its very coat."

Quincy: Any disorder of stomach or bowels attended with pain
1. Bilious colic—abundance of acrimony or choler that irritates the bowels so as to occasion continual gripes
2. Flatulent colic—bowel pain from flatules and wind pent up therein
3. Hysterical colic—arises from disorders of the womb
4. Nervous colic—convulsive spasms and contortions of the guts themselves, from some disorders of the spirits, or nervous fluid in their component fibers.

COLLICK, STONE

Quincy: "There is also a species of this distemper which is commonly called the *stone colic*, which is also, like the hysterical, by consent of parts from the irritation of the stone or gravel in the bladder or kidneys: and this is most commonly to be treated by nephretics and oily diuretics, and is greatly assisted with the carminative turpentine clysters."

CONSUMPTION

Borde: "Ptisis is the greke worde. In latyn it is named Consumpcio. In englyshe it is named a consũpcion or a wastynge, and there is .ii. kyndes, the one is natural and the other is vnnatural. The natural consumpcion resteth in aged persons in whom blode and nature dothe decrece and so consequtly wekenes foloweth, wherfor in old tyme old men were named wasted men consumed by age. An vnnatural consumpcion either it is with a feuer or without a feuer, yf it be with a feuer there is an other sicknes ronnynge in the body with it as the feuer hectycke or some other longe sicknes the whiche dothe consume the naturall moysture in man. Or els it doth come by some other feuer or sicknes the which dothe extenuate or make thyn the blode of man, so to conclude a consumpcion consumethe a man away out of this worlde. And some doth say that this empediment dothe come of an vlcerous matter in the longes."

Morton: "A Consumption in general is a wasting of the *Muscular* parts of the Body, arising from the Subtraction, or Colliquation of the Humours, and that either with, or without a Fever, and it is either Original, or Symptomatical.

An Original Consumption is that, which arises purely from a Morbid Disposition of the Blood, or Animal Spirits, which reside in the *System* of the Nerves and Fibres, and is not the effect of any other preceding Disease. Of which there are two sorts, to wit, an *Atrophy*, and a Consumption of the Lungs."

Quincy: To waste, signifies wasting of muscular flesh, frequently attended by hectic (*definition*: *slow and almost continual*) fever; and is divided by physicians into several kinds, according to the variety of causes, which must carefully be regarded in order to a cure.

CORNES

Lowe: "Of the little hard Tumour in the Feet, commonly called *Cornes*. Those hard callous tumours which commonly possesse the toes and soales of the feet, but chiefly the joynts and under the nayles, are called Cornes, and in Latine *Clavus*, of which there are three kindes, to wit, *Corpus*, *Callus*, and *Clavus*. The cause, is chiefly in wearing of strait shooes, superfluous excrements which cannot avoid, so remaineth in the nervous part, and requireth a certain hardnesse, according to the nature of the part where they are. The Signes are evident to the sight."

COUGH

Blancard: "*Tussis*, a Cough; 'tis a vehement Efflaition of the Breast, whereby that which is offensive to the Organs of Breathing is expel'd, purely by the Force of the Air."

CRAMP

Borde: "Spasmos is the greke worde. Spasmus is the barbarous worde. In latyn it is named Conuulcio or Contractio neruorum. In englyshe it is named ye crampe whiche is attraction of sinewes, and there be .iiii. kyndes the fyrste is named Emprosthotonos the which is whan the heed is drawen downeward to the brest. The second is named Thetanos, and that is whan the foreheed and all ye whole body is drawen so vehemently that ye body is vnmouable The thyrde is nameds Opisthotonos, & that is whan the heed is drawen backewarde or the mouth is drawen towardes ye eare, for these thre kyndes loke in there captyles. The fourth kynd is named Spasmos the which doth darwe [*sic*] the sinewes very strayt and sperusly in fete and legges."

"The .256. Capytle doth shewe of one of the kyndes of the crampe.
Opisthonos is the greke worde. In latyn it is named Conuulcio retrossa. In englishe it is named a crampe, the which doth draw the

heed backwarde towarde the shoulders, some latynest dothe name it Rigor ceruicis, and some doth name it Spasmus retrossus." (fol. ci)

"The .343. Capytle doth shewe of one of the kyndes of the crampe.

Thetanos is the greke worde. The barbarous worde is named Tetanus, out of whichd is vsurped a word named Tetanisi. Thetanos in englyshe is named a crampe the which doth pull ye head backewarde & dothe drawe the body so vehemently that for a space a man shalbe vnmouable, for this matter loke in the capytle named Spasmos, and vse the medecines that there be specified and beware of venerious actes after a ful stomake and beware of anger and feare."

"Tortura is the latyn worde. In englyshe it is named a drawynge vp of the mouth towarde the eare.

The cause of this impediment

This impedimente dothe come of a spasmouse cause, some dothe saye that it is a palsie, but it is a kinde of a crampe."

Paré: "*Of the flatulent convulsion, or convulsive contraction, which is common called by the French,* Goute Grampe, *and by the English, the Crampe.*

That which the French call *Goute grampe*, wee here intend to treat of induced thereto rather by the affinity of the name than of the thing, for if one speake truly, it is a certaine kinde of convulsion generated by a flatulent matter, by the violence of whose running downe or motion, oft-times the necke, armes, and legs are either extended or contracted into themselves with great paine, but that for a short time. The cause thereof is a grosse and tough vapour, insinuating it selfe into the ancles of the nerves, and the membranes of the muscles. It takes one on the night, rather than on the day, for that then the heat and spirits usually retires themselves into the entrailes and center of the body, whence it is that flatulencies may bee generated, which will fill up, distend and pull the part whereunto they runne, just as wee see lute-strings are extended. This affect often takes such as swimme in cold water, & causeth many to be drowned, though excellent swimmers, their members by this means being so straitly contracted, that they cannot by any meanes be extended."

Quincy: "Crampus so Helmont calls the cramp. It is a sort of convulsion, occasioning a sudden and painful rigidity of the muscle, which soon goes off; it principally affects the fingers, hands, feet, or legs."

DANDRIFFE

Borde: "Acor or Acoris be the greke wordes, Furfur is the latyn word, Acora is the barbarus word In englyshe it is named dandruffe or a skurfe in the heed lyke bran or otmell, the which doth penetrate the skyn of the heed makynge lytle holes, dyfferinge from an other infyrmyte in the skyn of the hed named Fauus."

DIGESTION

Borde: "Lienteria is the greke worde. In latyn it is named. In englyshe it is named the lyentery or imperfyte dygestion w^t egestiõ doth differ from Coleric passio. and from catastropha as it doth appere in theyr capy-tles . . . . This infyrmyte doth come of lubricite of slydinge of meat out of the stomake, the mawe & guttes without perfyte dycoction or digestion." (fol. lxxxi v.)

DIMNESSE AND DARKNESS OF SIGHT

Banister: "*Of the continuall dimnesse, diminishing, or hinderance of the sight, called in the Greeke*, amblyopia, *in Latine*, hebitudo, *or* cali-gato.

Amblyopia, is a continuall dimnesse and hinderance of the sight, with-out any appearance of any thing in the eye: notwithstanding the sight is darkened, and yet no hurt to be perceiued in the membranes, neither appeareth the apple of the eye, made lesser or greater, or hauing any other disorder."

"*Amaurosis* most commonly is a hinderance of the whole sight, with-out any appearance thereof in the eye: for the apple of the eye remaineth sound, and vnchanged, the sinew of sight onely is stopped. *Sauonarola* seemeth to name the beginning of this disease in Greeke, *Parorasis*, in Latine, *Hallucinatio*, or *Calligatio*, which we may name in English, the dim or deceitful sight, when we take one thing for another, which thing is forerunner & messenger of blindnes. These defaults befall to some suddenly, to others by little and little, but so, that either they see nothing, or very little. The causes of this which commeth by little and little, are like to that malady which is called in Greeke, *Ambliopia*, in Latin, *Hebetudo* . . . . The way to know the stopping of the sinew of sight, and that no spirit can pass thorow it, is this: Shut the other eye, and the apple of that eye which is stopped, will not appear to be inlarged, whidh it would be, if the spirit of sight were conueyed thereto by the sinew."

Borde: "Nyctalopis is the greke worde. In latyn it is named Nocturna excitudo. In araby it is named Amicalopes, or Sequibere, or Suberati, or Asse, or Tenebrositas. The barbarous worde is named Noctilopa. In englysh it is named darknes of the syghte for whan the sonne is downe and the euenynge in, a man can se nothynge in darknes, although other mẽ can perceiue and se somwhat that hath nat this impediment.

The cause of this imfyrmyte.

This impediment doth come of an humour the which doth lye before the syght, and it may come of dasshynge of a mannes eyes upon the sonne, or els of small prynted letters, or suche lyke." (fol. xxxxvia)

Blancard: "*Achlys*, a certain dark Distemper of the Eye, which is reckon'd amongst the Species of *Amblyopia*, or Dimness of Sight."

DREAMS, HORRIBLE DREADFULL

Borde: "Ephialtes is the greke word. Epialtes is the barbarous worde. In latyn it is named Incubus and Succubus. In englyshe it is named the Mare. And some say that it is an kynd of spirites ye which dothe infest and trouble whan they be in theyr beddes slepynge as Saynt Augustine sayth De ciuitate dei cap. 20 and Saynt Thomas of Alquine saytn in hs fyrsyte part of his diuinite. Incubus doth infest and troble women and Succubus doth infest men. Some holdeth opinion that Marlyn was begotten of his mother of the spirite named Incubus. Eldras doth speke of this spirite in Speculum exemplorum, and in my tyme at saint Albons here in Englande was infested an Ancresse of such a spirite as she shewed me, and also to credyble persons, but this is my opiniõ that this Ephialtes otherwise named the Mare the whiche doth come to man or woman whan they be slepynge shall thiynke that they do se. here and fele the thynge that is nat true. And in such troblous slepynge a man shal scarse draw breth . . . . This impediment doth come of a vaporous humour or fumosyte rysinge out from and from the stomacke to the brayne, it may come also thorowe surfetynge and dronkennes, and lyenge in the bed vpright, it maye also come of a rheumatyke humour suppressyng the brayne, and the humour descendynge doth perturbate the hert bryngynge a man slepynge into a dreame, to thick that the whiche is nothynge is somewhat, and to fele that thynge that he felyth nat, and to se that thynge he seyth nat, with such lyke matters." (fol. lii v.–liii)

DROPSIE (SEE ALSO **TYMPANY**)

Borde: "Hidrops, or Hidropis, or Hidropesis is deriued out of a worde of greke named Hidor, which is water, for the sicknes doth come of a wateryshe humour. The olde auncient grekes did name this sicknes Lencoplegmantia. In englyshe it is named the hiedropsy or the dropsy. There be .iii. kyndes of ye dropsies, the fyrst is named Ascites and some doth name it Alchites . . . . The seconde kynde of ye hidropsies is named Timpanites . . . . The thyrde kynde of ye hidropsies is named Sarcites, and some doth name it Iposarca and some doth name it Anasarca." (fol. lxxiv–lxxiv v.)

"Astites or Asclites be ye greke wordes. The barbarous men do name it Alchites or Alsclites. In englyshe it is one of the kyndes of the Hiedropsies, and in ingdredin the bely for the belyu wyll boll & swel, and wyl make a noyse as a botel halfe full of water."

Blancard: "Hydrops, a stagnation of a water Humour in the Habit of Body, or some particular cavity; and 'tis either *general*, as an *Anasarca* and *Ascites*, to which some add a Tympany, but falsly; or *particular*, confin'd to one Part, as a *Dropsy*, in the Head, Breast, Hand, Foot, &c. of which in their proper Places severally. A Dropsy."

Quincy: "Hydrops . . . a dropsy; thus named because water is the most visible cause of the distemper

Hydrops cysticus, the encysted dropsy. It is water enclosed in a cystis, that is in a hydratid.

Hydrops genu, a dropsy in the knee; when water is collected under the capsular ligament of the knee, this disorder is formed.

Hydrops ad matulam, from Matula, a chamber-pot or urinal, i.e. Diabetes, which see.

Hydrops medullae spinalis, i.e., spina bifida.

Hydrops ovariae, a dropsy of the ovaria.

Hydrops pectoris, i.e. Hydrothorax, or dropsy in the chest.

Hydrops pulmonum, dropsy of the lungs.

Hydrops sacculus lachrymalis, i.e., hernia lachrymalis

Hydrops scroti, i.e., hydrocele.

Hydrops testis vel testium, i.e., hydrocele.

Hydrops uteri, dropsy of the womb."

"Hydropic, one that is troubled with a dropsy; also a medicine contrived for that distemper"

DRUNKENESS

Borde: "Ebrietas is the latyn worde. In greke it is named *Mœthœ*. In englyshe it it named drõkinnes.

The cause of this impediment.

This impedimẽt doth come eyther by wekeness of ye brain or els by some great hurt in the heed, or of to much ryotte.

A remedy

Yf it do come by an hurt in the heed there is no remedy but pacience of all partes. Yf it do come by the debylyte of the brayne and heed, drynke in the mornynge a dysshe of mylke, vse a sirupe named *Sirupus acetosns de prunis*, and vse laxatiue maeates, and purgacions yf nede do requyre, and beware of superfluous drynkynge specially of wine and stronge ale, and beere, and yf any man do perceue that he is dronke, let him take a vomyt w^t water & oyle, or w^t a fether, or a rosemary braũche or else with his fynger, or els let him go to his bed to slepe." (fol. xlix v.–L)

DUGGS (SEE TEATS)

EARS, TICKLINGS AND NOISE OF THE

Goeurot: "Sometyme there chaunceth deafnes by wynde, whyche is in the eare, the whyche causeth tynklynge in the head."

Borde: "Tinnitus aureum be ye latin wordes. In englysh it is named syngynge or a sounynge in a mannes eares, and this doth prognosticate deefnes

The cause of this impediment

This impediment dothe come of a ventosyte or wynd the which is in the heed and in the eares and can nat get out."
Marginal index note: "Piping in the eare."

EMEROIDES

Borde: "Haemorrhoides is ye greke word. In olde tyme the latyns dyd use
this barbarous word named Emoroides. In englyshe it is named ye
Emorodes or pyles the which be vaynes in the extreme parte of the
longacion to whom doth happen by diuers tymes .ii. sondry passions,
the fyrsts is lyke pappes and teates, and they wyl blede, and be the
very Emerodes, ye other be lyke wartes and they wyll yche, and water
& smart, and they be named the pyles, and in the sayd place doth
brede other infyrmytes, as Ficus in ano, Fistula in ano."

Quincy: synonym of haemorrhoides.

EROSIONS IN THE CORNERS OF THE EYES

Borde: "Aegylops is the greke word. In englyshe it is a superfluous fleshe
in ye corner of the eye towarde the nose, where vnto corrupt humours
be gathered. And if this impediment do increase and a remedy by
tyme nat be had, it wyll fester and fystle the whiche is dangerous to
medle withall for it doth stande in a daungerous place.

The cause of this impedyment.

This impediment doth come thorow a reumatyke humour myxt with
corrupte blode or it maie come with a strype or hurt done in that
place." fol. x b

EYE, MATTER IN THE CORNER OF THE

Borde: "The 281. Capytle doth shewe of matter in the corner of the eye.

Piosis or Onix be the greke words. In latyn it is named Pus in cronea.
The barbarous wordes be named Sania in cronea. In englyshe it is
matter in the eye." (fol. cviii v.)

EYE LIDS, CORNS OF THE

Borde: "Ordiolus is the latyn worde. In englyshe it is named a corene in the
eye lydde much lyke a barly corne . . . . This impediment doth come
of a reume myxte with corrupt blode the which hath a recourse more
to that place than to any other place." (fol. ciiii)

EYES, SKARRES OF THE

Banister: "Although *oule* bee vsed generally for a cicatrice or scar in any
part: yet *Galen* taketh it for a white high scarre vpon the hornie membrane, because of a deepe vlcer: it may also happen in the white of the
Eye, but not so euidently to be seene. The kindes thereof are *aigis*, and
leucoma, when the scarre in the hornie membrane is thicker and higher
then the former, arising of a greater vlcer then the former, possessing
sometimes the circle *Iris*, or rainbow. Some assigne this default to the
chrystaline humour, which is wholly made white. *Paralampsis* is a
scarre on the blacke of the eye, mor hard, grosse, and shining then *aigis*.
In the cure, you must consider whether they be hollow, or standing vp."

EYES, SPOTS AND BLEMISHES OF THE

Banister: "*Aiglia*, is a white spotte resembling a cicatrice, gathered vpon
the membranes *coniunctiua*, and *cornea*. This commeth by a fleume,
which by little and little is heaped in the part. It may also proceed of
some piece of a webbe being left behinde, about the which some
humour may bee congealed, and in time come to a scarre. And where
these humours become very hard, there may bee seene a it were a knot
vpon the membranes *coniuntiua* and *cornea*, it is called *porosis*."

Borde: "Phlytanai is the greke worde. The barbarous worde is names
Vesice. In latyn it is named Pustule. In englyshe it is named pusshes or
whyte cornes vpon the eye, and some say it is a wheale or a lytle bladder in any place of the body . . . . This impediment dothe come of coleryke humours, boylinge vnder the skyn penytratyne the flesshe a
lytle, if it be as some do say it is a bladder than it dothe come of a
wateryshe humydyte, and than this impediment may come as well
thorowe standynge as by labour or any other waye, some doth name
this impediment Macula in oculo." (fol. cviii–cviii v.)

"Tarphati is the barbarous word. In latyn it is named Macula in oculo.
In englyshe it is named a spot or a pusshe in the eye."

EYES STANDING TOO FARRE FORTH OF THE HEAD

Banister: "*Exopthalmia*, is a standing out, a lifting vp, as it were, a casting
foorth of the eye from the hollownesse and circle wherein it is set and
placed, as a precious stone within his collet. This affection or disposition is sometimes meerely naturall, as wee may see in such as haue
great eyes, and to them it is not needfull to apply any thing. But if the

eye doe thrust out more and more, vntill it depart wholly out to the natural place, then, cometh *ecpiesmos*. In some it standeth so farre foorth, that it cannot be couered with the eye-lids, and is in such sort remoued out of the circle, that it hangeth without the bone ethmoides.

This disease commeth either of outward causes, as from falling from an high place, by a great stroke on the head, or about the eye with a ball or stone: it may grow also from strangling or choaking, as appeareth in them which vse wrastling, whereunto wee referre the great violent strainings which women suffer in hard trauels, and the stretching which they abide, that haue the disease called *tenesmus*. It is incident to them which are troubled with greiuous vomiting, straightness of breath, and vse blowing in great hornes. The inward causes amongst other are great inflamation and flowings, commonly called fluxes, which fall vpon the eye, because of the inflamation is called by *Celsus, proptosis*. It may be called also by an Aposteme, being in the substance of the braine, or in the skins and coates which couer the same, and from too much fulnessse and windinesse, which is heaped together and ingendred in the eye, as it commeth to passe in the child which dieth and putrefieth in the mothers woombe: and to these may bee added the loosing, and ouermuch mollifying of the muscles and membranes, which moue and turne the eye. According to these causes there are diuers signes whereby the disease is knowne. For when the eye falleth out through the aboundance of humors, it is greater and grosser then if it fell out by strangling and choaking, by straining or blowing (if there bee none other fulnesse of humors) albeit there is in both great stretching out of it: but if it arise from the softnesse and tendernesse of the muscles, and membranes, it is not so puffed up and swelled, yea scarcely can any stretching be perceiued."

FAINTNESSE ABOUT/AT THE HEART

Borde: "Cardiaca passio be the latin word. In englyshe it is named the Cardyacke passion, or a passion, about the hert, for the hert is depressed and ouercome with faintnesse."

FALLING OF HAIR FROM THE EYE-LIDS

Guillemeau: "*Of the fallng of haire from the eieliddes or* bauldnesse of them called in Greeke *Madarosis* and *Milphosis*, in latine *Defluuium pilorum*, or *Glabrithes palpebrarum*, also of thicknesse ioyned with baldnesse in the eyeliddes, called in greeke *Ptilosis* in latine, *Craisities callosa palpebrarum*.

Madarosis is onclye taken for the falling of hayre from the eyelids by a flovving of sharpe humours, and vvhere the hayres do simply fall avvay, and the vtmost part and banckes as it vvere of the eyelids are red like vuto leade the affection is called *milphosis* or *miltosis*. The cause according to *Auicen* is grosse salt matter, which maketh the eyeliddes redde, bringing vlceration to the parts where the haires take roote, the eye thereby being sometime impaired and corrupted. But if the edges and bankes therof growe thicke and hard in such maner that the haire cannot there bee fastened and perce thorough the disease is named *ptilosis* ioyntly mixed and compounded of *madarosis* and *xeropthalmia*." p. 48

FALLING SICKNESS

Borde: "Analepsia is the greke worde. The barbarous word is named Analencia. In latin is named Morbus caducus, and Morbus commicialis. In englyshe it is one of the kyndes of fallynge sicknes. And they yt hath this sicknes whã they do fall they do nat fome at eh mouth, but they do defyle tha self other by vryn or by egestiõ or both at ones.

The cause of this infyrmyte.

Many auctours in dyuers matters be of sondry opinions, but as for this matter I do say that for as much as it is one of the kyndes of the fallynge sicknes, it doth take his orygynall of a reumatycke humour, opylatyng ye celles of ye brayne and the brayne so opylated and stopped the paciet lyeth pytefully vnto the tyme that nature hath remoued the cause." (fol. xiiii).

"Epilepsia is the greke word. Epilencia is the barbarous worde In latyn it is named Conuulcio or, Morbus sacer, or Morbus harculeus, or Morbus caducus. And in diuers regions it is named Morbus Mahometus, for Mahomete (in whom the turkes dothe beleue) had the sayde sicknesse. In englyshe it is named the fallynge sicknes, or the foule yll. Also it is named in latyn Ira dei and some do name it Pedo and some do name it laracionen.

The cause of this infyrmyte.

This infyrmyte is ingendred either of a reumatyke humour, or els of a grosse & a colde winde or els of a melancoly humour the whidh is bred in the hinder part of te heed, or els of euy! humours abundynge in ye stomake, the whiche doth vapour and fume vp to the brayne opylatynge the vitall spirites. Galen sayth it is a cold humour the whiche doth opylate the celles of the brayne, vnto the tyme that naure hathe remoued the cause. There be .iii. kyndes of the fallynge sicknes, the fyrste is Epilepsia, the seconde is named Analepsia, and the thyrde is named Catalepsia. They the which be infected with Epilepsia in theyr fallynge shall foome at the mouth, and this is the comon fallyng sicknes and they the which hathe Analepsia whan they do fall they shal defyle them selfe and nat fome at the mouth. And they the which hathe Catalepsia whether they be take open eyed, or halfe closed, for the tyme they shall se nothynge, as it shall appere in the capytle named Catalepsis." (fol. lv a)

"Catalepsis or Cathocha be ye greke wordes. In latyn it is named Congelatio. The barbarus worde is named Catalencia. In englyshe it is named the Catalency, which is one of the kyndes of the fallynge sicknes.

The cause of this impediment.

This impediment doth come of a colde reume the whiche doth molest and troble the brayne and heeed, that it doth depryue one of his witte & doth fal to the grounde, & can nat moue nor stere, for as one is taken so shal he lye, otherwhile ope eyed and otherwhile close eyed. and although the eyes be open yet one shal nat see, heare, nor speake, nor scarse draw any wynd in or out yt can be perceiued for one shal lye as he were deed for a space." (fol. xxxii b)

Blancard: "*Analepsia*, or *Epilepsia*, Falling-sickness." "*Epilepsia*, or *Morbus Caducus*, or *Comitialis*, because that the persons affected fall down on a sudden. Or, *Hercules*, because it is hard to be cur'd; also *Lues Deifica*, *Sonicus*, *Sacer*, &c. And it is an interrupted Convulsion of the whole Body, which hurts all Animal Actions, proceeding from an Explosion of Animal Spirits in the Brain, whereby the Persons affected are suddenly cast upon the Ground. This explosion arises either from an irritation, or pricking in the Spirits, or when something *Heterogeneous* is intermix'd with the Animal Spirits. The *Epilepsy*, or *Falling-sickness*."

"*Cataptosis*, is not a Disease, but a Symptom of Epilepsies and Apoplexies, signifying a sudden or casual falling to the Ground, which is an involuntary Motion of some Organical Member, proceeding from a Palsie, and Relaxation of the Muscles and Tendons beyond Nature."

Quincy: "an epilepsia" "Epilepsia . . . it being sufficient to know that it is a convusion, or convulsive motion of the whole body, or of some of its parts, with a loss of sense."

FEAVER

Lowe: [Fever] "It is an extraordinary heat, beginning in the heart, sent through all the body with the spirit and blood, by the vaines and arteries." [p. 291]

Blancard: "*Febris*, a Fever, is an inordinate motion, and to great an Effervescence of the Blood, attended with Cold first, and afterwards with Heat, Thirst, and other Symptoms, wherewith the Animal *Oeconomy* is variously disturb'd. Fevers in general are divided in to Intermittent, Continued, Continent, and Symptomatical; as also into *Quotidien*, *Tertian*, *Quartan*, *Erratic*, &c. Agues or Fevers."

Quincy: "Fever, is an augmented velocity of blood. The almost infinite variety of causes of this distemper does so diversify its appearances, and indicate so many ways of cure, that our room here will not allow of any more than to refer to reverious, Willis, Morton, Sydenham, and Huxham for the practice, in all its shapes."

FEAVERS, CONTINUAL (SEE ALSO FEVER, SWEATING, AND FEAVERS EPIALES)

Borde: "Febris sinochos is the greke worde. In latyn it is named Febris sinochus or Febris continua. In englyshe it is named a continuall fever. Synochus is derived of .ii. wordes, syn that is to saye without, & choos whid is to say trauel, ant that is as much to say as a feuer without rest."

Harris: "FEAVER, is a fermentation or inordinate Motion of the Blood, and a too great heat of it, attended with Burning, Thirst, and other Symptoms, whereby the Natural Oeconomy or Government of the Body is variously disturb'd. . . . *Continual Feaver*, is that whole fit is continued for many Days, having its times of Remission, and of more Fierceness, but never of Intermission."

FEAVER, INTERMITTING

Blancard: "*Intermittens Febris*, is call'd a Fever or Ague that ceaseth and returns at certain times; 'Tis either Quotidian, Tertian, or Quartan, and some add the Quintan."

FEAVER, PESTILENTIALL

Borde: "Epidema is the greke worde. In latin it is named Pestilencia or Febris pestilencialis. In englyshe it is named the pestilence.

The cause of this infyrmyte.

This infyrmyte dothe come, either by the punyshment of g-d, either els of a corrupt and contagious ayre, and one man infected with this sicknes may infect may men, this sicknes may come also with the stenche of euyl dyrty stretes, of chanelles nat kept clene, of standynge puddels, of seges & stynkinge draughts of shedynge of mannes blode, and of deed bodies nat depely buried, of a great company beynge in a lytle or smal rome, of comõ pyssynge places, and of many such lyke contagious ayres as be rehersed in the dyetary of helthe."

FEAVER, QUARTAN

Borde: "Febris quartana be yᵉ latyn wordes. In englysh it is named a feuer quartayne the which doth infest a man euery thyrde daye, that is to saye.ii. dayes whole and one sicke, and theyr maye be a doble quartayne. . . . This impediment or feuer dothe come of melancoly, or els of coler adusted, and if the blacke Jawnes be concurrant with it, it is a dyffycyll sicknes to make on whole." (fol. lxi)

Blancard: "*Quartana febris intermittens*, a Quartan Ague, the which the Ancients call'd *Satum's* Daughter. 'Tis called this Day a Scandal to Physicians, because is so hard to be cur'd by those who follow the old way. 'Tis a preternatural Effervescense of the Blood, which seizes a Man every fourth Day, and then leaves him. 'Tis caus'd by an acid austere Blood and nutricous Juice, hinder'd in its Assimilation."

FEAVER QUOTIDIAN

Borde: "Febris quotidiana be the latyn wordes. In englysh it is named a cotidiane, the which doth infest a man euery day . . . . Every cotidiane is ingendred of a salt fleume or of swete fleume, or els of sower fleume. Yf it be ingendred of salt fleume the pacient shalbe in great heate, and wylbe thursty. Yf it do come of swete fleume the pacient wylbe sompnolent, dull and heuy, and his stomake wyll abhorre meates and drynkes, hauynge taste nor talege to comfort the palat of the mouthe. Yf it do come of sower fleume the paciẽt shal haue payne in the stomake and is euer disposed to vometynge, and the coldnes of the feuer wyle great and the heate lytle." (fol. lx)

FEAVER, SWEATING

Blancard: "Elodes, and Helodes, a continual Fever, attended with continued Sweats, wherein the Patients are almost melted through moisture. The Sweating Fever."

FEAVER, TERTIAN

Borde: "Febris terciana be yᵉ latyn wordes. In englysh it is named a feuer tercian the which doth infest a man euery second day, and there may be a doble terciane. . . . This feuer dothe come of coler, and it dothe dyffer frõ a feuer causon, for a feuer terciane doth operate or worke his malyce in the vaynes, and the feuer causon doth worke his malyce in the concauyte of the lyuer & the lunges & about the hert." (fol. lx verso.)

FEAVERS EPIALES

Borde: "Febris Epialtes is yᵉ greke worde. Febris Eipialia may be taken for yᵉ barbarus word & yᵉ latyn worde. In englyshe it maye be named the Epyall feuer, and some do name this feuer Febria Epiala Epi that is to saye aboue and Algor that is colde. . . . This feuer doth come of a grosse fleumatyke matter, causynge the interyall partes of the body to burne, and the exteryall partes of the body to be colde, oppylatynge the poores, the whiche doth prohibyte that the fume can nat be desolued, and this feuer causeth the paciẽt to be thyrsty, and the tonge to be rough and out of taste." (fol. lxiii v.)

Blancard: "*Epiala*, sive *Quercera*, a continued fever, wherein the patient feels both heat and cold at once."

FELLON (SEE ALSO **WHITLOW**)

Borde: "Antrax is the latyn worde. In englyshe it is named a Felon, and is like a Carbocle, but nat so great in quantyte or substance."

Blancard: "*Paronychia, Panarium*, or *Reduvia*, a preternatural Swelling in the Finger, and very troublesome. It arises from a sharp malign Humor, which can gnaw the Tendons, Nerves, the Membrane about the Bone, and the very Bone it self. A *Whitlow*."

Quincy: "Felon, so the paronychia is called when its seat is in the periosteum at the beginning. . . .

Paronychia, . . . , circum, about, and [greek], unguis, the nail is a tumor upon the end of a finger, commonly called a felon or whitlow." = =also name for plant used for medication of felons.

FISTULA

Borde: "Fistula is the latyn word. In greke it is named Seruix. In englyshe it is named a fystle, the which is a corrupt appostumacion in a vayne, or a fystle is a depe ulceracion, long, and strayt, and most comonly it wyl be in a mannes foundement." (fol. lxvii v.)

Blancard: "*Fistula*, a straight long Cavity, or a winding narrow and callous Ulcer, of difficult cure, proceeding for the most part from an Apostheme. *Fistula's* differ from winding Ulcers in this, that *Fistula's* are callous and hard, but Ulcers are not. Sometimes an Issue is call'd a *Fistula*."

Quincy: "so the Latins call a catheter." "Fistula, is any kind of pipe, and therefore, some anatomists call any parts that have any resemblance thereto in their figure, fistulae; . . . as the aspira arteria, fistulae pulmonis; the uretra, fistula urinaria . . . , but its common use is for ulcers that lie deep, and ooze out their matter through long, narrow, winding passages; in which cases the bone are frequently foul, and the extreme parts callous."

FISTULAES, AND HOLLOW ULCERS OF THE EYE

Banister: "*Aegilops* is a little *fistula* in th corner of the eye, neere to the nose, out of which issueth continually fleume, or a thin humor, arising of some former disease, as of *anchilops* suppurated, but either not speedily opened or negligently dressed: or rather it is procured of slimy matter, or moyst medicines, or the ayre which hath altered, and rotted the bone in that part. This maladie vexeth the eye without ceasing, being sometimes red, and piercing thorow euen to the nose. It hath in some, the nature and properties of a canker, an in those the veines are stretched forth, and crooked, the colour pale and blewish, the skin hard. If it bee touched as gently as possible, it stirreth vp inflamation in the parts adioyning. It is dangerous attempting the cure thereof, when it is of a cankrous or crabbed nature: for it hasteth the death of the Patient. And it is lost labour to take in hand the cure of it, when the apostume toucheth the nose, sith it will neuer bee perfectly healed: those which are in the corner of the eye, are curable, but yet the neerer their hole or mouth is to it, the greater difficulty is in the cure."

Borde: "The .10. Capytle doth shew of a fystulus impostume in the corner of the eye.
Algarab is the Araby word Auiven doth name it Algaras In englyshe it is an impostume in the corner of the eye.

The cause of this Apostumacion,

This Impostume doth come of a Reumatyke humour myxt with corrupt blode hauynge a recourse to the eye." margin index: "Apostume in the eye." fol. xi verso.

FLUX OF THE BELLY (SEE ALSO LASK)

Goeurot: "In al fluxes of ye belly, cause the excremtes to be dulye serched, for if the disease be seuche, that the meate commeth out, euen as it was receyued, or not half dygested, ye sayde fluxe is called lienteria. Yf great aboundace of waterye humours haue their issue by lowe, the sayde fluxe is named diarrhea, whyche is a moch to saye as fluxe humorall. And yf bloode of matter appeare wyth the excrementes in the syckeness, then they call it dyssenteria, which is a gret disease and a daungerous for to cure."

Borde: Extrauagantes "The .19. Capytle doth shewe of the kindes of fluxes. Fluxus ventris be the latin wordes. In englyshe it is named the flyxe, and there be .iii. kindes named in latyn Lienteria, Diarrhea and Dissiteria. In englyshe it is named the Lyentery, the Dyarrhy, and ye Dyssentery The Lientery egesteth or doth auoyde the meat in maner as it was eaten. The Dyarrhy is a common laxe. The Dyssintery is the blody flyxe, and some doth name these flyxes after this maner. Intestinal, Epatycall and Saguine. Intestinall cometh of day and nyght with fretynge in the bely. Epatycke or Epaticall flyxe cometh without paine prycking or fretynge. The blody or Sanguine flux maketh excoriacion of the guttes with payne prickynge and freatynge."

Blancard: "*Fluxus Alvinus*, the same with *Diarrhoea, Fluxus Hepaticus*, a kind of Dysentery, wherein black shining Blood, and too long roasted as it were, is driven out of the Guts by the Fundament, but without Pain. It is sometimes taken for a Dysentery, wherein serous sharp blood is evacuated, and is often the Consequence of it."

Quincy: "Fluxion, . . . It also signifies the same as Defluxion or Cattarrh, from fluo, to flow. For which reason likewise *Fluxus Alvinus* is a *diarrhaea*, *Fluxus Hepaticus* a *dysentery*, from the contents of the stools, and the like."

"Dysenteria, . . . a dysentery. It is a painful discharge from the bowels by way of stool. It is often called the **bloody flux**, because blood sometimes appears in the stools; but this is not a common symptom nor essential to the disease. Dr. Cullen defines it to be a contagious fever, in which the patient hath frequent stools, accompanied with much griping, and followed by a tenesmus."

Cullen: under discussion of dysentery: "the matter voided by the stool is very various. Sometimes it is merely a mucous matter, without any blood, exhibiting that disease which Dr. Roderer has named the *morbus mucosus*, and others the *dysenteria alba*."

FORGETFULNESS (SEE ALSO **LETHARGY**)

Borde: "Lethargos is the greke worde. And some grecions dothe name it the Syrsen. The barbarous me doth name it Litergia. In latyn it is named Lethergia or Obliuio. In englyshe it is named obliuious or forgetfulnes. . . . This impediment doth come thorowe colde reume the whiche doth obnebulate a mannes memory, and doth lye in the hinder part of a mannes heed witing the skull or brain panne." (fol. lxxxv)

FRECKLES

Borde: "Lentigo or Lentiginos be the latyn wordes. In greke it is named Phacos. In englyshe it is named frackles the which is in ones face and body. . . . This impediment doth come eyther by the calydyte of the son or els by the corrupcion of ye ayr or by some interyall cause in retaynynge some superfluous humour." (fol. lxxx v.)

"Pannus is the latyn worde. In englyshe it is named an impediment in the face, specially in the face of a woman whan she is with chylde, this impedimēt is like a sicknes named Lētigini, or Lētigo. . . . This impediment doth come either by heate of the sonne, or by heat the which doth fume from the lyuer and the stomake." (fol. cii)

FRENSIE

Borde: "Phrenitis is the greke worde. And some grecios doth name it after the arabyes, Syrsen or Karabitus. The barbarus word is named Frenisis.

The trewe latyns doth vse the terme after the grecions In englyshe it is named a phresyse or madnes the which absolutly is as an impostumacion bredde and ingendred in the pellycles of ye brayne named in latyn Pia mater the which appostumacion dothe make alyenacion of a mannes mynde and memory There is an other accident phrenyse the whiche is ioyned with an other sicknes, as a phrenyse with a feuer, or with a pleuryce & such other like sicknesses.

The cause of this sicknes

For the phrenyse the cause is shewed, how be it some holdeth opinion that a phrenyse doth come of a bylus humour oppressynge the brayne, and some say it is an inflacion of the brayne the whiche doth perturbate the reason and dothe make a man out of reason. The accident phrenyse doth come .ii. wayes the one is thorowe a hoote fume ascendynge from the stomake to the brayne. The other is thorowe collygacion of the nerues or sinewes the which the brayne hath with the mydryffe." (fol. C.vii verso–C.viii)

"Mania is the greke word. In latyn it is named Insania or Furor. In englyshe it is named a madnes or wooknes lyke a wylde beest, it doth differ from a phrenyse, for a phrenyse is with a feuer and lo is nat Mania this madnes that I dop rende to speke nowe of. . . . This infyrmyte doth come af a corrupt blode in the heed, and some doth say yt it doth come of a byluse blode intruted in the heed, and some saye it doth come of wekenes of the brayne the which letteth a man to slepe, and he that can nat ûrpe must nedes haue an yole brayne, and some say it is tyrnynge up so downe in the heed the whiche doth make the madnes." (fol. lxxxviii)

Blancard: *Phrenitis, Phrenetiasis,* or *Phrenesis,* a Dotage, with a continual Fever, often accompany'd with Madness and Anger, proceeding from too much Heat in the Animal Spirits, not from the Inflamation of the Brain, as the Ancients thought. *Willis* thus defines it, namely, an Inflamation of the whole sensitive Soul and Animal Spirits. A *Frenzy*."

FUNDAMENT (DISEASES OF)

Borde: "Anus is the latyn word. In greke it is named *Grans*. In englyshe it is a mannes ars let euery man kepe yᵉ place clene. And let no mã make no restryctions that nature wolde expell, other by egestion, or by ventosyte. In the aforesaid place is ingedred the pyles, or Emerodes, Fystles and Festures, Cankers, the Pockes, and *Ficus in Ano* and dyuers tymes the longacion which is the ars gut doth fal out fo the body, And otherwhyle many men can nat kepe theyr egestion by slepyng & waking they do defyle the self."

GANGRENE (SEE **SAINT ANTHONIES FIRE**)
GIDDINESS IN THE HEAD

Paré: *"Of the* Vertigo, *or Giddinesse.*

> The *Vertigo* is a sudden darkening of the eyes and sight by a vaporous & hot spirit which ascendeth to the head by the sleepy arteryes, and fils the braine, disturbing the humours and spirits which are conteyned there, & tossing them unequally, as if one ran round, or had drunk too much wine. This hot spirit oft-times riseth from the heart upwards by the internall sleepy arteries to the *Rete mirabile,* or wonderfull net; otherwhiles it is generated in the brain, its selfe being more hot than is fitting; also it oft-times ariseth from the stomack, spleen, liver and other entrals being too hot. The signe of this disease is the sudden darkening of the sight, and the closing up as it were of the eyes, the body being lightly turned about, or by looking upon wheels running round, or whirle pits in waters, or by looking down any deep or steep places. If the originall of the disease proceed from the braine, the patients are troubled with the head-ache, heavinesse of the head, the noyse in the ears and oft-times they lose their smell . . . . But if such a *Vertigo* be a criticall symptome of some acute disease affecting the *Crisis* by vomit or bleeding, then the whole businesse of freeing the patient thereof must be committed to nature." pp. 639–640

GOUT

> Borde: "Cchiragra is the greke worde. In englyshe it is the gout the which is in the handes & fingers of man. And it doth tunne from one ioynt to an other as other gouts doth.

The cause of this impediment.

> This impediment doth come of reume & euyll dyet. And there be .ii. kynds of the gout in ye hands the one is confyrmed and can nat be made whole for and it do come by kynde so that the ioyntes be broken the sicknes is vncurable. The other ye which is nat confyrmed may be made whole."

Lowe: "This disease (which commonly doth possesse the joynts, by the falling of some humor above nature betwixt the joynt bones) is called by the Latines *Morbus articularis*, and in vulgar the Gout, of the which there be divers kinds and names according to the joint which is diseased, as for example: that which occupieth the jawes, is called *Sciagonogra*: if in the Neck, it is called *Trahelagra*: in the Backe, it is called *Rachiagra*: that in the shoulders is called *Omogra*: that in the Clavicules, is called *Clersagra*: that in the elbow is called *Pethagra*, that in the hands is called *Cheiragra*, that in the foot is called *Podagra*, and that in the Haunch is called *Ischias*, and that in the knees is called *Gonagra*: here I shall content me to speak of he last two, because they be most common, the others I leave to the learned Physition, as matters more Physicall than Chyrurgicall. The disease which is called *Sciatica* proceedeth partly by the usage of such meats and ingendereth Phlegmatique humors, also a Defluxion of grosse congealed humor, which possesseth the joint of the hanch bone, which partly doth proceed for want of exercise, as also sometime by immoderate using of women, stopping of the hemorrhoides or monethly courses." pp. 264–5

Blancard: "*Arthritis*, or *Morbus articularis*, the Gout, which is a Distemper that exercises its Tyranny about two or three, or more Joints, and their Interstices, and it is defin'd to be a pain about the Joints, produced from an *Effervescence* of the Nervous acid Juice with the fix'd saline Particles of the Blood, whence the *Nerves*, *Tendons*, *Ligaments*, the thin membranes about the Bones are contracted, and miserably tormented; whence proceed Swellings, Redness, hard sandy *Concretions* in several Parts of the Body, and other Symptoms that accompany it. It is fourfold, *Chiragra*, the *Gout* in the Hands; *Ischias*, in or about the Bone that is connected to the *Os Illium*; *Gonagra*, in the Knees; and *Podagra*, in the Feet; almost and incurable Distemper."

"*Arthritis Vaga*, or *Planetica*, the erratic or wandring *Gout*; a Disease in the Joints that creates pain, sometimes in one Limb, sometimes in another. It is call'd *Vaga*, wandring, because 'tis not constant to one and the same place, as the true *Gout* is. Its Cause is owing to a Fermentation of the *Acid* and *Alcali*; which as it happens in one Joint or other vellicates the Nervous Fibres, and produces that Pain; and this is also sometimes call'd the *Rheumatism*."

"*Coxarius Morbus*, the Hip-Gout."

GRAVEL IN THE BODY; GRAVEL (SEE ALSO **STONE**)

Paré: Under heading "*Prognostickes in the stone*."

"Women are not so subject to the stone as men, for they have the neck of their bladder more short and broad, as also more straight; wherefore the matter of the stone by reason of the shortnesse of the passage is evacuated in gravell, before it can be gathered and grow into a stone of a just magnitude." p.666

HEAD, PAINES OF THE (SEE ALSO **HEAD-ACH**)

Borde: "Cephalargia is the greke worde. Soda is the araby worde. In englyshe it is named the Cephalarge or an vniuersal payne in the hed. Some auctours doth holde opinion that Soda and Cephalia is one infyrmyte.

The cause of this infyrmyte.

This infyrmyte doth come either by extreme labour, or by surfetynge or of the corrupcion of the ayer, or by some extreme heet, or els by extreme colde, or drynkynge of hote wines." Margin note: "Payne in the heed." (fol. xxxiiii A)

"Soda is ye latyn worde. In englyshe it is a paine in he heed, and there be .ii. kyndes, vniuersall and perticuler, vniuersal holdeth a mannes whole heed, and a perticuler is in a perticuler place in the heed in the which is payne." (fol. CXXV A)

"Cephalea is the greke word. In latyn it is named *dolor ingens in capite*. In englyshe it is named ye Cephale, the whiche is an extreme paine in the heed, tha a man can nat abide no lyght nor no noyse, and the pacient doth loue to be in darke places. And his heed he doth thynke doth go in peces, and a pylowe is beeter for the pacient, than a cote of defence.' (fol. XXXIIII v.)

HEAD, PAINS ARISING FROM COLD (COLD HUMORS ARE PHLEGME [FLEUME] AND MELACHOLY)

Goeurot: "Ye maye knowe that fleume is the cause of the peyne in the heed, when ye fele coldnesse with great heuynesse: specyallye in the hyndre parte: when one spytteth often, and hath hys face lyke sunne brent." (fol. v A)

"When peyne of the head procedeth of melancholie, the paciet feleth heuines of the heed, & hath terrible dreames, w^t great care & thought, or feare, and hys peyne is specyally upon the lefte syde." (fol. vi A)

HEAD, PAINS PROCEEDING FROM HEAT (HOT HUMORS ARE BLOOD AND CHOLER)

Goeurot: "Ye may knowe head ache when it commeth of bloude, for in the face and eyes there appeareth adarke rednesse, pryckyng and heuynesse with heate. . . .

One may know the head ache that procedeth of cholere, when in the face ther is a clere rednesse, enclynyng somwhat toward yelowe, holownesse of the eies and the mouth drye and hote: and somtymes bytternesse, small reste, greate heate with sharpe payne, chefely on the ryght syde of the head." (fol. iiiB–iiiiA)

HEAD-ACHE (SEE ALSO MEGRIM)

Goeurot: "Head-ache chaunceth often tymes, of dyuers and sondry causes as of bloud, cholere, fleume, or melancholye, or of ventositie, and somtymes of heat of the sunne, or of to great colde of the ayre.

Ye may knowe head ache when it commeth of bloude, for in the face and eyes there appeareth adarke rednesse, pryckyng and heuynesse with heate." (fol. iii B)

Borde: "As for aches in ye heed be many Fyrste there is an ache the which dothe come by extreme labour. Then is there an ache the whiche dothe come by extreme colde. There is an ache the whiche maye come by superabundance of reume. Then is an ache in the heed the whiche may come by acrydytie or drynes in the heed. Ther is an ache ye whiche may come by a bylus humour or by some appostumacion. There is an ache the whiche may come by or thorowe drokennesse. There is an ache in ye heed ye which may come by ventosyte. There is an ache the which may come by a blow, a strype or fal, or any great hurt in the heed. There is heed ache the whiche maye come by any maner of feuer and by other certeyne sicknesses. and besyde all these aches may be in the heed thorowe te calyditie or heate of the sone, or by intemporancy of ye ayer corrupted. And it may come by the euyll operacio of the planettes and signes." (fol. xxx B)

"Cephalea is the greke word. In latyn it is named *Dolor ingens in capite*. In englyshe it is named ye Cephale, the which is an extreme paine in the heed, that a man can nat abide no lyght nor no noyse, and the patient doth loue to be in darke places. And his heed he dothe thynke doth go in peces, and a pylowe is better for the pacient, than a cote of defence.

The cause of this impedyment.

> This impediment doth come either of extreme heet or els of extreme cold, or of some maliuolus humour." Margin note: "Cephaly heed ache." (fol. xxxiiii B)"

HOLY FIRE (SEE **SAINT ANTHONIES FIRE**)

IMPOSTHUME (SEE ALSO **ULCER**)

> Borde: "Flegmon is the greke word. In latyn it is named Appostema clidum or perticulare. In englyshe it is named an impostume or an inflacion ingendred in a perticuler place, and is very hote and burnynge, and doth swell."

> Blancard: "*Aposthema* . . . is an Exulceration left after a *Crisis*; but *Apostasis* and *Metastasis* sometimes differ in this, That the former is meant of an acute *Crisis* the latter of the Translation of a Disease from one part to another, an Apostume, an Imposthume."

IMPOSTHUME OF THE EYES

> Borde: "Algarab is the Araby word Auicen doth name it Algaras. In englyshe it is an impostume in the corner of the eye."

> "Bcthor is ye araby worde. In latyn it is named Pustula or Appostema. In englyshe it is named a pushe a wheale or an impostume in a mans eye And there be some auctours sayth that it is a lytle whyte whelke or wheale in the face named as I do thynke an ale pocke. And some auctours say it is a wheale in the mouth or tonge."

> "Ophtalmia or Hipophtalmia be the greke wordes The barbarus worde is named Obtalmia, and some say Hipopia. And the latyns doth name it Inflatio inconiunctiua of Apostema calidum in coiuctina In englysh it is named a hote impostume in ye eye. . . . This impediment doth come of a colde reumatike humour, or els of a corruput blode mixte with choler as autentike doctours dothe declare, but I saye it maye come accidentally as by a strype or a blowe with a mannes fyst or such like matter, for & if there were no cause of an infyrmite there shuld be no sicknes." (fol. ci v.)

INFLAMMATIONS OF THE EYE-LIDS

> Banister: "*Of the blowing or puffing vp of the Eye-lidde, called in Greeke,* Emphisema opthalmou, *in Latin,* inflatio

Emphisema is taken generally for a heape of windy spirits, which are gathered in the empty spaces of any part, as appeareth in *Galen*. But it is heere particularly vsed for a puffing vp of the vpper-most eye-lidde when it is lifted vp, losing his naturall colour with heauinesse and hard moouing, and in the end becommeth pale and wanne: and sometimes the white doth in part stand higher then the blacke. There is also a loose swelling without it, round about which being pressed downe with the fingers, is sodainely stayed, but presently is filled vp againe. And herein it differeth from the tumor called *Oedema*, because it being pressed with the finger, the marke and signe thereof remaineth afterward, and it proceedeth also from a stroke, which compassed the eye-lidde, which thing is not so to be seene in this windy swelling of it."

INFLAMMATIONS OF THE EYES

Banister: "*Of the inflamation of the Eye, called in Greeke*, opthalmia, *in Latine*, inflamatio adnatæ, *or* lippitudo: *also of the diuers kinds thereof, which are* chemosis *in Greeke, in Latine*, hiatus, *or* hiatulatio, phimosis, *or* præclusio, taraxis, *or* perturbatio, epiphora, *or* delachri-matio, opthalmia sphacelisousa, *or* inflatio ocularis in sphacelum degenerans.

Opthalmia, is an inflamation of the membrane in the eye, named *coni-unctiua*, ioyned with swelling, extension, paine, rednesse, heate, puff-ing vp of the eye-liddes, with doe hardly either open or shutte, and cannot suffer touching with the hands. *Taraxis*, is taken for a swift inflamation of the eye, being red and moist, but lesse grieuous than *opthalmia*, growing from outward causes, as smoake, dust, the sunne, the moone, oyle, rubbing of the eye. Some affirm, it commeth by the vse of strong wines, garlike, onions or mustard, *Chemosis* is, when the membrane called *coniuntiua*, is higher lifted then *cornea*, as if this were in a hole, which beside the rednes & heate, causeth the eye-liddes to be turned, so that they cannot couer the eye: contrary to this is *phimosis*, when by meanes of a great inflamation the eye-lids doe sticke fast each to other, & cannot be opened. Some impute this default to the eye-lids, but the hurt which they receiue, is but an acci-dent in this disease. *Epiphora* is taken genreally, for a sodaine streame of humours in any part, as *Pliny* calleth *epiphorum vteri, ventris*. Notwithstanding it is properly vsed for the affection in the eyes, when with great inflamation, graet quantity of humours flow vnto them. All these aforenamed affections doe accompany each other."

Borde: [Marginal term: "Payne in the eyes"] "Fpiphora is the greke worde. In latyn it is named Inflamacio oculorum. In englyshe it is named inflamacion of the eyes.

The cause of this infyrmyte.

This impediment doth come of some salt humour or els of corrupt blode myxt with reume." (fol. lv v.–lvi)

INFLAMMATIONS OF THE GROIN (OR SHARE)

Borde: "Altoin is the araby worde. In greke it is named Althaca. In latyn it is named Carbunculus. In englyshe it is named a Carbocle or a botch Carbunculus doth take his name of Carbo whiche is to say in englyshe a cole. For a cole beynge a fyre is hote, as so is a Carbocle . . . . This vlceration & infyrmyte most comonly doth brede in the emunctory places, there where ye .iii. pryncypal members hath theyr purgynge places the whiche be under ye eare or throte, or els about the arme holes or brest, or els about the secret partes of a man or woman, or in the share, or thyghe or flanke. And of Carbocles there be .iii. kyndes. The fyrst is blacke. The secde is reed. The third is of a glase or grenyshe colour. And the fourth is of a swarte or dym colour."

"Pauus is the latyn worde. In englyshe it is named a carnel in a mannes share, it may be also in other partes of a mannes body . . . . This impediment doth come of corrupcion of the lyuer and of a wateryshe blode or of coler." (fol. cvii)

INFLATIONS OF THE EARS

Borde: "Paristhomia is the greke worde. In latyn it is named Tonsille or Inflaciones aurium. In englyshe it is named inflacions of the eares . . . . This impediment dothe come of superaboundance of corrupte blode, or els of reume, or els of some hurte." (fol. cii v.)

ITCH (SEE ALSO **LEPROSY, SCAB, SCURF AND TETTER**)

Borde: "Prurigo is the latyn wode. In englyshe it is named itchynge of a mannes body skyn or flesshe . . . . This impediment doth come of corrupcion of euyl blode the which wolde be out of the flesshe, it may also come of fleume myxt with corrupt blode the which doth putryfy ye flesshe and so consequently the skyn."

"*Scabies*, the Itch; 'tis of two sorts, moist and dry; the moist is an inequality or roughness of the Skin, with moist and purulent Pustules, accompany'd with a constant itching. The dry Itch is fourfold, *Pruritis*, *Impetigo*, *Psora* and *Lepra*."

Quincy: Psora, a scab or tetter, a kind of itch.

ITCHING OF THE GENITALS

Borde: "Pruritis is the latyn worde. In englyshe it is a sprowtynge or burstyng out in ye secret places of a man and woman, an some dothe name it a ych for the pacient must crache and clawe . . . . This impediment doth come of greate humydyte in the inferiall partes of the body, specially in the oryfice of the matryx or els in the foundmente or to the partes adiacent to the sayd places."

JAUNDISE, BLACK AND YELLOW

Goeurot: "To the whiche there commeth oftentymes oppilations in the partyes about by the lyuer, or beneth in it selfe next tohe bowels, causyng great payne, by reason whereof the cholere turneth agayne vnto the lyuer, and there is me~gled with the bloode, and spred abrode into all the veynes of the bodye, and breedeth a disease named iaundys (ictericia in latin) whereof be thre kyndes, y^t is to saye, yelow iaundys that procedeth of cholere, and blacke iaundys that procedeth of blacke choler, which is called melancholye, an commonly cõmeth of the oppilation of the splene."

Borde: "Hictericia is the latyn worde. The barbarous worde is lctericia. In englyshe it is named the Jawnes or the gulsuffe, and there be .iii. kyndes of this infyrmyte which be to sayet he yelowe Jawnes the blacke Jawnes, and ye grene sicknes named Agriaca, and some do name it Penafeleon, & Melankyron or Melanchimon is ye black Jawnes

The cause of this infyrmyte

The cause of the yelow Jawnes doth come of reed coler myxte with blode, or els as I haue had experyence, the yelow Jawnes doth come after a great sicknes or a thought taken, the which hathe consumed the blode, and than the skyn & the exteryal parts must nedes turn to yelownes for lacke of blode, coler hauyng the dominion ouer it. The black Jawnes dothe come of coler adusted, or els of melacoly, the

which putrifieng the blode doth make the skyn blacke or tawny, and
comonly the body leane, for ye body or flesshe is arified & dryed up.
The grene Jawnes dothe come of yelow coler myxt with putrified
fleume, & corruption of blode." (fol. lxxiv)

Quincy: "Icterus, the jaundice. It is a vitiated state of the blood and humours,
from the bile regurgitating, or being absorbed into it, by which the functions of the body are injured and the skin is rendered yellow."

Dunglison 1839: Melæna entry; "*Black jaundice* . . . name given to vomiting of black matter, ordinarily succeeded by evacuations of the same
character. It seems to be often a variety of haematemesis . . . . Melæna
also signifies hemorrhage from the intestines."

KERNEL

Borde: "Amigdale is the latyn worde. In englyshe it is lytle cornels in the
rote of the tonge as some saye, but I do saye it be .ii. fleshly peces of
the whiche doth lye to ye .ii. vmiles lyke ye fashion of an almon." (fol.
xiii v.–xiiii)

"Cherade is the greke worde. Some auctours do call it Strume. And
some do call it in greke Antiades. The latyns call it Glandule. The barbarous people do name it Scrophule. In englyshe it is named Carnelles
in a mannes flesshe." (fol. xxxvi)

"Glandule is the latyn worde. In greke it is named Antiades or Cherade or Strume. In englysh it is named Carnelles in the flesshe. And
there be .ii. kyndes the one is harde and the other is softe . . . . The
cause of harde carnelles cometh of coloryke humours, and the softe
carnelles doth come of corrupte blode mixt with fleume." (fol. lxx)

"Parotides is the greke worde. In latyn it is names inflaciones. In
englyshe it is named Cornels about the eares . . . . This impediment
dothe come of a hote blode, or of a bylus humour and otherwile it
doth come of a melacoly humour." (fol. cv)

"Pauus is the latyn worde. In englyshe it is named a carnel in a
mannes share, it may be also in other partes of a mannes body . . . .
This impediment doth come of corrupcion of the lyuer and of a
wateryshe blode or of coler." (fol. cvii)

"The .317 Capytle dothe shewe of carnelles in the necke. Scrophule is
the latyn worde. In englyshe it is named knotts or burres which be in
chyldrens neckes."

KIBES OR KYBES

Borde: "Perniones is the latyn worde. Pernoni is the barbarous worde. In englyshe it it named ye kibes in a mannes heles."

Blancard: "*Pernio*, a preternatural Swelling caus'd by the Winter Cold, especially in the Hands and Feet, which at last break out. Kibes, or Chilblains."

KINGS EVIL

Borde: "Morbus regius be the latyn wordes. In englyshe it it named yᵉ kynges euyll, which is an euyl sicknes or impediment . . . . This impediment doth come of the corrupciõ of humours reflectyng more to a perticuler place than to vnyuersall places, and it is muche like to a fystle for & yf it be made whole in one place it wyl breake out in an other place." (fol. lxxxxvi)

Blancard: "*Morbus Regius*, the same with *Icterus*."

"*Icterus*, the Jaundice, is a changing the Skin into a yellow colour, from an Obstruction of the *Ductus Choledochus*, or Glandules of the Liver; or because the Gall abounds more than can be conveniently excern'd, so that it stays in the Blood. It taketh its name from ιχ/ιζ, a Ferret, whos Eyes are tinged with the like colour; or from a Bird call'd *Icterus*, of the same colour, which the *Latins* call *Galbulus*, which if one sick of the Palsie sees, says *Pliny*, the Pary is cur'd, but the Bird dies. The *Latins* call it also *Regius Morbus*, the Kingly Disease, because 'tis easily cured in Courts with the Pastime and Diversion there, which cheer the Mind. It is likewise term'd a Suffusion of the Gall."

LABOUR, WOMEN IN

Borde: "Partus is the latyn worde. In greke it is named Tocos. In englishe it is named whan a woman is redy to be delyuered the whiche delyuverance is very harde with many women and dothe put them in ieopardy of theyr lyues.

The cause of this matter.

The cause why it is more harder payne and ieopardy wt one woman than with an other, is whan they shulde be deliuered, is that one

woman is nat so stronge of complexion as an other woma is, and per-
auenture the chylde is turned in the mothers body, and that the heed
doth nat come fyrste, than there is great parell."

LASK (SEE ALSO **FLUX OF THE BELLY**)

Borde: Extrauagantes "The .19. Capytle doth shewe of the kindes of
fluxes.

Fluxus ventris be the latin wordes. In englyshe it is named the flyxe,
and there be .iii. kindes named in latyn Lienteria, Diarrhea and Dissiteria. In englyshe it is named the Lyentery, the Dyarrhy, and ye
Dyssentery. . . . The Dyarrhy is a common laxe. The Dyssintery is the
blody flyxe, and some doth name these flyxes after this maner. Intestinal, Epatycall and Saguine . . . . Epatycke or Epaticall flyxe cometh
without paine prycking or fretynge."

OED2: looseness of bowels, diarrhea.

LEPROSIE (SEE ALSO **SAWCIE FACE**)

Borde: "The .199. Capytle doth shew of leprousnes.

Lepra is the latyn word. In greke it is named Psora. In englysh it is
named leprousnes, and there be .iiii. kyndes of leprousnes which be to
say Elephcia, Leonina, Tiria and Alopecia. These .iiii. kyndes beestes,
for these .iiii. kindes of leprousnes hath the ppertes of ye bestes as it
appereth playnly in ye captytles of ye sicknesses."

"Alopecia is the greke worde. Ophiasis, both ye grekes and the latyns
dothe use that worde The barbarous worde, is Alopecia. The Araby
worde is Albaras. In englyshe it is a sod fallyng of a mans here of his
heed & berde hauynge growynge upon the skynne under the here an
humour lyke brane or otemel and betwyxt the fynger is a white
drynes, it is named Alopocia for as muche as ye worde is deryued of a
worde of greke named Alops which is in englyshe a Fox, for a Fox
ones a yere hath that infyrmyte shedynge his here hauynge also a lytle
skurfe under ye here up ye skyn. . . . And then the skurfe is lyke
otmel, but some loketh whytyshe & other blackyshe."

"Elephas or Elephantia be the greke wordes. In latyn it is named Cancer vniuersalis. In englyshe it is named the Elephancy, or the
Olyphant sicknes, for an Olyphant is sturdy & hathe no ioyntes, and
who so euer that hath this kynde of leprousnes c not moue his ioyntes
& is starke wherefore he is bedred and can nat helpe him self."

"Leonina is the greke worde. In englyshe it is named the lyons propertie, for this worde is deriued out of Leo Leonis whiche is in
englyshe a lyon for as ye lyon is most fercest of al other bestes so is
this kynd of leprousnes most worst of al other sicknesses, for it doth
corode and eat the flesshe to the bones, and the desine doth rotte
away."

"Tiria is the latyn worde. In englyshe it it named the tyre or the prop-
erty of an adder whiche is full of skales, so is this kynde of leprousnes
ful of skales and skabbes corodynge the fleshe."

Lowe: "This disease which is called *Elephantiasis*, if it be universally
throughout all the body, it is called Leprosie, and by the Arabians
Malum sanctæ manus: but if it be particular, it occupieth only one
member, which spoyleth the form, figure and disposition thereof, and
maketh it rough, scurfie, red and unequall, like the skinne of the Ele-
phant, for the which it is called *Elephantiasis*: if it possesse the skinne
and not the flesh, it is called *Morphæa*. . . . The Signes, is great tumor
possessing the whole member or some part thereof, and doth augment
by little, and little unsensible, not dolorous, sometimes inflamed, the
eyes troubled, the breath evill savoured, the skinne rough, knotty and
unequall, hard and scurffy; at last the body becometh atrofied and
leane, the bones tumified, the hands and fingers become swelled, and
the feete deformed" pp.270–271.

Blancard: "*Lepra*, the Leprosy, a dry Scab, whereby the Skin becomes sca-
ley like Fish. It differs *Leuce* and *Alphus*, in that a Leprosy is Rough
to the Touch, and causeth an itching, for the Skin is the only part
affected, and therefore it being flea'd off the Flesh, underneath
appears sound and well."

"*Lepra Græcorum*, or *Impetigo Celsi*, is the highest degree of
scabbedness; but it must be observ'd (left any should be gravel'd in
the reading of Authors) that we here speak of the *Leprosy of the
Greeks*, not the *Arabians*; for that which the *Arabians* call a Leprosy
is the *Elephantiasis* of the *Greeks*, and is nothing else than a universal
Canker of the whole Body. A Leprosy is a Disease proceeding from
black Bile diffused thro' the whole Body, whence the Temperature,
the Form and Figure, and at last the very Continuity of the Body is
corrupted, and becomes a Canker thro' the whole Body. The *Arabians*
call the Leprosy of the Greeks *Albaras Nigra*, which is the same with
a kind of Ring-worm or Tetter that flea's the Flesh, and is a rough violent Scab in the Skin, accompanied with Scales like Fish, and an itch-

ing. There's a greater Corruption of the Humours in a Leprosy than in a Scabbedness, and from the latter there only fall little Flakes like Dandriff from the Head, but from the former as it were Fish-Scales, so that one passes from Itching to a Leprosy by the Scab; for *Pruritus*, or Itching, is a certain small Asperity of the Skinm wherein (unless you scratch very hard) nothing falls from thence; when it is grown to a Scab the Humour is more apparent, and certain little Particles like Dandriff fall off, whether it be scratch'd or no, for in a Scab the Matter is thinner, and at last preys upon the surface of the Skin, but in a Leprosy 'tis thicker, and not only feeds upon the surface, but the inner part of the Skin. *Celsus* doubtless meant this Leprosy of the *Greeks* by the word *Impetigo*, but not the *Lichen* of the *Greeks*, which some call *Impetigo*. The *Leprosy of the Greeks*."

"*Elephantiasis*, five *Lepra & Leprosis*, is a cutaneous Distemper, appearing first of all with *Pustules* in the Face, Forehead, Breast, Arms, about the Hips. They are of a bluish colour, like a *Canker*, but without pain. *2dly*, Such like Pustules appear on the Tongue, and in the Throat. *3dly*, These exulcerations are broad, but not deep, never reaching below the skin, but their Extremities or Edges are hard; they are most frequently on the Fingers, Toes and Joints; and if they are remov'd from one place, they break out in another. *4thly*, By degrees they seize also on the Nose, which is often eat up, Bones and all, and at last fix on the Palate and Wind-pipe. *5thly*, there is a Swelling near the Extremity of the Nose and Ears. *6thly*, A thin Skin grows over the Apple of the Eye. *7thly*, The Skin is very rough, and chapt in many places, and covered with Scales. *8thly*, The Hairs fall off, the Nails grow crooked, like the Talons of Birds of Prey. The muscles appropriated to Inspiration lose part of their use, by reason of the many exulcerations, and in process of time the sanguiniferous Vessels are so straightened, that when you prick 'em with a Pin no Blood ensues, but you may see a purulent Matter. The *Leprosy*."

LETHARGY (SEE ALSO **FORGETFULNESS**)

Borde: "The. 63 Capytle doth shew of the pryvation of mannes wytte.

Caros is the greke word. Subeth and Sabara be the araby wordes. In latyn it is named Dormitio vigilatiua. In englyshe it is named pryua-cion of a mannes wyt, it doth dyffer from a sicknes named the letherge, for Caros doth drawe ye breth in, and expelleth it out and so doth nat ye letharge that can nat be perceyued. And the pacient ye hath this infyrmyte named Caros yf any man do aske him a question he wyl answere. And the letharge pacient can nat. Also it doth differ from an infyrmyte named Apoplexia, for the Apoplexy is euer with vehement aspyracions and drawyng deeply the breth. And so is nat Caros . . . . This infyrmyte doth come of a colde humour perturbatynge the brayne." (fol. xxxiia–b)

"Lethargos is the greke worde. And some grecions dothe name it the Syrsen. The barbarous me doth name it Litergia. In latyn it is named Lethergia or Obliuio. In englyshe it is named obliuious or forgetfulnes. . . . This impediment doth come thorowe colde reume the whiche doth obnebulate a mannes memory, and doth lye in the hinder part of a mannes heed witing the skull or brain panne." (fol. lxxxv a)

Blancard: "*Caros, Carus,* or *Sopor,* is a loss of Sense and Motion in the whole Animal Body, ye the Faculty of breathing remains, buth the forepart of the Brain, and the Muscles of the Temples are seiz'd, whence profound Sleep succeeds, and the Eyes are perpetually shut. The *Carus* is a sleepy Affection greater than the Lethary, much less than the Apoplexy, but so nearly allied, that it frequently ends in the latter."

"*Lethargus,* a Lethargy; 'tis a Drowsiness causing a heavy Sleep call'd *Coma,* accompanied with a Fever and Delirium; and 'tis nothing else but a heap of too much incongruous moist Matter within the Pores of the barky Substance of the Brain. This distemper doth not seem to come of itself, but rather from the degeneration of Fevers."

LIGHTS, CORRUPTION OF THE (SEE PHTHISIS)

LIVER, COOLING OF

Goeurot: "Yf the lyuer be colde, for the phlegmatyke matter that is in it, the pers hath his water white, out of coloure, the face pale, and his mouth watry, lytle bloode, and feleth heuynesse aboute his lyuer." Fol. li.

LIVER, HEAT OF

Goeurot: "Yf the lyuer [liver] be to hote, bycause of to moch blood, the person hath red vrine hasty pulse, his veines great & full, and he feleth his spattle, mouth and tonge sweter then it was wont to be, wherfore it is good to be let blood of ye liuer veine on the ryghte arme. . . . Yf the lyuer be ouer hote by cholera the pacient hathe hys vryne cleare and yelowe, without measure, great thyrst without appetyte, & feleth great burnyng in his bodye, and cmonly hath his bellye rounde, and hathe the face yelowe."

Borde: "Eper is the latyn worde. . . . If the liuer be hote, payne and heat is felt in the ryght side."

LIVER, OBSTRUCTION (STOPPING) OF (SEE ALSO **KING'S EVIL**)

Goeurot: "Oppilation or stoppyng cmeth sometyme in the holownesse of the lyuer [liver], and it is knowen by cpasson [compassion] and payne of the stomacke, and is healed by medicines laxatiue, as it is declared before.

And sometyme the oppilation is in the veynes of the holowe parte of the lyuer, and is perceyued then by ye grefe which the pacient feleth in his backe, & in his reynes" Fol. lii.

Borde: "Eper is the latyn worde. . . . If the liuer be opylated the face wyl swel, and payne wyl be in the ryght side."

LOATHING OF MEATE OF WOMEN WITH CHILDE

Borde: "Abhominatio stomachi, or els fascidium stomachi, be the latin wordes. In englyshe it is named the abhorryng of the stomake, for many men & women beyng sicke or defeated, theyr stomakes doth abhorre the sight of meat, or the sauer of meates and drynkes.

The cause of this impediment

This impediment doth come of debylyte of the stomake and wekenes of the brayne. And diuers tymes it doth come by corrupt humours the which be in the stomake. And otherwhile it doth come by replecion, and otherwhile by ouer muche and wylfull fastynge, but as for fastynge, that rule nowe a days nede nat be spoken of, for fastyng prayer, and almes dedes, of charyte, be banyshed out of al regions & prouinces & they be knocking at padyse to go in wepynge and waylynge for the Temporaltie and Spyrytualtie the whiche hathe exyled them."

LUNGS, STOPPING OF THE

Goeurot: "Shortness of the wind procedeth oftentymes of fleume, that is tough and clmishe, hangynge vpon ye longes [lungs] or stoppinge ye

conduits of ye same, being in the holowenes of the brest, or of catarrous humours yt [that] droppeth downe into the longes, and thereby
cmeth straitnesse in drawing of the breth, whych is called of phisitions
dispnoea or asthma, & when a pacient can not bend his necke down
for drede of suffocation it is callsed orthopnoca." Fol. xxviii

Borde: "Orthopnoisis is the greke worde. In latyn it is named Recta spiracio. In englysh it is named an euyl drawynge of a mannes brethe, for
yf he do lye in his bedde he is redy to sound, or the brethe wylbe
stopped. . . . This impediment dothe come either of the malice of the
lunges or of opilacions of the pypes or els it may come thorowe viscus
fleume."

Blancard: "*Dyspnoea*, a difficulty of breathing, which proceeeds from vitiated, obstructed, or irritated Organs."

MATRIX

Goeurot: "Fyrst agaynst superfluous fluxe of the mother, in the which ye
must cosider whether it doo come of to greate quantitye of bloode,
and the it is good for to open the veyne saphena, and abstayne fro all
thynges that multiplye the bloode, as egges, wyne and flesshe. Or
whether it cometh of cholere."

Borde: "Matrix is the latine worde. In greke it is named Mitra. In englyshe
it is named the matryx or the moder, or the place of concepcio the
which hath divers tymes many impedimentes as suffocacios,
lubrycyte, the mole of the matryx, the rysyng of the matryx, and the
fallynge out or descendyng downe of the the matryx the which no
mayd can haue for the orifice of that place in a mayd is very strayt
considerynge there be .v. vaynes the which doth breake whan a maid
doth lese her maydenheed." (fol. lxxxviii v.–lxxxix)

Blancard: "*Mater*, the same with *Matrix*, or *Uterus*; it signifies also a
Woman who hath brought forth a Child."

MATRIX, SUFFOCATION OF THE

Borde: "Svffocatio or Strangulacio be the latyn wordes. In englyshe it is
named a suffocacion, ye which doth come .ii. wayes the one is a suffocacion of the matryx, and the other is a strangulacion, for ye suffocacion of the matryx looke in the capytle named *Isteruchi puiux*."

"*Isterici puiax* be the greke wordes. In latyn it is named *Suffocacio vteri*. In englyshe it is named the suffocacion of the bely or matryx.

The cause of this impedyment

This impediment doth come of ventosyte and coldnes taken, this sickness in women is named the suffocacion of the matryx." (fol. lxxviiiv.)

Blancard: "*Hysterica passio*, or *Suffocacio hypondriaca*, *Uterina*, *uteri ascensus*, &c. Fits of the Mother, a Convulsion of the Nerves of the *Par Vagum* and Intercostal in the *Abdomen*, proceeding from a pricking irritation or explosion of *Spirits*. This Distemper does not always depend on the Womb, as is commonly thought; we have seen it more than once in Men, because the *Spleen*, *Pancreas*, and other adjacent Bowels, are often the cause of it."

MEGRIM

Borde: "Hemicrania is a compode of .ii wordes, of Hemi which is to say in englysh the mydle, and of craneum which is to say the skulle. In englyshe it is named ye megryme, which is a sicknes that is in the heed kepynge ye mydle part of the skull descendynge to the temples, and doth fetche a compas lyke a rayne bower, and ye diuers tymes it wyl lye more at the one syde than ye other, the barbarus men doth name his sicknes Emigrania."

Paré: "*Of the* Hemicrania, *or Megrim.*

The Megrim is properly a disease affecting the one side of the head, right, or left. It sometimes passeth no higher than the temporale muscles, otherwise it reacheth to the tope of the crowne. The cause of such paine proceedeth eyther from the veynes and externall arteryes, or from the *meninges*, or from the very substance of the braine, or from the *pericranium*, or the hairy scalp covering the *pericranium*, or lastly, from putrid vapours arising to the head from the ventricle, wombe, or other inferiour member. Yet an externall cause may bring this affect, to wit, the too hot or cold constitution of the encompassing ayre, drunkennesse, gluttony, the use of hot and vaporous meates, some noisome vapour or smoake, as of Antimony, quick-silver or the like, drawne up by the nose, which is the reason that Goldsmythes, and such as gilde mettals are commonly troubled with this disease. But whence soever the cause of the evill proceedeth, it is either a simple distemper or with matter: with matter, 1 say, which againe is either simple or compound." (p. 640)

Quincy: "a headache that affects only one part of the head at a time."

MELANCHOLY (MELANCHOLICK)

Lowe: "Pe. What is Melancholy?
Jo. It is an Humour cold and drye, thick in consistence, sour tasted, proper to nourish the parts that are cold and drye, and is compared to the earth or Winter."

Borde: "Melancholia is deriued oute of .ii. wordes of greke whichbe to saye of Molon whidhe is to say in latyn Niger. In englyshe it is named blacke and of Colim whidh is to say in latin Humor. In englyshe it is named an humour, the deriuacion of this worde is as well referred to this sicknes as to the humour whiche is one of the complexions. This sicknes is named the melacoly madnes whiche is a sicknes full of fantasies, thynkyng to here or to se that thynge that is nat harde nor sene, and a man hauynge this madnes shall thynke in him selfe that thynge that can neuer be for some be so fantasticall that they wyll thynke them selfe good or as god, or suche lyke thynges pertaynynge to presumpcion or to desperacion to be dampned the one hauynge this sicknes doth nat go so farre the one way but the other doth dispayre as much the other way.

The cause of this impediment

The orygynall of this infyrmyte doth come of an euyl melacoly humour, and of a stubburne hert and runnynge to farre in fantasies or musynge or studienge upon thynges that his reason can nat comprehende, such persons at length wyll come & be very natural foles, hauynge gestes wt them, or els peuyshe fantastical matters nothynge to ye purpose & yet in theyr conceyt do thinke the selfe wise." (fol. lxxxxib)

Blancard: "*Melancholia*, a Sadness without any evident Cause, whereby Peoa[p]le fancy terrible, and sometimes ridiculous things to themselves. It proceeds from the degeneracy of the Animal Spirits from their own Spirituous saline Nature into an acid, like the Spirit of Vitriol, Box-tree, Oak, &c. Also 'tis called black Choler, or black Blood, Adust, and *Salinosulphureous*."

Quincy: ". . . thus called, because supposed to proceed from a redundance of black bile. But it is better known to arise from too heavy and too viscid a blood, which permits not a sufficiency to spirits to be separated in the brain to animate and invigorate the nerves and muscles. Its cure is in evacuation, nervous medicines and powerful stimuli."

Paré: Heading "*Of the Spleene or Milt.*" p.111

OED2: lists quote for obscure usage: "To knock down, properly by a stroke in the side, where the [melt] or spleen lies."

MONTHLY PURGATIONS, WOMANS

Borde: "Menstrua is the latyn worde. In greke it is named Roufgynechios. In englyshe it is named a womans termes, the which most comonly euery woman and mayden hath, yf they be in good helth and nat with chylde, nor geuynge no chylde sucke, from, xv. yeres of there age to .I. nat .ii. yeres vnder or aboue, and where I dyd saye that the womans termes in latyn is named Menstrua that worde of latyn is deriued out of a worde named Mensis whiche is a month, for euery month they ye hath theyr helth hath theyr termes or flowers. And there be iiii. kyndes of womans flowers, reed, tawny, white and blackyshe, the reeed is natural, and the other be unnatural and nat perfyte and they betoken infyrmyte or sicknes to come whan they be nat reed." (fol. lxxxx v.)

MORPHEW

Borde: "Mophea is the latyn worde. In Englyshe it is named the morphewe. And there be .ii, kynds of the morphewe, the white morphewe, and ye blacke morphewe. The white morphewe is named Alboras for is loke in the capytle named Alboras." (fol lxxxxiv v.–lxxxxv)

"Alboras is an Araby worde & some do name it Albaras, it is named in latyn Morphea alba. In englyshe it is named the whyte Morphewe."

Blancard: "*Alphus*, or *Vitiligo*, is thus described by *Celsus*; A Distemper wherein the white Colour of the Skin is somewhat rough, not continued, but rather like so many several Drops: sometimes it disperses it self wider, but with some Interstices. *Alphus* is likewise call'd *Morphæ*. It differs from *Leuce*, in that it penetrates not so deep."

NOLI ME TANGERE

Goeurot: "For as much as Noli me tangere chaunceth often in the nose or about the face, begynnynge of a lytle harde and round kyrnel, or knobbe, and ful of payne, declyning towarde a pale and leady colour, ye may iuge that disease verye peryllous, notwithstading it is good to annoynt it as hereafter followeth."

Borde: "Noli me tangere be ye latyn wordes. In englyshe it is named tuch me nat, and some doth name it an ale pocke, which is a whele about the nose, or the lyppes or chekes or in some place in ye face, and why it is named tuche me nat, for yf one do nyppe or brose him, or do make him to blede, he wyll ryse and breake out in an other place, or els it wyll festure and brede a further displeasure." (fol. lxxxxvii v)

Blancard: "*Noli me tangere*, a sort of Cancer in the Face, especially above the Chin. There arises a Tumor or Ulcer about the Mouth like an exulcerated Canker, which grows slowly at the beginning, like a little Pimple; it remains a whole Year, else 'tis less troublesome than a Canker, which gnaws and eats more in one Day than a *Noli me tangere* doth in a Month."

NOSE, DROPPING AND DISTILLATIONS OF THE (SEE ALSO **CATARRHE AND RHEUMES**)

Borde: "Coriza is the barbarous worde. In greke it is named Corriza. In latyn it is named Rupia or grando. In englyshe it is named ye pose, or reume stoppinge and opylatynge the nosethrylles that a man can nat smell.

The cause of this infyrmyte.

This infyrmyte doth come of reume the which doth dystyl from the heed to ye nose or nosethrilles And this reume is ingendred thorowe inperfyte digestion and thorowe fumosyte or vaporous humours. And diuers tymes it is ingendred of cold taken in ye fete, and it may come of late drynkynge or surfetynge."

PAINES OF THE SIDES WITHOUT A FEAVOUR (SEE **STITCH**)

PAINES OF THE STOMACH

Borde: "Lepus marinus be the latyn wordes. In englishe it is named a paine in the bely and wyl cause a man to vomyte, and will cause the patient to sweate for paine . . . .This impediment doth come of colde, and of ventosyte, and it doth differ from the Colycke and the Iliacke."

PALSIE

Borde: "Paralisis is the greke worde. In latyn it is named Dyssolucio. In englyshe it is named ye Palsey, and there be .ii. kindes, the one is universal and the other is perticuler. The universal palsey doth take halfe the body either the ryghte syde or ye lefte syde. And what syde so ever is taken the sayd sicknes doth take away halfe the memory, the one eye is dymme, and halfe the spech or al is taken away the one legge and the one arme is benommed or astonned that can nat do thyr office, and the proper name of this palsey, amonges ye grekes is named Hemiplexia, and some grekes & latyns dothe name it Semiapoplexis. The barbarous worde is named Semiapoplexia. The perticuler palsey doth rest in a perticuler member or place whiche is to say, in the tonge, heed, arme, legge, and such lyke membres. Ignorant persons doth say ye is wh a mannes heed, handes, or legges dothe shake trymble or quake, that it is the palsey for suche matter loke in the capytle named Tremor."

Skilful Physician: "This shaking is a continual strife of natural powers, which are raised with out ceasing. It hapneth; first by looking from a great height, by sudden fear or sudden joy, or much cold or great heat, or much bleeding."

Quincy: "is a privation of motion, or sense of feeling, or both, . . . joined with a coldness, softness, flaccidity, and, at last, wasting of the parts. . . . the internal senses, and the motion of the heart and thorax, or the pulse and respiration, are not necessarily destroyed. It is wont to be called a particular paralysis."

"There is a three-fold division of a palsy worth taking notice of in practice: the first is a privation of motion, sensation remaining. Secondly, a privation of sensation, motion remaining. And, lastly, a privation of both together." Definition includes paralysis, hemiplegia, paraplegia and apoplexy.

PHLEGME

Lowe: "Pe. What is Flegme?
Jo. It is an Humour cold and humide. thinn in consistence, white coloured, when it is in the vaines it nourisheth the parts cold and humide, it lubrifieth the moving of the joynts, and is compared to water."

Blancard: "*Phlegma*, or *pituita*, a slimy Excrement of the Blood, caused often by too much nitrous air. 'Tis likewise a watery distill'd Liquor, opposite to Spirituous Liquor; also those Clouds which appear upon distill'd waters. *Hippocrates* uses it often for an *Inflammation*. 'Tis also the Disease of Hens, call'd the Pip, and is sometimes taken for a viscous Excretion."

PHTHISIS

Goeurot: "Pthisis is an ulceration of the longes, by the which al the body falleth into consption, in suche wyse that is wasteth al saue the skyn. Ye maye knowe hym that hath a pthisicke, for from day to day he waxeth euer leaner and dryer, and hys hear falleth, and hath euer a cough, a spitteth somtyme mater and bloody stringes wythal. And yf yt [that] whyche be spytteth be put to a basyn of water it falleth to ye bottome, for it is so heauye." (fol. xxix)

Borde: "Phthisis is the greke word. In latyn it is named Tabes. In englyshe it is named an vlceraction in the lunges, and some say it is a spetyng of blode and some dothe name it Emoptoica passio, and use the medecines that there is specified, & be ware of straynyng, or lyftyng, or great coughyng." (fol. cix-cix v.)

Blancard: "*Phthisicus*, a Man in a Consumption, whose Lungs are spoil'd or corrupted."

"*Phthisis*, a Consumption of the whole Body, rising from an Ulcer in the Lungs, accompany'd with a slow, continu'd Fever, smelling Breath, an a Cough."

PIMPLES OF THE NOSE (SEE SAWCIE FACE)

PIN AND WEB (SEE ALSO WEB (IN EYE))

Quincy: "*Pin and Web*, is a horny induration of the membranes of the eye, not greatly unlike the *Cataract*."

PISSE WITH DIFFICULTY AND PAINE

Borde: "Disuria is the greke word. In latyn it is named *difficultas mingendi*. In englyshe it is named the disury, which is whan a man or a woman that can nat well make water but with payne.

The cause of this infyrmyte.

This infyrmyte doth come many wayes, fyrst it may come by the coly-cke & the stone, or yᵉ gravel stoppynge the condites of the vryne, or els an anpostume, or a lompe of flesshe may growe or be ingendred in the condites of the vryne, or els it may come of congelacion of blode, or of matter yᵉ whiche doth stoppe the cundites of the vryne, or else of long holdynge of the water." (fol. xlviii)

PISSING

Borde: "The .98. Capytle doth shewe of them that can nat kepe theyr water but doth pysse as much as they do drynke.

Diabete is the greke worde. And some grekes doth name it *Dipsacos* or *Sipho*. The latyns do name it Afflictio renum. The barbarus men do name it *Diabetica passio*. In englyshe it is named an immoderate pyssinge." (Marginal printed notation: "Inordinate pyssinge", fol. xlv)

"Mictus or Mictura be ye latyn wordes. In greke it is named Vria. In englyshe it is named pissinge, and there be many impediments of piss-ing for some can nat holde theyr water & some can nat pysse or make water, some doth pysse blode, & some in theyr pyssinge doth auoyde gravel & some stones, and som whan they haue pyssed it doth burne in the issewe as well in woman as in man." (fol. lxxxxii v.)

"Diampnes is the greke worde, and the Latyns dothe vse the sayde worde, In Englishe it is named a passion of the bladder, out of whiche inuoluntarily doth pass or issueth out of the vrine of some men that they can nat kepe their water neither wakynge nor slepynge, and some men hauynge this passion in their slepe shall thinke and dreame that they do make water against a wal, a tree, or hedge or such lyke, and so dreaminge they do make water in their bedde. . . . This impediment dothe come of great debilitie and wekenes of the bladder, or els thorowe greate frigiditie or coldness of the bladder, or els of too much drinkinge, and sloughfulnesse."

PLEURISIE

Goeurot: ". . . apostemes called pleuresie, & it may be knowen by iiii. manner of signes. Fyrst the pacit [patient] hath a great burnyng feuer [fever]. Secondly, the ribbes are so sore within, as if thei were prycked continually wt nedylles. Thirdly, the pacient hath a shorte breathe.

> The .iiii. sygne is a strg cough, wherewyth the sycke is vexed, and by
> these sygnesmaye ye surelye knowe a ryght pleuresie, that is the skyn
> vnder the rybbes wythin the bodye.
>
> But there is an other kynde of pleuresie wythout vpon the rybbes
> apostemed, but in that is nothyng so greatte daunger nor the fyeuer
> [fever] is not so strõg as is the other aforerehearsed." (fol. xxvii.)

Lowe: "*Plurisie* is an inflammation and tumor, or a masse of blood, which
turneth into a bilious matter, in divers parts, but chiefly of the membraines and muscles, which knit and cover the ribs, wherof there are
two sorts, the false and true: the false is outward in the muscles of the
short ribs, and the true, is that which happeneth in the membraines,
which knitteth the ribs,

The Cause, is externe and interne: externe, is great heat or cold:
the usage of strong wine or very cold water, viloent exercise, and cold
ayre after great heate: the internall cause, is great repletion of all the
foure humors, but chiefly the blood and choller, which maketh the
most subtill part of the blood ascend from the cave vein into the vaine
Asygos, thereafter in the vaines and membrainee intercostalles.

The Signes are great dolour, from the shoulder unto the nether-
most rib, punction in the side, continual fever, difficulty of respyring,
coughing, hard pulse, great alteration, with want of appetitie, evil
favored breath, heavines, and ponderosity of the sides, great fever
chiefly in the night, little sleep, some sweats which happen through
great pain." pp. 220–221.

Borde: "Pluritis is the greke worde. And some do name it Anaxia. In latyn
it is named Lateralis dolor. The barbarous worde is named Plurisis. In
englyshe it is named a pluryse the which is an impostume in the ten-
eryte of the bones, but there be .ii. kyndes, the one ins inwarde, and
the other is in the grystelles of the bones, and the other is in lacertes in
the breste, and isaacke saythe that it is a hote impostume that is ingedred in the mydryffe named Diafragma, and comonly feuer is concurrant with this sicknes . . . . This infyrmyte doth come of a fumyshe
blode and of an hasty hert the which doth perturbate eythe the ioyntes,
or els of the hert & stomacke with the brest, it may also come of great
heat or extreme colde by the northe wyndes, and it may come by
dronkynnesse." (fol. cx)

Blancard: "*Pleuritis*, a Pleurisy, an Inflammation of the Membrane *Pleura*,
and the intercostal Muscles, attended with a continual fever and
Stitches in the Side, difficulty of Breathing, and sometimes spitting of

Blood; an it is either a true Pleurisy, this which we have describ'd, or a bastard Pleurisy."

PLEURISIE, HOT

Skilful Physician: ". . . a pricking pain about the ribs with a cough and an Ague . . ."

PUR-BLINDE

Banister: *"first, of such as see best downeward, or things that bee neere them, commonly called pore blind, in Greeke,* miopiasis, catopsis, *in Latin,* lusciositas, misciositas, propinqua visio.
Myopiasis, myopia, catopsis is when one cannot see one thing, but such as bee very neere and euen, offered vnto his eyes with great dif-ficultie, pearcing those which are farre off. They which haue this default, are constrained when they read, to looke very nigh, imagining oftentimes that they behold little bodies, like to flies, or motes which flie in the aire, as wee see it happeneth to those which haue looked very long on their bookes, or haue viewed any thing diligently."

PUSHES

Borde: "Bothor is ye araby word. In latyn it is named Pustula or Appostema. In englysh it is named a push a wheal or an impostume in a mans eye.

"Epynictides is the greke worde. In latin it is named a whele, or a pushe the which doth ryse in the skyn the which is ingendred in the nyght . . . . This impediment doth come of euyll dyet, or els of an euyl humour procedynge from the liuer or drynkīg late, or els of some ven-emouse worme." (fol. lv v.)

"Escara or Essare or Essara be the latyn wordes. In greke it is named Aegineta or Epinictides. In englyshe it is named a harde pushe or whele much lyke to styngynge of a waspe, a hornet, or a nettle, and some saye it is the place where a man is burnt with a hote yron and nat made whole. . . . This infyrmyte dothe come of a salt fleumatyke humour or els of adusted coler, or melancoly." (fol. lvi)

"Formica is the latyn worde. In greke it is named Mirmichia. In englysh it is named a little wheale growynge out of the skyn, some doth call this sicknes in latyn Formica milliara as who shuld say briefly bytinge of Amytes or Pysmars or Antes, for this infyrmyte dothe take his name of an Ante or a Pysmare, or Emyt al is one thynge, & why this sickenes is so called is because the similitude is lyke the bytynge of an Ante &c. And there be .iii. kyndes of this infyrmyte, the fyrst is runnynge, the seconde is corodynge or eatynge and the thyrde is named Formica milliaris the whiche I do take it for the syngles." (fol. lxviii v.)

"Pustule is the latyn worde. In englyshe it is named wheals or pushes."

QUINZIE

Blancard: "*Angina*, an Inflammation of the Jaws or Throat, attended with a continual Fever, and a difficulty of Respiration and Swallowing. It is twofold, either *Spuria* or *Exquisita*, a bastard or a true *Squincie*."

Harris: ANGINA, a *Quinsy* or *Squinancy*, is an Inflammation of the Jaws or Throat, attended with a continual Feaver and difficulty of Respiration and Swallowing, and it is two-fold; either *Spuria* or *Exquista*, a Bastard or a True *Squinsie*: The latter is again four-fold, *Synanche, or Parsynanche, Chynanche* and *Parchynanche*: of all which in their proper places.

REINES (OR RAINS) OF THE BACK

Goeurot: "Against disease of the raynes of the backe, and the loynes.
Payne of the reynes is called nephretica passio, & cmeth of some one or grauel, & it is most lyke vnto the colicke in cure, but in causes they be cleane contrarie: for the colicke beginneth at the lower partes on the righte side, and goeth vp to the hyer partes on the left side, of the belly, and it lyeth rather more forwarde then backewarde, but nephretica passio begynneth contrarywise aboue, descendyng downewarde, and euer lieth more towarde the backe.
Also nephretica is paynfuller afore meat, and the colicke is euer more greuous after. And often the colicke chaceth sodenlie, but nephretica contrarie, for commonlie it commeth by litle and litle, for euermore before, one shal fele payne of ye backe wt difficultie of vrine.
Item there is more difference, for the colicke sheweth vrynes [urines] as it were coloured, but nephretica in the begynuinge is cleare, and white like water, & after waxeth thycke, and then appeareth at the bottom of the vessel leke red sande or grauel." (fol. lxiii)

Borde: "Renes is the latin worde. In greke it is named Nephroi. In englyshe it is named the raynes of the backe ye whiche may haue many impedim tes as indacions, the stone, ache and such like. For this matter loke in the capitles of these infyrmites and in the Extrauagates in the ende of this boke."

(from Extrauagantes) "Renes is the latyn worde. In greke it is named Nephroi. In englyshe it is named the raines of a mannes backe the whiche may haue diuers impedumentes as ache, the crycke, and straininge &c."

Paré: "*Of the Kidneyes, or Reines.*" p. 117

Blancard: Kidneys from entry for "Urine" "We known Reins are affected by Caruncles, Blood, and *Pus*, coming away with the Urine."

RHEUMES

Skilful Physician: "Rheume is nothing else but a defluxion that falls from the head into the throat or brest, which doth otherwhiles so stop the pipes of the Lights and throat that its ready to choak, also these Rheumes fall into the nose, and cause the pawse.

These Rheums are caused divers waies; as from gross meats which cause vapours, or of cold, or from a sharp North wind which bloweth suddenly after a South wind.

The cold Rheumes are knowne by these signes following, as wearinesse, heavinesse of the whole body, sleepiness, heavinesse of the head and forehead, palenesse with full vaines, stuffing of the head or nose, swelling of the eyes, pain in the throat, motion to vomit, swelling of the Almonds . . .

Hot Rheume, the signes thereof are these, viz. the face is red, mixt with a pale or black colour, great heat in the nose with itchings, when the mouth and the throat is full of bitterness and sharpnesse, and if the head be hot in feeling." p. 135

Blancard: "*Rheuma*, Rheum, a defluxion of Humours from the Head upon the Parts beneath, as upon the Eyes, Nose, &c."

Harris: "CATARRHUS, is a Defluxion of Humours from the Head towards the Parts under it, as the Nostrils, Mouth, Lungs, &c. Some distinguish it by the Name of *Loryza*, when it falls on the Nostrils, by that of *Bronchus* when on the Jaws; and by the word *Rhume*, when it falls on the Breast."

RHEUMES OF THE EYES

Banister: *"Of the moist, running, or weeping Eye, called in Greeke,* Reuma opthalmou, *in Latine,* Fluxus oculi, delacymatio.

Rheusma opthalmou, is a flowing of thinne humors, which in such sort, against the will, fall downe into the eyes, that there cannot be any meanes found to stay them. It commeth to some by nature, as wee haue seene some from their childhood neuer hauing drie, but alwayes moist eyes, with a thinne pearsing humour, which alwayes was painefull to them. And it will soone stirre vp and inflamation, and blearednesse, in many tormenting them all their life, without admitting an cure. Those also which haue great and grosse heads, are subiect to it, and scarcely doth any medicine at any time profit them. It may also arise from some outward causes, as from a Feuer, from some medicine, or sharpe thing which hath beene put into the eye, or falne into it, from great weaknesse either in the facultie which retaineth, or that which digesteth the nourishment in the eye, by the vnskilfulnesse of the Chirurgian, which in curing the disease of the eye called *vngula,* did cut away more of the flesh in the corner of the eye than hee ought, whereof wee will speake in the proper place, for a full discharge of all the head, touching this part."

RING-WORM

Borde: "Impetigo is the latyn word. And some latyns do name it zerna or zarma, this sicknes doth dyffer in the more and lesse, the grekes dothe name this sicknes Lichen, the barbarous word is Lichena. In englyshe it is named roughnesse of the skyn or scabbes in ye skyn, and there be .ii. kyndes the one is a dry scabbe and the other is wete or an vlcerous scabbe named in englysh a rynge worm or beynge of that sort." (fol lxxvii–lxxvii v.)

Paré: *"Of the* Herpes; *that is Teatars, or Ringwormes, or such like."*

Blancard: *"Herpes,* a spreading and winding Inflammation; 'tis two-fold, either *Miliaris* or *Pustularis,* like Millet-seed, which seizes the Skin only, and itches; or *Exedens,* consuming, which not only seizes the skin, but the *Muscles* underneath. The cause of it is, that the *Glandules* of the Skin are too much stuff'd with salt *Particles,* which, if the peccant Matter abount, grow into a Crust, and eat the *Parts* they lie upon. A *Ring-worm* or *Tettar."*

RUPTURE AND WINDY RUPTURE

Borde: "Ruptura is the latyn worde. In greke it is named Epigozontay-
menon. In englyshe it is named a rupture, and that is whan the Siphac
wich is a pellicle or skyn that doth compasse about the guttes is
relaxed or broken then ye guttes doth fal into the codde. And there be
.iii. kyndes of ruptures, the first is zirbale, the second is intestinall,
and the thirde is naterall, for he dothe take his originall of both the
other. . . . A rupture doth come of cryeg, or els of a great lyfte, or of a
great fall or brose, or lepynge unesely upon an horse, or clymynge
ouer a highe hedge or style, or by a great strain or vociferation."

"Hernia or ramex be the latin wordes. In greke it is named Kyli. In
englyshe it is a posthumacion in the coddes, and there be .iii. kyndes
named in latyn Hernia aquosa, Hernia uentosa, Hernia carnosa,
whiche is to say in englyshe a wateryshe hernye, a wyndye hernye, a
flesshy hernye. . . . These impediments be ingendred in the codde
either of a grosse flesshely humour, or of a grosse wateryshe humour,
or els of a wyndy humour."

"Ramex is the latyn word. In greke it is nameb Kyli. In englyshe it is
named hernies or swellinge in the cod. Hernia is the comon name to
thre diseases, which be to say Enterocela, Epiplocela, & Hidroocela.
Fyrst, Enterocela is whan the guttes do fal out of the bely into the cod
where the stone lie. Epiplocela is when the guttes doth fal into the cod
with the oment or siphac which is a pellicle ye which doth compasse
and doth bere up the guttes. Hidrocela is a humour the which hath a
confluence to the stones as Celsus sayth. Ramices doth some what
differ from Ramex, for it hath also .iii. sondry kindes, the which be to
say Parocela, Sarcocela, Cirsocela. Parocela is whan the matter is
harded in ye cod or about the stones. Sarcocela is whan there doth
growe a flesshe in the cod or about the stones Circocela is whan the
vaynes in the cod doth swel inflatynge the stone. Also there is an other
kind named Bubocela which is whan the bowelles do fall no further
than the share. For this matter and for a remedy loke in the capytles
named Hernia and Ruptura."

SAINT ANTHONIES FIRE

Goeurot: "In Greke herisipela, and of the Latines Sacer ignis, our
Englysshe women call it the fyre of Saynt Anthonye, or chingles, it is
an inflammatiõ of membres wit excedyng burnynge and rednesse,

harde in the feelynge, and the most parte crepeth aboue the skynne or but a lytle depe within the flesshe.

It is a greuous payne, and maye be lykened to the fyre in consumyng." (The Booke of chyldren)

Borde: "Ignis santi Anthonij, Ignis persicus and Pruna be the latyn wordes. In englyshe it is named saynt anthonyes fyer, the be lytle wheales the whiche doth burne as fyre, how be it Ignis periscus or saint anthonyes fyer is nat so vehement as is the infyrmyte named Pruna, for Pruna is more grosser and greate, and dothe burne more than dothe saynte anthonyes fyer."

Paré: *"Of a Gangreene and Mortification.*

Certainely the maligne symptomes which happen upon wounds, and the solutions of Continuity are many, caused either by the ignorance or negligence of the Chirurgion; or by the Patient, or such as are about him; or by the malignity and violence of the disease; but there can happen no greater than a Gangreene as that which may cause the mortification and death of the part, and oft times of the whole body; wherefore I have thought good in this place to treate of a Gangreene, first giving you the definition, then showing you the causes, signes, prognostickes, & lastly the manner of cure. Now a Gangreene is a certaine disposition, and way to the mortification of the part, which it seaseth upon, dying by little and little. For when there is a perfect mortification, it is called by the Greekes *Sphacelos*, by the Latines *Syderatio*, our countrymen terme it the fire of Saint *Anthony*, or Saint *Marcellus*." p. 452.

Lowe: "We must here consider the difference betwixt Gangrene and Sphasell, and know that Gangren is the latin word, [i]t is a mortification of the parts it happeneth in, except the bones, and is curable: but Sphasell or sideration, is a mortification both of the soft and solid parts, which is no way remedied but by amputation, som do call it S. Anthony or S. Martials fire. . . . The signes are these, the member weareth black, like as it were burnt, afterwards it becometh rotten, and in that time it overthroweth the whole body, in such sort that the skin both come from the flesh." p. 88.

Blancard: *"Erysipelas,* . . . St. *Anthony's* Fire, is a Swelling in the Skin or any fleshy or membranous Part, red, broad, not spreading high, not beating with a Pulse, but attending with a pricking sort of Pain, arising from a sharp and frequently sulphureous Blood. I take the cause of it not to be the Blood so much a serous Sweating, which is sharp and sulphureous, and flows from the Fibres themselves."

SAWCIE FACE

Borde: "Salsum flegma be the latyn wordes. In englyshe it is named a saucefleume face which is a tok or preuy signe of leprousnes."

"Gutta rosacea be the latyn wordes. In englysh it is named a sauce fleume face, which is a readnes about the nose and the chekes with small pymples, it is a preuy signe of leprousnes."

Blancard: "*Gutta rosacea*, a Redness with Pimples, wherewith the Cheeks, Nose and the whole Face is deformed as if it were sprinkled with red Drops; these Pimples or Wheals often increase, so that they render the Face rough and horrid, and the Nose monstrously big."

SCAB (SEE SCURF, WHITE AND LEPROSY)

Borde: "Psora is the greke worde. In latyn it is named Scabies. In englyshe it is named skabbes whiche is an infectiouse sicknes, for one man maye infect an other by lienge togyther in a bed, and there be .ii. kyndes the drye skabbes and ye wete skabbes or moyst skabbes.

The cause of this impediment,

Yf ye skabbes be drye it dothe come of coler adusted, yf they be moyst it dothe come of the corrupcion of blode."

"Lichen is the greke worde. Lichenais the barbarous worde. In latyn it is named zarna or Impetigo, and some doth name it Mentagra, & some grecions doth name it Psora. For this matter loke in the capytles of the aforesayd names. But Psora in greke is taken for one of the kyndes of leprousnes which is a perylous sicknes & is infectiouse and so be at maner of kindes of skabbes wherfore I do aduertise al maner of persons ye which be vnfected nat to lye in bed w and person or psons the which be infected w these infyrmites or any other diseses lyke, as the pestylence, the sweatyng sicknes, or any of ye kyndes of the agewe or feuers, or any of the kyndes of the fallynge sicknes & suche lyke, and Meutagra is engendred of a grosse melacholy humour." (fol. lxxxiii)

"Scabies is the latyn worde. In greke it is named Psora. In englyshe it is named skabbes. And there be .iii. kindes named in latin Scabies lupinosa[,] Scabies Furfuria, and Scabies sabina. In englyshe it is named skabbes like hoppes, and skabbes like bran, and skabbes like benes." Extrauagantes, Capytle .61.

Blancard: *"Impetigo Celsi,* the same with *Lepra Græcorum. Celsus* makes four sorts: The most harmless, says he, is that which is like a Scab, for it is red and hard, and exulcerated and gnaw'd; but it differs from it, in that it is more exulcerated, and is accompanied with speckl'd Pimples, and there seems to be in it certain Bubbles, from which after a certain time there falls, as it were, little Scales, and it returns more certainly. Another sort is worse, almost like a sort of Meazles, or hot Pimples in the Skin, but more rugged and redder, and of different Figures: In thie Distemper little Scales fall from the surface of the Skin, and it is call'd *Rubrica.* The third sort is yet worse, for it is thicker and harder, and smells more, and is cleft on the top of the Skin, and gnaws more violently; 'tis Scaly too, but black, and spreads broad and slow; 'tis called *Nigra.* The fourth sort is altogether incurable, of a different Colour from the red; for 'tis something white, and like a fresh Scar, and has pale Scales, some whitish, some like the little Pulse call'd *Lentil*; which being taken away, sometimes the Blood follows. Otherwise, the Humour that flows from it is white, the Skin hard and cleft, and spreads farther. All these sorts arise especially in the Feet and Hands, and infect the Nails likewise. *Impetigo* some reckon the same with *Lichen.* See *Lepra Græcorum."*

SCAB, FILTHY

Borde: "Malum mortuum be ye latyn wordes. In englysh it is named a fylthy skabbe the which moste comonly is in the armes and legges.

The cause of this impediment

This impediment doth come most comonly of a menstrouse woman, and it may come by corrupcion of blode, and diuers tymes doth come of a melancoly humour adusted." (fol. lxxxvii)

SCAB, WILD

Borde: "Acria is the greke worde, Celsus doth name it in latyn Fera scabies. in englysh it is named a wylde or rynnynge skabbe, the which doth infest a ma more in one tyme of the yere tha in an other.

The cause of thys infyrmyte.

> This infyrmyte cometh to man, after his coplexion, by superabundant humours, or by lyenge wt infectiouse persos hauynge the sayde infyrmyte or by arydyte or drynesse of coler or melancholy the whiche doth ingender a drye skabbe whiche is the worste amonges all the kyndes of scabbes."

Blancard: "*Psora*, a wild Scab that makes the Skin scaly. A Scurf."

SCABBED HEAD (SEE **SCALD HEAD** AND **SCURF**)

SCALD HEAD (SEE ALSO **SCAB** AND **SCURF, WHITE**)

Borde: "Fauus is ye latyn worde. In englyshe it is scabbes in the skyn of ye heed like to an impediment named Acor, but the holes of Fauus is much more bygger than Acor is. . . . This impediment doth come thorowe greate hymidite I˜ the heed, or it may come of a salt humour." (fol. lix)

Paré: "*Of the* Tinea, *or Scalde Head.*

> The *Tinea* . . . or scald head, is a disease possessing the musculous skin of the head or the hairy scalpe, and eating thereinto like a moth. There are three differences thereof, the first is called by *Galen* scaly or branlike for that whilst it is scratched it cast many branlike scales: some practitioners terme it a dry scall, because of the great adustion of the humour causing it. Another is called *ficosa*, a fig-like scall, because when it is despoyled of the crust or scab which is yellow, there appear graines of quick and red flesh, like to the inner seeds or graines of figs, and casting out a bloudy matter. *Galen* names the third *Achor*, and it is also vulgarly termed the corrosive or ulcerous scall, for that the many ulcer wherewith it abounds are open with many small holes flowing with liquid *sanies*, like the washing of flesh, stinking, corrupt and carrion like, somewhiles livid, somewhiles yellowish. These holes, if they be somewhat larger, make another difference which is called *Cerion* or *Favosa* (that is, like a hony comb) because as *Galen* thinks, the matter which floweth from these resembleth hony in colour and consistence." p. 638

Quincy: "Scalled head, see Crusta Lactea"; "Crusta Lactea, when the Tinea affects the face it is thus named. In the hairy scalp only it is called Tinea only, or scalled."

"Tinea, a sore or tetter that discharges a salt lymph. Tinea Capitus, scalled head, this and the Crusta Lactea are commonly described as distinct and unconnected diseases."

SCIATICA (SEE ALSO **GOUT**)

Borde: "Siatica passio is the barbarous worde. In latyn it is named Dolor scie. In greke it is named Ischias, the of whiche worde dothe come Ichiadici, and some doth name this infyrmyte Coxendrix or Coxendricis morbus.

The cause of this infyrmyte

This infyrmyte doth come of harde lyenge on the hokyll bones or lyenge on the grounde, or up a forme, or such lyke harde thinges, it may come by a stripe or a great fall, and it wyll ronne from ye hokyll bone to the kne, and from the kne to the ancle and from the ancle to the lytle too, & than it is past cure, and otherwhile this gout wyl haue a reflection to the raynes of the backe, and to ye flankes, and it may come of a grosse fleumaryke humour."

Paré: "*Of the* Ischias, *Hip-gout, or* Sciatica.

For that the hip-gout in the greatnesse of the causes, bitternesse of pain, and vehemency of the symptomes, easily exceeds the other kindes of Gout, therefore, I have thought good to treate thereof in particular. The pain of the *Sciatica* is therefore the most bitter, and the symptomes most violent, for that the dearticulation of the hucklebone, with the head of the thigh-bone, is more deepe than the rest, because also the phlegmaticke humour which causeth it is commonly more plenteous, cold, grosse and viscid, that flowes down into this joint, and lastly because the *Sciatica* commonly succeeds some other chronicall disease, by reason of the translation and falling down thither of the matter, become maligne and corrupt by the long continuance of the former disease. But the paine not only troubles the hippe, but entering deepe, is extended to the muscles of the buttocks, the groines, knees, and very ends of the toes, yea often times it vexeth the patient with a sense of paine in the very *vertebræ* of the loines, so that it makes the patients, and also oft-times the very Physitians and Surgeons to thinke it the wind or stone Collicke." pp. 719.

SCIRRUS

Borde: "Scirrus is the greke worde. In latyn is named Tuber. In englyshe it is an harde swellynge aboue nature."

"The .357. Capytle doth shewe of swellynges of wartes and agnelles.

Tvber is the latyn word. In englyshe it is named every swellynge or tilinge in the flesshe. Tubercula is a dymynytiue of the latyn word Tuber, and in englyshe is named a wert or an agnell growynge in the fete & toes, and in latin they hath many kyndes and termes, as Mellicerides, Gangilia, Athoromata, and Stratomata."

SCURF, WHITE (SEE ALSO SCAB AND SCALD HEAD)

Borde: "Acor or Acoris be the greke wordes, Furfur is the latyn word, Acora is the barbarus word In englyshe it is named dandruffe or a skurfe in the heed lyke bran or otmell, the which doth penetrate the skyn of the heed makynge lytle holes, dyfferinge from an other infyrmyte in the skyn of the hed named Fauus."

"Lvce or Leuci be the greke wordes. In latyn it is named Vitiligo. In englyshe it is named a skurfe in al the body. . . . This infyrmite doth come of colerike & melacoly humours." (fol. lxxxv)

"The .290. Capytle doth shewe of a lytle skurfe in the heed.

Porrigo or Porre or Furfures some latenyst dothe use these termes. The grecions dothe use this worde named Pitariasis. In englyshe it be smal skales bygger than the skales of dandruffe sprowting out in latitudes and longitudes lyke ye heed of a leke."

Blancard: "*Crusta lactea*, a Species of *Achor*, a Scurf, or crusty Scab, only with this difference, that an *Achor* infects only the Head, but this, not only the Face, but almost the whole body of an Infant, at the time of its first sucking. *Crustea lactea* turns white, but *Achors* have another colour."

"*Psora*, a wild Scab that makes the Skin scaly. A Scurf."

Hooper: "Scurf small exfoliations of the cuticle, which take place after some eruptions on the skin, a new cuticle being formed underneath during the exfoliation."

SEED, NATURAL

Borde: "Natura is the latyn word. In greke it is named Physis. In englyshe
it is named the nature of man, the which is the chefest blode in man,
and it doth chaunge into whitenesse whan it doth come in the
cundytes by the stones. The nature of man doth dyffer from the sede
of man, although they be coniuncted togyther, for the sede of man is
like the sedes of ryce whan it is soden, but it is nothynge so bygge,
and that is in the nature of man, which is whitishe and thycke, without
the whiche can be no procreacion, and it may waste and consume, or
be putrified." (fol. lxxxxvii v.)

Blancard: "*Semen*, Seed, a white, hot, spirituous, thick, clammy, saltish
Humour, which is made out of the thinnest part of the Blood in the
Testicles and *Epidiymides*, and by proper Passages is ejected into the
Womb of the Female. There is also in the Female a Matter that is
call'd *Seed*, which proceeds from the *Prostates*, and frequently in their
Lechery is emitted forth. The Use of this is to raise Titillation, and
render the Coition more pleasant; for the rest of the Female Seed (if it
may be so call'd) lies in their *Ovaria* or Testicles. The word Semen
relates also to the Seed of Vegetables, which each produces its own
kind."

SHARPNESSE OF THE EYES, AND EYE-LIDS (SEE BLEAR-EYEDNESS)

SHARPNESSE OF THE THROAT

Skilful Physician: "Hot Rheume, the signes thereof are these, viz. the face
is red, mixt with a pale or black colour, great heat in the nose with
itchings, when the mouth and the throat is full of bitterness and sharpnesse, and if the head be hot in feeling." p. 137

SHINGLES

Goeurot: "In Greke herisipela, and of the Latines Sacer ignis, our
Englysshe women call it the fyre of Saynt Anthonye, or chingles, it is
an inflammatiõ of membres wit excedyng burnynge and rednesse,
harde in the feelynge, and the most parte crepeth aboue the skynne or
but a lytle depe within the flesshe.

It is a greuous payne, and maye be lykened to the fyre in consumyng."
(The Booke of chyldren)

Borde: "Formica is the latyn worde. In greke it is named Mirmichia. In englysh it is named a little wheale growynge out of the skyn, some doth call this sicknes in latyn Formica milliara as who shuld say briefly bytinge of Amytes or Pysmars or Antes, for this infyrmyte dothe take his name of an Ante or a Pysmare, or Emyt al is one thynge, & why this sickenes is so called is because the similitude is lyke the bytynge of an Ante &c. And there be .iii. kyndes of this infyrmyte, the fyrst is runnynge, the seconde is corodynge or eatynge and the thyrde is named Formica milliaris the whiche I do take it for the syngles." (fol. lxviii v.)

"Herisipulas is the greke worde. In latyn it is named Apostema calidum. Some latyns do name it Ignissacer. Auicen doth name it Spina bycause it doth prycke & burne. In englyshe it is named the shyngles or the shyngylls, and the barbarous worde is named Erisip-ule." (fol. lxxii v.)

Quincy: "It consists of small pimples, which soon form little vesicles that dry and become scaly. This disorder usually spreads farther than its first limits."

SINEWS

Borde: "Neruus is the latyn word. In greke it is named Neuron. In englyshe it its named synewew the which may haue diuers impedimentes . . . . The impedimentes the whiche doth fortune to the sinewes may come by cuttynge of a sinew, or by straynynge, or by sterknesse, or by the crampe, or such lyke matter or causes." (fol. lxxxxvii)

SINGING IN THE BRAIN (SEE EARS, TICKLINGS AND NOISE OF THE)

SPASM (SEE CRAMP)

SPLEEN AND STOPPING [OPPILATION] OF THE SPLEEN

Goeurot: "The splene is a mbre lge softe, and spongy, beinge in ye lefte syde ioyned unto the holownesse of ye stomacke, and to the thycke endes of ye rybbes, & to ye backe, the whiche is ordeyned fo to receyue the melcholy humours, & to cleanse the blood of the same, for by that meane ye blood remayneth pure & nette. Wherfore it is good nourishyng for al the membres, and is the cause that maketh a bodye merye, but oftentymes there happeneth oppilati or debilitie wherof commeth the blacke iaundys.

And somtymes it is greater, fuller, or grosser then it ought to be, by ouermuche melancholie that is not natural, caused of the dregges of the blood engendred in the lyuer, & doth hyndre generacion of good blood, wherethrough the membres become drye, for defaute of good nourishynge. And therfore the pacient is called splenetycke, which ye maye knowe by that, that after meate they haue payne in theyr left syde, and are alwayes heuye, and hath theyr faces somwhat enclyning unto blaknesse." fol. lvi.

Blancard: "*Splenetica*, such Medicines as are good against the Disease called the Spleen."

"*Hypochondriacus Affectus*, or *Affectio Hypochondriaca*, a pure flatulent and convulsive Passion, arising from flatulent and pungent Humours in the Spleen, or Pancreas, which afflicts the Nervous and Membranous parts. The Hypochondriack Disease."

Dunglison 1839: "Hypochondriasis ... *Spleen* ... This disease is probably so called, from the circumstance of some hypochondriacs having felt an uneasy sensation in the hypochondriac regions."

SQUINANCIE (SEE QUINZIE)

STENCH OF THE NOSE, STINKING NOSTRILS AND STINKING BREATH

Borde: "The .154. Capytle dothe shewe of the stenche or euyl savour that may come out of a mannes mouth or nose or the arme holes.
Fetor oris or Fetor narium or Fetor assellarum be the latyn wordes. In englyshe it is named stench of the mouth, stench of the nosethrilles, and stench of the arme holes . . . . This infyrmyte dothe come diuers wayes, yf it do come out of the mouthe or nosethrylles, either it do come out fro the heed or stomake, or by some roten tothe." Printed margin note: "Stynkynge breth." (fol. lxvi v.)

STITCH

Quincy "Pleurodyne, pains in the pleura, usually a rheumatism" "Pleurodyne rheumatica, rheumatism in the muscles of the thorax, or bastard pleurisy."

Dunglison 1839: "Pleurodynia"
"A spasmodic or rheumatic affection, generally seated in the muscles of the chest."

STONE: STONE IN THE KIDNEYES (REINES); STONE IN THE BLADDER (SEE ALSO **COLIC, GRAVEL,** AND **STONE**)

Borde: "Lithiasis is the greke word. In latin it is named Calculus in vesica and Lapis is takē for all the kyndes of the stones. In englyshe Lithiasis is the stone in the bladder, and some doth say that Nephesis is the stone in the raynes of the back, therfore loke in the capytle named Nefresis.

The Cause of this impediment

Thisse infyrmytes dothcome either by nature or els by eatyng of euyl and viscus meates & euyl drynkes, as thycke ale or beere, eatynge broyled or fryed meates, or meates ye be dryed in ye smoke as bacon, martynmas befe, reed herynge sprotes and salt meates, and crustes of breed, or of pasties and such lyke," (fol. lxxxiiiib)

"Nehpresis or Nephritis be the greke wordes. Nefresia is the barbarous worde. In latyn it is named Dolor renum, and some doth say it is Calculus in renibus. In englyshe it is named the stone in the raynes of the backe.

The Cause of this impediment

This impediment doth come of many wayes, as by great lyftynge, or great straynynge or to much medlynge with a woman, and it may come by kynd of eatynge of euyl meates ingendrying ye stone."

Of the causes of the stone.

Paré: "The stones which are in the bladder have for the most part had their first originall in the reines or kidneys, to whit, falling down from thence by the ureters into the bladder. The cause of these is two-fold, that is, materiall and efficient. Grosse, tough, and viscide humours, which crudities produced by the distempers of the bowels and immoderate exercises, chiefly immediately after meat, yeeld matter for the stone; whence it is that children are more subject to this disease than those of other ages. But the efficient cause is either the immoderate heate of the kidneyes, by meanes whereof the subtler part of the humours is resolved, but the grosser and more earthy subsides, and is hardened as we see bricks hardened by the sun and fire; or the remisse heat of the bladder, sufficient to bake into a stone the *fæces* or dregges of the urine gathered in great plenty in the capacity of the bladder. The straightnesse of the ureters and urinary passage may be accounted as an assistant cause. For by this meanes, the thinner portion of the urine floweth forth, but that which is more feculent and muddy being stayed behind, groweth as by scaile upon scaile, by addition and collection of new matter into a stony masse. An as a weeke often-times dipped by the Chandler into melted tallow by the copious adhesion of the tallowy substance presently becomes a large candle, thus the more grosse and viscide fæces of the urine stay as it were at the barres of the gathered gravell and by their continuall appulse are at length wrought and fashioned into a true stone." p. 664

Quincy: "Is an aggregate of many of the harder parts of the urine, pent up by reason of the straightness of the ducts."

The Skilful Physician: Differential diagnosis of stone and colic.

For the Stone in the Kidneyes.

There is great pain in the raines of the back, which draweth downwards; stirring encreaseth the pain, they are much inclined to vomiting, the body is bound, Urine raw and watrish, often provoking to pisse, but not without pain, the Urine avoids with gravel, sand and slime, yea sometimes mixt with blood.

To know it from the Chollick, first its not so sharp as the paine of the Chollick.

Secondly, The Chollick doth appear beneath on the right side, and stretcheth from thence upwards toward the left side, but the pain of the Kidneyes begins above, and stretcheth downwards, and a little more towards the back.

Thirdly, the pain is most of the Kidneyes fasting, the Chollick otherwise.

All Saxifrage and other things good for the Stone, are good for the Kidneyes, but not for the Chollick.

Lastly, there is found in the Urine gravel or sand, and not in the Cholick or pain of the guts."

STRANGURY (STRONGURION)

Borde: "Stranguria is the greke word. In latyn it is named Stillicidum vrine. In englyshe it is named the strangury, the which is a dystyllynge or droppynge of a mannes water diuers tymes in one houre with great payne & burnynge in the issewe of man o woman, or els it is an opylacion in the necke of the bladder, and thorowe the stone ore elles by some imposthumouse humour . . . . This infyrmyte doth come of some ulceracion in the bladder or raynes of the backe, or els it may come thorowe acredyte or sharpnes fo the water, as it may come also of to much heat or to much coldnes in the backe and bladder."

Blancard: "*Stranguria*, the Strangury; a difficulty of Urine, when the Urine comes away by Drops only, accompany'd with a constant inclination of making water."

STROKES OR STROAKS

Lowe: in a description of the causes of luxation, wrote:

"PET.   Which are the Extern [causes of luxation]?
JOH.   Falls or stroaks, and too violent extending of the member violently against the figure naturall." p. 362.

SWEAT

Borde: "Sudor is the latyn word. In greke it is named Hydros. In englyshe it is named sweat, & there be diuers sweates the one doth come by labour, the other may come by sicknes and payne, and those be hote or colde, and there is an other sweat the which is vehement, and that sweat is named ye sweatynge sicknes, and some sweates dothe stynke and some dothe nat. . . . The cause of sweates either it doth come of heat or corrupcion of the ayer, or it may come by one person infectynge another or as I sayde by labour or some sicknes."

SWELLING, WHITE

Dunglison 1839: "The French surgeons apply the term hydrarthrus to dropsy of the articulations. White swelling is an extremely formidable disease. It may attack any one of the joints, but is most commonly met within the knee, the haunch, the foot, and the elbow, and generally occurs in scrofulous children. It consists, at times, in tumefaction and softening of the soft parts and ligaments which surround the joints, at others, at swelling and caries of the articular extremities of bones; or both these states may exist at the same time."

SWELLINGS

Borde: "Cancrena is the latyn worde. In englyshe it is a swellynge the which may ve in euery member in man hauynge a grenyshe colour or elles a blacke coloue." (fol. xxviii v)

"Edema is the greke worde. In latyn is named *Tumor mollis*. In englyshe it is named a swellynge the which is soft." (fol. l)

"Icterus is the greke worde. Bilis is ye latyn worde and Celsus doth name it Aurigo, and some latyns dothe name it Arquatus. In englyshe it is named a puffing or swellyng of the flesshe puffynge vp the skyn as one were poysoned or stonge with some venemous worme or beest, and some grekes say that licterus is he the which hath any of the hernyes in the codde, loke in the captyle named Hernia." (fol. lxxvii)

"The .191. Captyle doth shewe of inflacions or swellynges.

Inflacio is the latyn worde. In englyshe it is named an inflacion, or swellynge, or bollynge, or rysynge of humours in the flesshe. . . . This infyrmyte dothe come, or is ingendred many wayes, as by reumatyke humours, corrupcion of blode, or by ye admyxtyon of euyl humours And where many doctours in phisicke doth holde diuers opinions in this infyrmyte, sayenge that inflacions doth dyffer from appostuma-cions, consyderynge that al inflacions doth appeare exteryally and appostumacions most comonly be interyal I do day al inflacions and appostumacions be nuters, for they may be as well exteryal, as interyal." (fol. lxxviii)

Blancard: "*Inflatio*, the distention of a Part from flatulent Matter."

SWELLING ABOUT THE EARS OR BEHIND THE EARS (SEE ALSO KERNEL)

Blancard: "*Eparmata*, any kind of Tumor, or Tumors of the Glandules, cal-l'd *Parotes*, behind the Ears."

"*Satyriasis, Priapismus, Satyriasmus*, or *Salacitas*; is an immoderate desire of Venery, which upon *Coition* vanishes. . . . 'Tis likewise us'd for the swelling of the Glandules behind the Ears."

"Parotides is the greke worde. In latyn it is names Inflaciones. In englyshe it is named Cornels about the eares. . . . This impediment dothe come of a hote blode, or of a bylus humour and otherwhile it doth come of a melacoly humour." (fol. cv)

SWOUNDINGS OF THE HEART (SEE FAINTNESS OF THE HEART)

TEATS

Borde: "Mamille is the latyn worde. In greke it is named Mastos or Mazion. In englyshe it is named a womans brestes the which may have diuers impedimentes as lackynge of mylke, curdynge of mylke, inflamynge of the brestes, and otherwhyle they may be ouer longe and great, and otherwhile the skyn may go of from the nipples. . . . These impedimentes doth come diuers wayes it may come for lacke of suckynge or drawynge of the mylke, it may come by grosnes of the bloude, it may come fo debylyte & wekenes or opylacions as whan a woman doth lacke mylke it maye come by to much handlynge of them, and it maye come by nature or grosnes of humours." (fol. lxxxvii v.)

TETTER

Borde: "Herpes or Herpethe be the greke worde. In latyn it is named Herpera and some do name it Flaua bilis. In englyshe it is named a tetter, and some doth name it Lupus or Lupie bycause a wolfe hath oftymed such impedimentes, it dothe crepe and corode and eateth the skyn and waxeth broder and broder. . . . This infyrmyte doth come of putrified blode and of coler, or els by corrupt blode only, or of coler only, and Lupus or Lupie is ingendred of a fleumatyke matter the whiche do make a dyfference." (fol. lxxiii v.)

"Serpigo is the latyn worde. And some auctours doth name it Ignis volatilis. And some saythe that this sickness doth by lytle dyffer from a sicknes of skabbes named Impetigo, but that the one is bygger than the other, and some doth name Impetigo zarna as it doth appere more playnlyer in this boke before this matter and after as it is spec[i]fied in the capytles of these infyrmytes, but I do saye that this sickness or disease named Serpigo is a burnynge skabbe, and doth ronne in ye skyn infesctynge it more or lesse, and is named in englyshe a tetter."

Blancard: "*Herpes*, a spreading and winding Inflammation; 'tis two-fold, either *Miliaris* or *Pustularis*, like Millet-seed, which seizes the Skin only, and itches; or *Exedens*, consuming, which not only seizes the skin, but the *Muscles* underneath. The cause of it is, that the *Glandules* of the Skin are too much stuff'd with salt *Particles*, which, if the peccant Matter abount, grow into a Crust, and eat the *Parts* they lie upon. A *Ring-worm* or *Tettar*."

TISICK (SEE CONSUMPTION AND PHTHISIS)

TYMPANY

Of the Dropsie.

Paré: "First that Dropsie which fils that space of the belly, is either moist or dry. . . . The dry is called the *Tympanites*, or Timpany, by reason the belly swolne with winde, sounds like a (*Tympanum*), that is, a Drum."

Blancard: "*Tympanites*, *Tympanias*, or *Aqua intercus Sicca*, a Tympany, is a fix'd, constant, equal, hard, resisting Tumour of the *Abdomen*; which being beat, sound. It proceeds from a stretching Inflammation of the Parts, and of the Membraneous Bowels, whose Fibres are too much swoln with animal Spirits, and hinder'd from receding by the Nervous Juice which obstructs the Passage; to which Distemper there is consequently added, as the complement of all, an abundance of flat-ulent Matter in the places that are empty."

Quincy: "Tympanites . . . is the particular sort of dropsy that swells the belly up like a drum and is often cured by tapping."

UVULA (FALLING OF THE UFULA/UVULA)

Lowe: "Of the Inflammation and relaxation of the *Uvula*, or *Columella*.

Nature hath placed and hung in the roof of the mouth, a piece of spongious flesh named by the Greeks, Gargarion, and by the Latines, Gurguleo, in vulgar the pape or chap of the mouth, the which being augmented, and lengthened above Nature, through dis-tillation of humors, is caled Schion in Greek, and in Latine Col-umella, and Uva, for it being tumified in length, it is like a pillar, or collume, somtime the nether part of it is round, and then it is called Uva, through the similitud it hath with the blacke vine berrie: it is placed in the roofe of the mouth for divers reasons: First, it helpeth to pronounce the sound, and to speak cloer by dividing the ayre which cometh from the lights, for the which it is called *Plectrum vocis*: Also that the ayre which cometh by the Mouth and Nose, entreth not in the lights by the Trahe-Arterie, till the coldnesse of it be correded, so that the lights be not offended by cold. Such as want the pape or pellet, hath ordinarily deformitie in speech, with refrig-eration of the loines: it doth impath that neither dust nor rhume enter the trahe arterie with the ayre.

The Signes are evident to the sight, by pressing down of the tongue, accompanied with dolour, feaver, difficulty to swallow the meat. The sick thinketh ever to have something in his mouth redie to go over with great hast by the continuall distilling of the humor, impassing to sleep but with open mouth; Sometime it hangeth so long that it falleth on the tongue, and so grieveth the sick, that sometime he is con-strained to put his finger in his mouth to help the over-going of the meat, as saith Avicen." pp. 206–207

Blancard: "*Cion, collumella, gargareon, gargulio, uva, uvula, uvigena, uvigera, epiglottis, sublinguium, pensilis de palato lsthmus, gutturis operculum*, the Palate which hangs betwixt the two glanules call'd *Amygdale*, above the chink of the *Larynx*. . . . Sometimes this *Uvula* sticks out too far occasioned by the Humours that fall upon it, which can't return by the Lymphatick Vessels, whence proceeds the Fall of the *Uvula*, which we call Roof of the Mouth."

ULCER

Borde: "Aphtæ is the greke worde. Alcola is the barbarous worde. And Ulceratio in palato be the latyn wordes. In englyshe it is named a hote ulceration in the rough or palat of the mouth.

The cause of this infyrmyte

This byle, or vlceration in the palace or the rough of the mouth, is ingendred of a hote stomake fumynge and metynge w^t reume at the vnels in the roughe of the mouthe and that is the cause of this impedyment."

Lowe: *Pet*. What are those six kindes of Ulcers?

Jos. The first is sanious, 2. virulent, 3 filthie, 4 cancrous, 5. putrid or stinking, 6 corrosive or rotten away. . . . p. 326.

Blancard: "*Exulceratio*, a Solution of continuity proceeding from some gnawing Matter, and in soft Parts of the Body, attended with a loss of their substance. It differs from an *Abscess* in this, that an *Abscess* is occasion'd by a *Crisis*. An Exulceration is either great, little, broad, short, narrow, straight, transverse, winding, equal, unequal, deep, &c. An Exulceration."

ULCER, EVIL

Borde: "Metasincrisis is the greke worde. In latyn it is named Mala vlceratio. In englyshe it is named an evyll ulceration. . . . This impediment doth com of corrupcion of blode and fleume." (fol. lxxxxii)

ULCER OF THE NOSE

Borde: "Ozenai is the greke worde. In latyn it is named Vlcera narium. In englyshe it is named an vlcer or sere in the nose. . . . This impediment

dothe come of a fylthy and an euyl humour the which doth come frō the
brain and heed engendred of reume and corrupte blode." (fol. ciii v.)

ULCERS OF THE EYES

Banister: "*Elos*, is taken generally, for any ulcer in any part: but *Galen*
applyeth it to the eye. The old Phisicions haue made seuen kinds of
them, whereof foure are in the ouermost part of the horny membrane,
which may be named outward, and three are inward in the bottome of
the same membrane. The first of these outward vlcers is called *achlis*,
which resembleth smoke, or a mistie ayre, of a sky-colour, relying
vpon the blacke of the eye, possessing a great part of it, and when it
hath gained the apple of the eye, the partie seeth very little. Some suppose it to bee a blacke scarre, which beginneth to obscure and make
dim the sight. The second is called *nephelion*, like to the former, but
more deepe and white, occupying lesse roome, because it is not so
stretched, nor lifted vp, yet it hindereth the sight. The third is called
argemon, which is a round vlcer in the white of the eye, neere vnto the
circle named *iris*, or the raine-bow: it is white, neere to the apple of
the eye, and redde in the membrane *coniunctiua*. *Galen* affirmeth it to
be an vlceration appearing white in the blacke of the eye, and redde in
the white of it. The fourth is called *epicauma*, which is a fiery boiling
vlcer, rough, in colour like vnto ashes, lying vpon the apple of the eye,
as if it were a flock of wooll. Notwithstanding *Ægineta* taketh it for a
deepe, filthy, and crustie vlcer. Beside these, there are three other
inward and deepely settled. The first is named *bothryon*, which is a
straite deepe vlcer, like to a pricke without filthy matter. The second is
coiloma, like to the former, but greater, yet not so deepe. The third is
encauma, which is a filthy and crustie vlcer, out of which commeth
most vile, stinking slimie matter, which cannot hardly be kept cleane."

Blancard: "*Achlys*, a certain dark Distemper of the Eye, which is reckon'd
amongst the Species of *Amblyopia*, or Dimness of Sight."

"*Argemon*, a little Ulcer of the Eye in that Circle of it which is call'd
Iris, comprehending part of the white and black."

"Encauma, seu Inustio, a burning in any Part of the Body. It also signifies an Ulcer in the Eye, with a filthy Scab, which often follows a
Fever."

"*Epicauma*, a crusty Ulcer that sometimes happens to the Black of the
Eye."

ULCERS WHICH GROW ON THE ENDS OF THE FINGERS, AND DIVIDE THE SKIN FROM THE NAYLES (SEE FELLON AND WHITLOW)

URINE, STOPPING OF THE (SEE ALSO PISSING AND STRANGURY)

Borde: "The .192. Capytle doth shewe the suppression of a mannes vryne. Ischuria is ye greke worde. In latyn it is named a Suppressio vrine. In englyshe it is named supression of the urine, that is to saye that whan a man wolde pysse and can nat. . . . This infyrmyte doth come many wayes, either by oppylacion or stoppynge of the stone, or some grosse humour, or els thorowe some euyl humour growynge in the condyte of ye vrine, or els it may come thorowe long retencion or longe holdynge in of a mannes water." (fol. lxxiii v.)

VERTIGINOSITIES (SEE ALSO GIDDINESS IN THE HEAD)

Borde: "Scotoma is the greke worde. Scotomia is the barbarous worde. In latyn it is named Vertigo. In englyshe it is named the scotomy or musyng or swymyng in the fore part of the heed.

The cause of this infyrmyte

This infyrmyte doth come of a vaporous humour, the which doth perturb the animal powers." (fol. C.xix)

Paré: "The *Vertigo* is a sudden darkening of the eyes and sight by a vaporous & hot spirit which ascendeth to the head by the sleepy arteryes, and fils the braine, disturbing the humours and spirits which are conteyned there, & tossing them unequally, as if one ran round, or had drunk too much wine. This hot spirit oft-times riseth from the heart upwards by the internall sleepy arteries to the *Rete mirabile*, or wonderfull net; otherwhiles it is generated in the brain, its selfe being more hot than is fitting; also it oft-times ariseth from the stomack, spleen, liver and other entrals being too hot. The signe of this disease is the sudden darkening of the sight, and the closing up as it were of the eyes, the body being lightly turned about, or by looking upon wheels running round, or whirle pits in waters, or by looking down any deep or steep places. If the originall of the disease proceed from the braine, the patients are troubled with the headache, heavinesse of the head, the noyse in the ears and oft-times they lose their smell. . . . But if such a *Vertigo* be a criticall symptome of some acute disease affecting the *Crisis* by vomit or bleeding, then the whole businesse of freeing the patient thereof must be committed to nature." pp. 639–640

VOMITING

Borde: "Vomitus is the latyn worde. In greke it is named Emitos. In englyshe it is named vometynge, or a vomyt or parbrekynge. . . . This impediment doth come either voluntary or inuoluntary, yf it be voluntary it dothe come by prouocacion, as by puttynge the fynger into the throte, or els to put a fether or a brānche of rosemary or such like into the throte. Or els it may come by takynge some pocion, or by some herbe, or some other medicine, yf it do come inuoluntary, then it dothe come of the malyce of the stomake."

"Lepus marinus be the latyn wordes. In englishe it is named a paine in the bely and wyl cause a man to vomyte, and will cause the patient to sweate for paine . . . . This impediment doth come of colde, and of ventosyte, and it doth differ from the Colycke and the Iliacke."

WARTS (SEE ALSO SCIRRUS)

Borde: "The .357. Capytle doth shewe of swellynges of wartes and agnelles.

Tvber is the latyn word. In englyshe it is named every swellynge or tilinge in the flesshe. Tubercula is a dymynytiue of the latyn word Tuber, and in englyshe is named a wert or an agnell growynge in the fete & toes, and in latin they hath many kyndes and termes, as Mellicerides, Gangilia, Athoromata, and Stratomata."

WATER, CAN NOT KEEP THEIR

Borde: "Diampnes is the greke worde, and the Latyns dothe vse the sayde worde, In Englishe it is named a passion of the bladder, out of whiche inuoluntarily doth pass or issueth out of the vrine of some men that they can nat kepe their water neither wakynge nor slepynge, and some men hauynge this passion in their slepe shall thinke and dreame that they do make water against a wal, a tree, or hedge or such lyke, and so dreaminge they do make water in their bedde . . . . This impediment dothe come of great debilitie and wekenes of the bladder, or els thorowe great frigiditie or coldness of the bladder, or els of too much drinkinge, and sloughfulnesse."

WEB (IN EYE) (SEE ALSO PIN AND WEB)

Borde: "Lencomata or Lencoma is the greke worde as some do say. In englyshe it is a webbe the whiche is rooted in and upon the eye or eyes . . . . This infyrmyte is ingendred of a viscus humour or reume, and it maye come of a strype or some great brose." (fol. lxxxi)

"Pterygion is the greke worde. In araby it is named Sebel. In latyn it is named Vnguis. The barbarous word is Vngula. In englyshe it is named the webbe in ye eye, whidh is a neruus matter bred upon the eye, and dothe couer the pupyle of the eye."

Banister: (1) *"Of the naile of the Eye, commonly called the webbe, in Greeke,* pterugion, *in Latine,* vngula, *or* angulus.

Pterygiũis, when the white of the eye, called *coniunctiua,* is increased aboue measure, or when in it is ingendred a superfluous growing of flesh, after a continuall recourse of humours or scabs, or an inflamed itching. This maladie most commonly beginneth to increase at the great corner of the eye, nigh vnto the nose, seldome at the lesse, and most rarely it is seene to begin at the higher or lower eye-lidde. It is stretched vnto the horny membrane, growing greater and greater, vntill it couer the apple of the eye, and darken the sight. The ancient writers haue made three kindes of it. The first is nameed *membraneus,* that is, skinny, which is a finewish skinne, beginning at the great corner, by little and little stretching and growing outward. The second is called of *Guido, adipeus,* that is, fatty, which is as a congealed humour, that becommeth round, when it is touched to bee pulled out: it groweth in the same place with the former. The third is called of the *Arabians, Sebel,* in Latine, *panniculus,* which is worse than the others, being interlaced with grosse red veines, and arteries, resembling a thin cloth or webbe: vpon this appeareth oftentimes inflamation, rednesse, and itching. Some of them sticke not to the eye in euery place, but hold onely by their edges, so that between the naile and the eye an instrument may be put thorow."

(2) *"Of the webbe or cataract, called in Greeke,* hypochyma, *in Latin,* suffusio, gutta, aqua, imaginatio.

Hypochyma is a heape of superfluous humours made thicke, like to a little skinne betweene the horny membrane and the crystalline humour, directly upon the apple of the eye, swimming aboue the waterish humour in that place which *Celsus* affirmeth to be void and empty. It hindreth the sight, or at least, the discerning & iudging of such things as are before our eyes. *Fernelius* appointeth the place of it betweene the membrane and the *Vuea,* and the Crystalline humour. The differences of it, are borrowed frõ the quantity or quality. From the quantitiy, when it is whole, couering all the compasse of the apple of the eye, in such sort that the partie cannot see any thing. Sometimes it couereth onely halfe of the apple of the eye, or some part of it, either aboue or beneath, or in the middest, in such manner, that that onely part of the thing before our face can be discerned, which is placed against the part of the eye which is free from this disease, whereby it falleth out oftentimes, that either the partie seeth nothing, or onely some part of things. For if that which is offered to the sight bee set before the part affected fully, he seeth nothing, but if hee prie at it with that part of the eye which is sound, he may see clearely. Now if the spot or webbe be in the middest of the eye, not touching the edges or borders thereof, euen as a pricke in the middest of a circle, then the partie seeth onely the extermitie and edges of things, in the middest thereof supposing there is a window, or couering, or some darke place. The differences which are drawn from their qualities, are either from their essence and substance, sith some are thin, slender and clear, thorow the which, the light of the Sunne may bee discerned: others are thicke and grosse, or from their colous, sith some are like brasse: others white, like Plaster or Pearles: others pale-coloured, mixed of greene and white, or greene and yellow: others like golde, others blacke, others resembling ashes. Amongst the *Arabians, cataracta, suffusio, aqua, gutta, imaginatio*, are used for the same things: herein onely is the difference, that *imaginatio* is called by *Auicen, gutta zala*, as it were the beginning of a webbe or cataract, because we image we see that which indeed we see not, when the cataract is as thin and slender as a spiders webbe. It is then named *aqua* and *gutta*, when the cataract beginneth to receiue some forme, inlarging and running abroad like water: but when it is thicke and ripe, and harder, it is called a cataract, and of *Auicen, gutta obscura* . . . . Now when the webbe or cataract beginneth, thes signes and tokens are incident to the diseased: They imaging there are before their eyes little darke things resembling flies: other suppose they see haires, other threads of wooll, other spiders webbes, other thinke they behold a circle about the candles when they are light, and sometime two candles for one. When these things doe thus fall out, if you looke vpon the apple of the eye, it appeareth cleare and pure: but if you behold and view it more neerely, it will seeme somewhat troubled: and if you compare it with the other eye which is sound, it will appeare somewhat appalled."

Paré: "The *Ungula, Pterygion* or Web is the growth of a certaine fibrous and membranous flesh upon the upper coate of the eye called *Adnata*, arising more frequently in the bigger, but sometimes in the lesser corner towards the temples. When it is neglected, it covers not onely the *Adnata*, but also some portion of the *Cornea*, and coming to the pupill it selfe hurts the sight thereof. Such a Web sometimes adheres not at all to the *Adnata*, but is onely stretched over it from the corners of the eye, so that you may thrust a probe betweene it and the *Adnata*: it is of severall colours, somewhiles red, somewhiles yellow, somewhiles duskish, & otherwhiles white. It hath its originall either from externall causes, as a blow, fall, and the like; or from internall, as the defluxion of humours into the eyes." p. 647.

Lowe: "Of the web in the Eye, called *Suffusio Cataracta* and *Hypochyma*.

Suffusio is a maladie called by the greeks *Hypoxima*; and by the Arabs *aqua* and *gutta*; in english, the Cataract or Tey, which is an abstruction of the Prunall, by a gathering together of a thick hardned of congealed humour betwixt the membrain *Cornea* and humour Christalline, directly upon the prunall empassing the sight . . . . The Signes when it beginneth, the sick both imagine to see before his Eyes little things like flies or moats, like the dust of the sunne, threads of wool, haires, spiders webs, or as it were a circle about a candle when it is lighted, thinking one candle to be two." p. 166.

Blancard: "*Hypochyma*, a depraved Sight, whereby *Gnats*, *Cobwebs*, little *Clouds*, &c. seem to swim before the Eyes. The cause of it seems to consist in turbid Humours, or sometimes in the Optick Nerves, whos little pores are obstructed by the Matter that is thrust into them."

"*Cataracta* is two-fold; either *beginning*, or a *Suffusion* only, or con-firm'd, or a Cataract properly so call'd; the *incipient* is but a *Suffusion* of the Eye, when little clouds, motes, and Flies seem to fly the Eyes, but the confirm'd Cataract is when the Pupil of the Eye is either wholly or in part cover'd and shut up with a little thin Skin, so the the Sunbeams have not due admittance to the Eye."

Quincy: "Wen, a soft, insensible and movable tumour under the skin."

WHEAL (SEE PUSHES)

WHITLOW (SEE ALSO FELLON)

Borde: "Pannaricium is the latyn worde. In englyshe it may be an impostu-macion in the fyngers and the nayles of a mans hande, and some soth say it is a white flawe vnder the nayle." (fol. cii)

"Perioniche is deriued out of .ii. wordes of greke of Peri which is to say about, and Onix which is to say a naile which is an impediment about nayle. I do take it for a white flawe or suche lyke do name it Paronichius."

from Extrauagantes:

"The .56. Capytle dothe shewe of a white flawe or blowe. Reduuie is the latyn worde. And some dothe name it Rediuia. The barbarous worde is named Redimie. In englyshe it is named a white blowe, or a white flawe, the which doth grow about the rote of the nayle, the grekes dothe name in Paranochia, medecines may be had in this cause but my counsel is nat to medle with no chirurgy matters, for as muche as phisicions wyl nat medle with it."

WIND

Borde: "Lectigacio is the latyn word. In englyshe it is named a wynde the which may be in many mēbers of a man specially and most comonly under the skynne . . . . This impedimt doth come of a vaporous ventosyte or winde intrused vnder the skynne and can nat gette out, it may also be in many other members."

WORMS

Borde: "Astarides is the greke worde. In englyshe it is lytle small wormes the whiche most comonly doth lye in ye longacion other wyse named the ars gutte. And there they wyll tycle in the fundement."

"Cvrcurbiti is the latyn worde. In englyshe it is square wormes in a mannes mawe and guttes.

"Sirones is the latyn worde. In englyshe it be wormes that doth brede under the skyn. And there be .ii. kyndes the one kynde doth brede in the handes and wrestes, and the other dothe brede in the fete and they be named degges."

WORMS, LONG

Borde: "Lumbrici is the latyn worde. In greke it is named Elmthia. In englyshe it is named longe white wormes in the maw of the stomake and guttes." (fol. lxxxv v)

YARD, STANDING OF

Borde: "*Satiriasis* is the greke worde. In latyn it is named *Desiderium erigendi virgam*. In englyshe it is named a desyre of standynge of a mannes yerde and some doth say it is a continuall standynge of a mannes yerde.

The fyrst cause why it can nat stande.

A man that is in great age, or spent, or beynge in sicknes, or grace workyng aboue nature in man unmaried shall have no erections of his flesshe to exercyse any venerious act, yf any maried man the which wold haue this matter or desyre and can nat thorowe unbecyilyte, use the act of matrimony, I will shewe my mynde to them in the capytle named *Concepcio*, and in the capytle named *Coitus*."

"*Priapismus* is the greke word. In latyn it is named *Erectio inuoluntaria virge*. In englyshe is tis named of an inuoluntary standynge of a mannes yerde.

The cause of this impedimente.

This impediment doth come thorowe calidite and inflacions from the raynes of the backe, or els it doth come of inflacions of the vaynes in ye yerde and stones, it may come by the usage of venerious actes." (fol. cix)

Blancard: "*Satyriasis, Priapismus, Satyriasmus*, or *Salacitas*; is an immoderate desire of Venery, which upon *Coition* vanishes. 'Tis sometimes also a convulsive Erection of the manly Yard, not attended with Venereal Appetite, and not ceasing after *Coition*; unto this may also be refer'd the *Nocturnal Erection* and *Pollution* in the time of sleep. 'Tis taken sometimes for the Leprosy, because in that Disease the Skin acquires the roughness of a Satyr, and they are much addicted to Venery. 'Tis likewise us'd for the swelling of the Glandules behind the Ears."

YEXING

Borde: "The .325. Capytle doth shewe of yexynge or the hycket.

Singultus is the latyn worde. In greke it is named Alexos ligmos. In araby Alsoach. In englyshe it is named the yexe or ye hycket, and in some the dronken mannes coughe. . . . This impedimēt doth come of a colde stomake or some euyll humour aboute the herte, it may also come of to much drynkynge, & therefore many men doth name it the dronkyn mannes coughe." (fol. cxxiii)

Blancard: "*Singultus*; see *Lygmus*, the Hick-cough, which is sometimes attended with a Fever, and then is very severe."

"*Lygmos*, the Hickup, a convulsive Motion of the Nerves which spreads up and down the Gullet, returning after short Intermissions. It proceeds from some troublesome Matter that vellicates the *Oesophagus*."